STUDIES OF THE RESEARCH BUREAU
OF THE WELFARE COUNCIL

NUMBER FIVE

Chronic Illness in New York City

IN TWO VOLUMES

CHRONIC ILLNESS IN NEW YORK CITY

BY

MARY C. JARRETT

VOLUME II

The Care of the Chronic Sick by Different
Types of Voluntary Agency

PUBLISHED FOR

THE WELFARE COUNCIL OF NEW YORK CITY

BY COLUMBIA UNIVERSITY PRESS

1933

PRINTED IN THE UNITED STATES OF AMERICA

THE COMMONWEALTH PRESS, WORCESTER, MASS.

Contents

VOLUME II:

The Care of the Chronic Sick by Different Types of Voluntary Agency

CHAPTER 1

THE CARE OF THE CHRONIC SICK IN PRIVATE HOSPITALS

SECTION A

THE CHRONIC SICK IN PRIVATE HOSPITALS

CHAPTER 2

MEDICAL SOCIAL SERVICE IN RELATION TO THE CARE OF THE CHRONIC SICK

CHAPTER 3

THE CARE OF THE CHRONIC SICK IN PRIVATE HOMES FOR THE AGED

SECTION A

THE CHRONICALLY ILL PERSONS FOUND BY A CENSUS IN PRIVATE HOMES FOR THE AGED

SECTION B

FACILITIES OF PRIVATE HOMES FOR THE AGED IN RELATION TO THE CARE OF THE CHRONIC SICK

CHAPTER 4

CONVALESCENT HOMES IN RELATION TO THE CARE OF THE CHRONIC SICK

SECTION A

The Chronic Sick in Convalescent Homes

CHAPTER 5

CARDIAC AFTER-CARE SERVICES

CHAPTER 6

THE CARE OF THE CHRONIC SICK BY NURSING SERVICES

SECTION A

The Chronic Sick under the Care of Nursing Services

xi

CHAPTER 7

VISITING DOCTOR SERVICE IN RELATION TO THE CARE OF THE CHRONIC SICK

CHAPTER 8

THE CARE OF THE CHRONIC SICK BY FAMILY SERVICE AGENCIES

SECTION A

THE PROBLEM OF CHRONIC ILLNESS IN RELATION TO THE WORK OF THESE AGENCIES

SECTION B

THE FACILITIES OF FAMILY SERVICE AGENCIES IN RELATION TO THE CARE OF THE CHRONIC SICK

CHAPTER 9

AGENCIES FOR SHELTERED WORK IN RELATION TO THE CARE OF THE CHRONIC SICK

Appendices

Tables in the Text

CHAPTER 1

CHAPTER 2

CHAPTER 3

CHAPTER 4

CHAPTER 7

CHAPTER 8

CHAPTER 9

Tables in the Appendix

CHAPTER 1

CHAPTER 3

CHAPTER 6

CHAPTER 8

Charts

The Care of the Chronic Sick by Different Types of Voluntary Agency

CHAPTER 1

The Care of the Chronic Sick in Private Hospitals

SECTION A

THE CHRONIC SICK IN PRIVATE HOSPITALS

HOSPITAL CARE IN CHRONIC ILLNESS

HOSPITAL care for the chronic sick is one of the urgent problems of medical organization today. These patients with conditions often obscure in origin, progressing slowly, and requiring treatment for many months cannot be cared for advantageously in the same hospital wards with the acutely ill, whose conditions as a rule can be diagnosed and treated within a few weeks. Patients who remain in a hospital for months and for the most part are not suffering acutely should be in a different atmosphere from those who are extremely and often dangerously ill. Since the general hospital must be conducted in the interests of the acutely ill, the chronically ill are out of place there. In case of an attack of acute illness, they are admitted and kept until a diagnosis has been made; but for further care they should be in a hospital where a general unified plan of treatment is possible that covers the patient's whole future life and can be carried out over as long a period as necessary.

The General Hospital

It is well known that the medical and surgical staff of general hospitals look upon chronic patients as a nuisance; and very often the nurses also share this attitude. The chronic patient by his presence keeps out some more interesting case, and it is difficult if not impossible to find another place for him. The indifference of the physician is no doubt due not only to his greater interest in other types of disease, but also to a feeling of helplessness in attempting to aid these patients. Even if he should arrive at a promising plan of treatment, the chances are that it would be unsuccessful without social and economic adjustments that are beyond his function. The assistance of a competent social worker will sometimes change the physician's point of view in such a situation. In most instances, however, the social workers of a general hospital are called upon in behalf of chronic patients only in order to make provision for them upon discharge.

If the chronically ill are refused admission to a general hospital, either because of an expressed or generally accepted policy to exclude them or because of lack of capacity, the hospital is met with the problem of its social responsibility to direct these persons elsewhere for care. What each hospital does is apt to vary with the adequacy of the staff provided for the work to be done, their knowledge of community resources and recognition of community problems, and the hospital's policy of service to the community as a whole.

Although general hospitals do not intend to admit chronic patients, they are obliged for various reasons to accept them; and sometimes a hospital filled to capacity because of the chronic sick, who remain for a long time, is forced to refuse acutely ill patients. In the census of the chronic sick in private general hospitals made for the study, from 4 to 34 per cent of the ward beds in different institutions were occupied by patients with chronic diseases. Only four of the fifty-seven institutions for the sick in which the census was taken reported no chronic patients at that time; and these were four general hospitals having only 3 per cent of all ward beds in the hospitals studied. The census was taken in the spring, when the number of chronically ill persons requiring hospital care is probably somewhat larger than at other seasons; so that the census figures perhaps represent the maximum provision for hospital care for the chronic sick. A fifth of all the ward beds in general hospitals, as shown in Chart 1, were being used for chronic patients. (See p. 17 for details.) It may be supposed that about a fifth of these patients were there for a legitimate reason—admitted in an emergency, under temporary observation for a special condition, or receiving treatment for an acute phase of the chronic illness. It may be expected that between 3 and 5 per cent of general hospital beds will be required for chronic patients admitted for such reasons as the above, which would account for about a fifth of the 1,000 patients found by the census in private general hospitals. In the general hospital wards of public hospitals, 20 per cent of the beds were occupied by 747 chronic patients, or about 600 more persons than might have been expected.

There were 1,400 patients, therefore, found by the census in public and private general hospitals who could have been more suitably cared for in a chronic hospital. To this number should be added an estimate of about 500 persons in the private general hospitals not included in the sample studied. It would appear then, that in all the general hospitals of the city there were at least 1,900 chronic patients for whom chronic hospital facilities should have been available.

The Modern Hospital for Chronic Diseases

The modern hospital for chronic diseases is a comparatively recent type of medical institution. Persons with chronic ailments and those interested in their welfare are gradually coming to realize that many of the chronically ill have a right to expect such medical care as only a well-equipped modern hospital can furnish. The "homes for incurables" are a survival of the old attitude toward chronic disease. In the past, chronic patients were not individualized and the medical and nursing services that each required were

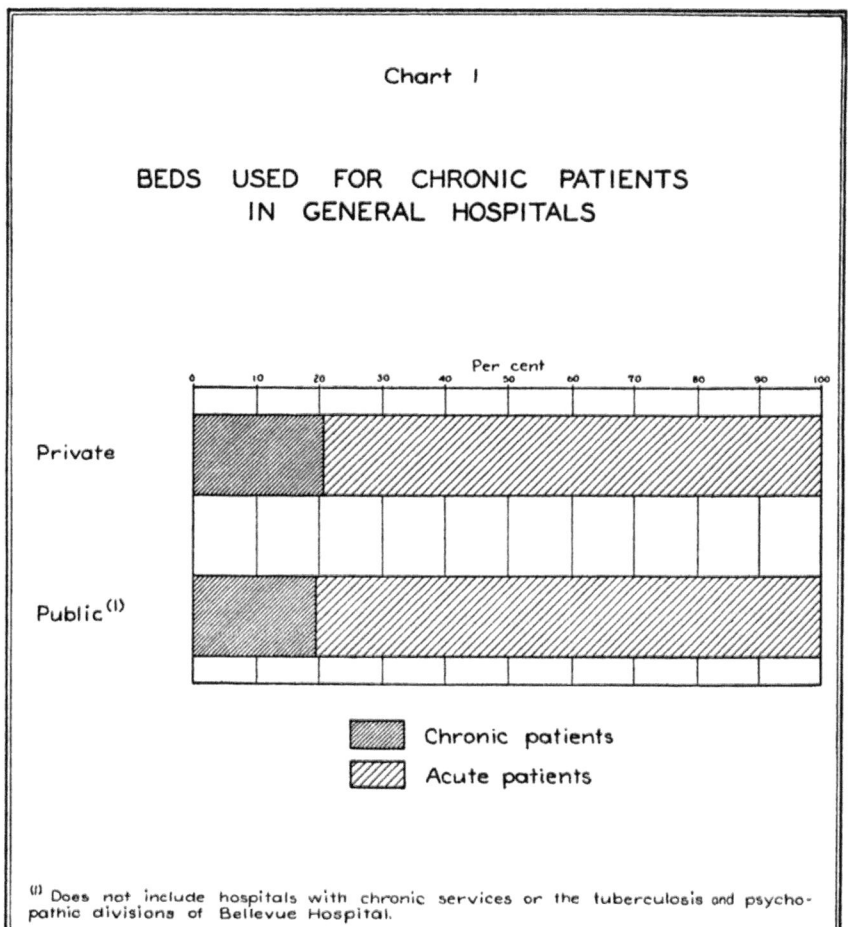

Chart I

BEDS USED FOR CHRONIC PATIENTS
IN GENERAL HOSPITALS

not clearly defined. Once labeled "incurable," it was assumed that a patient needed only simple custodial care.

With the progress of medical science, the conception of chronic disease as "incurable" is dying out. Physicians are recognizing the ineptitude of calling a condition incurable because they are unable to discover its cause. It has been said: "In the present state of medical knowledge, the pronounce-ment of the sentence (incurable) on a patient places a serious responsibility on the physician and implies, at times, a greater knowledge than he posses-ses."[1] Even when it is not possible to restore the patient to health and nor-mal activity, skillful medical care seldom fails to relieve his discomfort and increase his activity.

New York has in Montefiore Hospital the first hospital for chronic dis-eases to be opened in this country. It was founded in 1884 as a "Home for Chronic Invalids" and gradually developed into a modern chronic hospital.[2] It now serves other communities as a model for institutions of this type. It has a hospital department to which all patients are first admitted, where they receive medical care for diagnosis and treatment. In addition, it has a custodial pavilion to which patients may be transferred after a period of treatment in the hospital department. Apart from its tuberculosis service, it now has a capacity of 700 beds, of which a few are private or semi-private.

The chronic hospital of the modern type is a research center offering special opportunities for study of the etiology and treatment of chronic diseases. At Montefiore Hospital, a completely equipped research labora-tory is devoted to the study of chronic diseases and every year members of the staff publish numerous papers on their researches.

There are only a few other instances of modern hospitals for chronic diseases throughout the country. Among the best known are those in Boston and Cleveland. Cincinnati recently opened the first unit of a municipal hospital for chronic diseases, built upon the grounds of the county alms-house. In Boston, following a survey of the Boston City Hospital, a recom-mendation to establish a special unit for chronic diseases in connection with this hospital was submitted to the city government, but no action has yet been taken.

The census of the chronic sick found nearly 2,900 patients who needed the type of care given in a hospital for chronic diseases but who were not so placed. Nearly 2,000 of them, as mentioned above, were in general hos-pitals. There were also 791 persons ill at home who should have been in a hospital and 170 persons in institutions where they could not receive ade-quate medical attention who also needed hospital care.

Different Forms of Care

For the three types of care needed by the chronic sick, different types of institutions are required. For those who need active medical study and treatment or "A" care, either a hospital or an institution with full hospital

[1] Boas, Ernst P., M.D., and Michelson, Nicholas, M.D., The Challenge of Chronic Diseases. New York, The Macmillan Company, 1929, p. 9.
[2] *Ibid.*, Chapter 6, The Hospital for Chronic Diseases, pp. 82–171.

facilities is required; for skilled nursing or "B" care, a hospital organization is usually required but not necessarily one with extensive laboratory facilities; for custodial or "C" care, the institution need have only general oversight by a physician and hospital facilities necessary for emergency treatment, although it should have close working relations with a hospital of the "A" type. The custodial institution should be planned with a view to giving patients care over long periods in comfortable surroundings; and, therefore, it should have recreation rooms, adequate facilities for rest during the day, and a location that would make it possible for the patients to get out-of-doors every day.[3]

In the whole census, 60.5 per cent of the patients required active medical, or "A," care; but as over two thirds of them could receive such care outside an institution, about a fifth of all the chronic sick in the study, or 3,850 persons, were in need of "A" care in hospitals or institutions with hospital facilities. Three and a half per cent, or 714 patients, required "B" care—600 of them in a hospital and the remainder in their homes. Thirty-six per cent, or 7,342 patients, needed "C" care—6,780 in an institution of the custodial type and the rest at home.

Different Kinds of Institutions Caring for the Chronic Sick

The attitude formerly held by the medical profession that chronic patients were hopelessly incurable brought about the establishment of the institutions known as "homes for incurables" to provide a refuge for those who were indigent and homeless. Some of these institutions have endeavored to keep abreast of modern medical practice and to provide medical service, but they have not been equipped or organized as hospitals and usually cannot give adequate care to patients who require active medical attention. Their function is the custodial care of permanently disabled patients for whom medical skill has done all that is possible. Of the 14,248 adult chronic patients in the census, 46 per cent, or 6,609 persons, required custodial care in an institution. In this number were 4,641 persons sixty years of age or over, to many of whom a home for the aged should be able to give suitable care. (See also p. 114.)

The study and care of certain diseases that have become medical specialties has led to the establishment of special hospitals devoted to this purpose. Among the chronic diseases with which this study is concerned, there are three instances of such specialization—cancer, orthopedic diseases, and neurological diseases. For the first time, in Boston, a special chronic hospital has been devoted almost entirely to the study and treatment of arthritis; and a program for prevention of the disability caused by this disease is being considered by the Massachusetts Department of Public Health.

In New York City, the institutional facilities for cancer consist of one private hospital with about 100 beds, one public hospital with nearly 200 beds, and three custodial homes for incurable cancer having altogether

[3] *Ibid.*, pp. 14–20.

about 300 beds. Other private hospitals have about 150 beds for cancer patients. About 100 new beds have been added since the study was made. The hospitals now have a total of nearly 500 beds for cancer, and the custodial homes for cancer have over 300 beds. The census found about 400 patients in cancer institutions, over a third of whom were in homes for incurables. These patients represent 7 per cent of all hospital patients in the census and 10 per cent of all patients in chronic hospitals.

Orthopedic facilities consist of more than 1,200 beds in six private hospitals and one public hospital, besides the State Reconstruction Home and St. Agnes Hospital outside the city, each of which cares for some New York City children. In addition, Seaview Hospital accepts bone and joint tuberculosis, the wards for which were included in the study. The 599 patients found in orthopedic hospitals were 11 per cent of all hospital patients and 15 per cent of all those in the hospitals intended for chronic diseases.

The subject of convalescent institutions is so closely related to hospital care that it should be mentioned here although another section of the report deals with it. Convalescent care should not be confused with care for chronic conditions, although a chronic patient may need a period of care in a convalescent home after an acute attack. Convalescence, in general, implies a capacity to return to a normal state of health after a temporary illness; and the convalescent home is intended for this type of patient. The special convalescent homes restricted to patients with heart diseases or orthopedic diseases are indeed serving chronic patients. Cardiac homes, however, are for the convalescent period following acute phases of heart disease. Orthopedic homes, particularly the country branches of the orthopedic hospitals, are not strictly speaking convalescent homes, as they are for long-time treatment; and therefore they must have special educational and recreational facilities and should be conducted according to the standards developed for other child-caring institutions. (See pp. 156-157.) The four cardiac homes for children reported 104 patients in the census; the eight orthopedic homes, 501 patients. A fourth of the beds in general convalescent homes were occupied by chronic patients.

The care of the aged suffering from chronic diseases as well as from infirmities that normally accompany senescence has fallen largely to the private homes for the aged and the public homes for dependents. Nearly half of all the guests of private homes for the aged and two thirds of those in the public homes were chronically ill. Twenty-two per cent of all the chronic sick in the census were in homes for the aged—14 per cent in private homes and 8 per cent in public homes. A larger number of chronically ill persons were found in private homes for the aged than in private hospitals. Of the chronic sick in these homes, 8 per cent required hospital care; but over a third of those who needed it were not receiving it. A few of the homes maintain a department equipped as a hospital. Among the private homes for the aged, discussed in another section of the report, four with hospital departments have a total of nearly 700 hospital beds, or one third of their capacity. Three of the four care only for those who become ill after admission, but one, the Brooklyn Hebrew Home and Hospital, with 218 hospital beds, admits the chronically ill aged. This institution has recently extended its medical service in order to accept more chronically ill aged than heretofore, in accordance with the policy recommended in the Jewish Communal Survey that certain of the Jewish homes for the aged should expand their facilities for the care of the aged chronic sick.[4]

Of the chronic sick who needed hospital care, shown in Table 1, 69 per cent were in hospitals, the other 31 per cent were distributed as follows:

TABLE I

CHRONIC PATIENTS REQUIRING HOSPITAL CARE IN VARIOUS TYPES OF
INSTITUTIONS AND AT HOME, EACH AGE GROUP

Age group	Total needing hospital care	INSTITUTIONS						At home
		Hospitals			Homes for the aged	Convalescent homes	Reported by non-institutional agencies	
		Total	General services	Chronic services				
Total	3,852	2,649	1,423	1,226	229	22	161	791
Under 16 years .	1,035	589	299	290	...	18	78	350
16–39 years . .	783	578	420	158	...	3	41	162
40–59 years . .	1,084	869	466	403	7	1	34	173
60–69 years . .	497	370	163	207	57	0	7	63
70 years and over	424	227	69	158	163	0	1	33
Not reported . .	29	16	6	10	2	0	1	10

at home, 21 per cent; in homes for the aged, 6 per cent; in various institutions reported by non-institutional agencies, 4 per cent; and a few persons in convalescent homes. Of those who were receiving hospital care, 84 per cent were reported by hospitals, and the other 16 per cent were in hospital departments of homes for the aged or were reported by non-institutional agencies as being temporarily in various institutions.

Of those needing skilled nursing, or "B" care, who were 3.5 per cent of the patients in the total census, 35 per cent were in hospitals, about a fourth in orthopedic convalescent homes, nearly a fifth in homes for the aged, and nearly a fifth at home under the care of nursing agencies. Of those who received nursing care, 37 per cent were in hospitals.

Of the patients needing custodial, or "C" care, one fifth of whom required only the simplest form of attendant care suitable for the infirm aged not suffering from disease, 27 per cent were in hospitals. Of the 6,750 persons who received "C" care, 22 per cent were in hospitals.

Public Responsibility

Governmental responsibility for public health has been directed in the past mainly toward preventive efforts; and it has been expected that cura-

[4] Jewish Communal Survey of Greater New York: Report of Executive Committee, The Bureau of Jewish Social Research, New York, October, 1929, p. 37.

tive activities should be supported by private resources including philanthropy. The two large disease groups that are exceptions, tuberculosis and mental disease, are both a serious menace to the community if not brought under control. In the case of both, furthermore, private philanthropic resources would be insufficient to cope with the large number of persons needing treatment and unable to pay for it. The expense of hospital provision for these diseases is also as a rule too great to be borne entirely by county or municipal governments. Better medical service, moreover, can be given in large well-equipped hospitals than in numerous small local units; and the larger institutions also offer more opportunity for research. The result is that hospitals for mental diseases are for the most part state institutions, approximately 80 per cent of the hospital beds of this kind being in state hospitals;[5] and hospitals for tuberculosis are maintained by both local and state governments. Large cities, with populations close to a million or over, can afford to conduct such hospitals under municipal auspices and may find it advantageous to do so. The City of New York cares for more than half of its tuberculosis patients in municipal institutions, a small percentage in state institutions, and the remainder in private institutions. It provides hospital care for acute phases of mental disease and for the rest of the service required depends upon state institutions.

The care of crippled children and of the blind are also responsibilities that have usually been assumed to some extent by state governments. In New York State, a recommendation of the Governor's Special Health Commission advises that both "state and local services be extended for the discovery and care of crippled children." For the blind, in communities outside of New York City, the New York State Commission for the Blind does whatever is not already provided for by local agencies. It may give outdoor relief to needy blind to the amount of $300 annually. In New York City, the Commission does no case work among the blind but shares with the local private agencies in coördinating the program of care for blind persons and educational activities for the prevention of blindness. Outdoor relief to the amount of $300 a year is given through the Department of Public Welfare.

Other chronic diseases have not been regarded as the responsibility of the state. Local responsibility of cities and counties for the care of the chronic sick has been recognized as a rule only to the extent of providing a minimum of medical service and care for the destitute infirm when they are forced to seek refuge in the almshouse. In some communities, particularly in New York City, cancer has been an exception to the usual method of dealing with chronic diseases. The Department of Hospitals now has a special Division of Cancer. The first municipal cancer hospital was opened here in 1923. The old building is now unfit for use as a hospital and the amount of service provided is inadequate, but the medical service is good. Plans have been made in the Department of Hospitals for adequate provision for this

[5] Rorem, Rufus C., The Public's Investment in Hospitals. Chicago, The University of Chicago Press, November, 1930, p 21.

group of chronic patients. The state of New York has conducted a cancer research hospital for a number of years; and as the result of a recommendation by the Governor's Special Health Commission a division of cancer control has been created in the health department. State responsibility for prevention and cure of cancer has recently been accepted in Massachusetts to an unprecedented extent. A state-wide attack against cancer was undertaken by the State Department of Public Health about six years ago, when the Legislature directed that an investigation of this disease be made. The result was a state hospital for cancer patients, cancer clinics organized in coöperation with local medical societies in various localities and aided by state funds, and an extensive program of public education.[6] In addition, the whole problem of chronic disease is being studied intensively with the expectation that the state will assume a similar responsibility for other chronic diseases. Heart disease and rheumatism will probably be the next diseases to receive attention, since the first is the most fatal and the second the most crippling of chronic illnesses.

For some years there has been a decided movement to replace the old type of almshouse by a modern institution equipped as an "infirmary" with facilities for medical care. In Albany County, New York, a modern almshouse building was built in 1929, with a good infirmary service. About the same time, a new infirmary building was added to the almshouse in Erie County. Plans for a model almshouse with ample provision for the sick are now going forward in Westchester County. The recent transfer of the municipal homes for the aged and infirm in New York City from the Department of Public Welfare to the Department of Hospitals is a recognition of this trend.

In Massachusetts for some years, the Department of Public Welfare has been endeavoring to get the city homes in all the larger centers to establish wards for the chronic sick. The term "almshouse" was replaced by the term "infirmary" in 1927. When the city of Cambridge built a new city home, the plans called for a building primarily of the hospital type with provision also for well inmates.[7]

In New York City, it was originally intended that two municipal hospitals on Welfare Island, City Hospital, and Metropolitan Hospital, should care exclusively for chronic patients. But as a result of pressure from the attending medical staff and nursing schools of these hospitals for an acute service, the policy was changed in 1910.[8] Both are now general hospitals, but each maintains a chronic service. Some attempt was made to segregate the chronic patients, but as both hospitals were continually overcrowded it was unavoidable that chronic patients should be placed wherever there

[6] Bigelow, George H., M.D., The Cancer Program of Massachusetts. The Committee on the Costs of Medical Care, Miscellaneous Contributions, No. 6, Washington, D. C., December 10, 1930.

[7] Bardwell, Francis, The City and Town Almshouses and Statistics of Poor Relief. The Commonwealth of Massachusetts, Annual Report of the Department of Public Welfare for the Year Ending November 30, 1926, Part III, p. 113.

[8] Wright, Henry C., Report of the Committee on Inquiry into the Departments of Health, Charities, and Bellevue and Allied Hospitals in the City of New York, Board of Estimate and Apportionment, 1913, p. 763.

was room for them. It was not until the summer of 1931 that, in response to requirements of the State Board of Regents for nurse's training schools, a definite number of beds were set aside for acute and chronic services respectively. Now, 65 per cent of City Hospital's 1,060 beds are for chronic service; and 39 per cent of Metropolitan Hospital's 1,620 beds, more than two thirds of which are for tuberculosis service. The two hospitals now have a total of 893 beds for chronic patients aside from the tuberculous. These hospitals have the equipment and surroundings necessary for a chronic hospital but these advantages are only partly utilized. The care of the chronic patients is incidental to the main purpose that the institutions as general hospitals now serve.

The two special municipal institutions for chronic patients, the Cancer Institute and the Neurological Hospital, are both housed in ancient and unsavory buildings unfit for use as hospitals. In the city homes for the aged and infirm, which lack facilities for the care of chronic patients, two thirds of the inmates were found to be chronically ill. In all, the city was found to be maintaining over 4,500 chronic patients: 1,258 in general hospitals with chronic services; 680 in the three special hospitals for neurological and cancer patients; 137 in orthopedic hospitals; 27 in other special hospitals; 1,720 in the homes for the aged; and 747 in general hospitals with acute service only. All the public agencies, including correctional institutions, reported a fourth of all the dependent chronic sick in the census. Less than half of all those needing institutional care were in public institutions.

Besides the chronic sick in municipal institutions, there were 829 chronic patients in private hospitals who were "city charges," for whose care the hospitals expected to be partly reimbursed by the City. When patients are unable to pay for their care and cannot be provided for at the time in public institutions, private hospitals and custodial institutions may charge the city a certain amount per day for their care. For chronic patients, the amount paid by the City is $3.00 a day in general and certain special hospitals, and $1.15 a day in custodial institutions. If a hospital continues to keep a patient whose condition requires only custodial care, it receives from the city only $1.15 a day. (See footnote on p. 41 for details.) In private general hospitals, the daily costs per patient are usually between $3.00 and $6.00; so that the amount paid by the city in the majority of cases does not meet the full cost. A Private Hospital Committee estimated that, in the year 1930, fifty-five private hospitals of the city suffered a total loss of over $2,500,000 in caring for patients recognized as city charges. The average amount allowed by the city was $2.09 per day per patient and the average daily cost per patient was $4.54. Montefiore Hospital for Chronic Diseases in the same year expended more than $450,000 beyond the payments received for the care of patients acknowledged to be the responsibility of the city.[9]

There were approximately 3,000 patients at the time of the study in

[9] News release, United Hospital Fund of New York, September 25, 1931.

private hospitals and homes who were "city charges," of whom 27 per cent were chronically ill. The amount paid by the city did not equal the ward rate in the case of two thirds of these chronic patients who were the city's responsibility. Moreover the hospitals were giving free care to over 600 other chronic patients who could not claim aid from the city. Although the hospitals are obliged to make a contribution to the care of "city charges," they are often glad to receive these patients for whom some payment at least is made by the city rather than have empty beds or admit more free patients.

From the standpoint of the number of patients under care, the public and private hospitals were found to be sharing the burden of the chronic

TABLE 2

NUMBER AND PER CENT OF BEDS USED FOR CHRONIC PATIENTS IN GENERAL HOSPITALS

Hospitals	Ward beds	CHRONIC PATIENTS	
		Number	Per cent
Total	15,465	3,632	23.5
Public	7,494	2,005	26.8
General	3,785[1]	747	19.7
General with chronic services	3,709[2]	1,258	33.9
Private	7,971	1,627[3]	20.4

[1] Omitting beds in the tuberculosis, psychopathic, and drug experiment divisions.
[2] Omitting beds in the tuberculosis and psychopathic divisions.
[3] Includes an estimated number in hospitals not included in the census.

sick in New York City about equally. The public hospitals had a somewhat larger number of chronic patients and a larger percentage of all the facilities of the public hospitals were used for chronic care. The public hospitals are inclined to keep their patients under care for a longer time than the private hospitals, since in most cases there is no other hospital to which they can discharge them. In private hospitals, 50 per cent of the chronic patients reported had been under care for less than three months; in public hospitals, only 36 per cent. Two thirds in private hospitals had been under care less than a year; 59 per cent, in public hospitals. However, the proportion of those under care by the hospital for five years or longer was slightly larger among private than among public hospitals.

The chronic patients cared for by private hospitals were in special hospitals for chronics to a greater extent than those cared for by public hospitals. Of the total patients in private hospitals, 37 per cent were in general hospitals; and in public hospitals, 70 per cent were in general hospitals, the majority to be sure in hospitals with chronic services. Although the public hospitals maintain chronic services in three general hospitals, about the same proportion of general hospital beds were being used for chronic patients in public as in private hospitals, which is shown in Table 2 above.

Besides the chronically ill needing hospital care, there were 6,780 persons in the census who needed institutional care of the custodial type; 48 per cent of them were in public institutions, 48 per cent in private institutions, and 4 per cent at home. In addition, institutional care was probably required for several hundred persons needing "C" care whose home conditions were not reported. Many other chronically ill persons besides those known to the welfare agencies studied were also unquestionably in need of such institutional care.

Most of the chronic patients who need institutional care require such care for long periods—the majority for the rest of their lives. Among the adults in the census, 37 per cent had been under care for two years or longer; 16 per cent for five years or longer; and nearly 6 per cent for ten years or longer. Children, on the whole had required long-time care as frequently as adults. In chronic hospitals and private homes for the aged, about a fourth of the patients had been under care five years or longer. The average period of care for the patients reported by all private hospitals and homes for incurables was two years.

The expense of caring for a chronic invalid is likely to be an impossible burden for the family with a small income. Seventy-one per cent of the families in the census with five or more members, for whom the amount of income was reported, had incomes of less than $2,150 a year, which the Labor Bureau, Inc., estimated to be, in 1928, a minimum standard of health and decency for a family of five persons. Only 8 per cent had as much as the standard budget for a skilled workman's family. The average income of families in the census of the chronic sick was $6.67 weekly per person. At this income level, there is no margin for the cost of prolonged illness. The length of time that the patient had been disabled averaged 5.8 years.

Even if the family has moderate resources beyond the minimum required for living expenses, they are quickly exhausted in the effort to obtain medical care for the patient. If an individual is without family resources, when incapacitated for work he uses up his savings even more quickly in paying for medical services. The cost of chronic illness must be borne largely by the community. As Dr. Boas has said, "Chronic sufferers will not receive a square deal until there is general acceptance of the fact that they too are a proper charge on the organized community and that it is necessary to apply intensive effort and enlightened study to the many problems involved in their care, as has been done in the case of the mentally ill and of the tuberculous."[10]

Costs of Hospital Care

The care of the 2,700 chronic patients in private hospitals in which the census was taken was costing approximately $11,800 a day. The 626 persons with chronic diseases estimated to have been in the general hospitals

[10] Boas, Ernst P., M.D., How the Community Can Adequately Serve Its Chronic Sick. Reprinted from *The Modern Hospital*, vol. 36, No. 5, May, 1931, p. 2.

not included in the sample studied would have added $3,500 to this amount. As the average stay in the hospital was over two years, the total cost of institutional care alone, in private hospitals, had already been about $6,000,000. For approximately a fourth of their chronic patients, the hospitals were receiving payment to the extent of their ward rates, which do not cover the cost of medical service nor even the entire cost of hospital care; and over a third of these patients were city charges. For two fifths, over half of whom were city charges, the hospitals received part payment. Over a fourth were receiving free care.

The expense of care for these 2,700 patients would have been even more than the estimated $6,000,000, if all of the hospitals included had been modern medical institutions. In homes for incurables, the daily cost per patient was sometimes as low as $2.50 a day.[11] In Montefiore Hospital, the average cost was nearly $4.00 a day including the custodial division. The average per capita cost in orthopedic hospitals was nearly $5.50; and in general hospitals over $5.50. Moreover, as it is customary to calculate the per diem cost per patient on the basis of operating expenses only and not to include interest on investment nor depreciation of property and equipment, the total cost has been greater than the above estimate shows, since it is based on published figures for daily costs per patient.

The old conception that chronic patients were "incurable" led to the conclusion that hospitals for the chronic sick should be less expensive to maintain than hospitals for the acutely ill. On the contrary, a hospital equipped to give chronic patients the benefit of whatever medical knowledge can contribute to their improvement must have practically all of the facilities of a general hospital and in addition requires more elaborate services for physiotherapy and occupational therapy than are usually necessary in a general hospital. The dietary budget also should be higher in a chronic hospital than in a general hospital, since few chronic patients require less than an average amount of food, which is often the case with acutely ill patients, and as many require special diets.[12] In hospitals where children remain sometimes for years, particularly the orthopedic hospitals, special facilities must be provided for their education and training.

The nursing service required for patients in chronic hospitals giving complete medical care is little less expensive than nursing service in general hospitals. A study of seven representative patients in Mt. Sinai Hospital showed that each received on an average 4 hours and 49 minutes of nursing care in each twenty-four hours.[13] Seven typical patients selected for study at Montefiore Hospital received an average of 5 hours and 20 minutes nursing care in each twenty-four hours. A further study of twenty-three patients at Montefiore Hospital, ranging from the easiest to the hardest cases on the ward, reduced the average to 4 hours and 14 minutes, without

[11] Based on the figures of two that reported to the United Hospital Fund of New York in 1928.
[12] Boas, Ernst P., M.D., and Michelson, Nicholas, M.D., The Challenge of Chronic Diseases. New York, The Macmillan Company, 1929, p. 138.
[13] Greener, Elizabeth, R.N., A Study of Hospital Nursing Service. The Modern Hospital, vol. 16, No. 1, January, 1921, pp. 28–31.

baths or special tests.[14] For Dr. Corwin's study of hospitals in New York in 1924, thirty-three cases were studied by ten hospitals; and the average time required to perform every function of the nurse in attendance was found to be 5 hours and 5 minutes.[15]

There is no basis for estimating the cost of the social service in chronic and acute hospitals respectively, for few hospitals of any kind have a sufficient staff for adequate social service. The demand for social service in chronic hospitals depends to a great extent upon the number of patients who can be discharged to the care of an out-patient department and require supervision in their homes. Generally speaking, chronic patients under medical treatment are more likely to require social guidance and assistance in adjusting themselves and their circumstances to their illness than patients with acute diseases.

On the whole the cost of maintaining a modern hospital for chronic diseases is only slightly less than the maintenance costs for a well-equipped general hospital. A factor in reducing the cost somewhat is the lower turn-over in a chronic hospital.

The future cost of hospital care for the chronic sick will depend to a large extent upon the development of clinic service for chronic diseases. The medical apathy in regard to chronic illness commonly found in hospitals also prevails in most clinics. Even when the interest of the clinic doctor is engaged, the successful treatment of chronic patients outside of institutions calls for a development of medical social service and home nursing service not often found. Dr. Bigelow referring to the inevitable increase in the volume of chronic disease to be expected with the increasing average age of the population, says, "Certainly to offer hospital care alone would seem economically short-sighted, since wholesale hospitalization, particularly of advanced cases, is the most expensive solution of any sickness problem to-day."[16]

PROPORTION OF PRIVATE HOSPITAL FACILITIES
IN USE FOR THE CHRONIC SICK

For the discussion of the care of the chronically ill by private hospitals that follows, the hospitals are divided into three groups—institutions for the chronic sick including chronic hospitals and "homes for incurables"; orthopedic hospitals; and general and other special hospitals. The last group includes in addition to the sample of thirty-two general hospitals covered by the census nine so-called special hospitals. Six of the nine are essentially general hospitals and special only in the sense that they serve entirely children or entirely women and children. Three others, although special in function, treat acute rather than chronic conditions. Appendix

[14] Constantine, Mildred, R.N., The Nursing of Chronic Diseases: What It Demands and What It Offers. *The Modern Hospital*, vol. 27, No. 5, November, 1926, p. 128.

[15] Corwin, E. H. L., The Hospital Situation in Greater New York. New York, G. P. Putnam's Sons, 1924, pp. 216–217.

[16] Bigelow, George H., M.D., The Cancer Program of Massachusetts. The Committee on the Costs of Medical Care, Miscellaneous Contributions, No. 6, Washington, D. C., December, 1930, p. 8.

Table 1 shows the number of chronically ill patients reported by each hospital studied together with the bed capacity and daily cost per patient in each hospital.

Institutions for the Chronic Sick

Of the sixteen private institutions for chronic diseases studied, nine were equipped for full hospital care and seven were homes for incurables equipped to give only "B" or "C" care. The former had 54 per cent of the patients, one half of them in six hospitals for orthopedic diseases, nearly two fifths

TABLE 3

CHRONIC PATIENTS IN RELATION TO CAPACITY AND AVERAGE OCCUPANCY IN PRIVATE CHRONIC HOSPITALS AND HOMES, 1928

Institution	Capacity	Average occupancy, 1928	CHRONIC PATIENTS		
			Number	Per cent of capacity	Per cent of occupancy
Total	1,946	1,612	1,244	63.9	69.9[1]
Memorial Hospital	104	96	40	38.5	41.7
New York Skin and Cancer Hospital	98	56	18	18.3	32.1
St. Francis' Home	250	250	193	77.2	77.2
St. Rose's Free Home	89	. . . . .	63	70.8	. . . . .
Montefiore Hospital	614[2]	589[2]	393	64.0[2]	66.7[2]
Beth Abraham Home for Incurables	224	177	160	71.4	90.4
Home for Incurables	307	295	184	59.9	62.4
House of Calvary	100	86	74	74.0	86.5
House of the Holy Comforter . . .	100	63	65	65.0	101.6
St. Joseph's Hospital	60	. . . . .	54	90.0	. . . . .

[1] Based on the chronic sick in the institutions for which average occupancy was known.
[2] Includes the tuberculosis service for which average occupancy is not shown separately.

in one general chronic hospital for all types of chronic diseases, and the remainder in two cancer hospitals. Of the 46 per cent in seven homes for incurables, approximately a fifth were in two homes for incurable cancer and the remainder in five general homes.

At the time of the census, chronic patients occupied 64 per cent of the 1,946 beds, excluding the orthopedic hospitals, in ten[17] private institutions caring for the chronic sick, although not in every instance limited to chronic patients. The beds in use for chronic patients in the New York Skin and Cancer Hospital,[18] which is not limited to cancer, represented 18 per cent of the bed capacity; and in Memorial Hospital, which receives suspected

[17] In one institution, Faith Home for Incurables, arrangements for taking the census could not be made.
[18] Early in 1931, this hospital changed its name to Stuyvesant Square Hospital and its purposes to those of a general hospital. The original name will be used throughout this report, in which the hospital appears as it existed in 1928.

as well as true cases of cancer, 38 per cent. In the other hospitals, the proportions ranged from 60 per cent in the Home for Incurables to 90 per cent in the chronic ward of St. Joseph's Hospital for Consumptives and 91 per cent in Montefiore Hospital exclusive of the tuberculosis service. It should be noted that these percentages are modified by the percentage of total occupancy in the institutions; for example, the chronic patients of the New York Skin and Cancer Hospital represented 32 per cent of its average occupancy but 18 per cent of its capacity; those at the House of the Holy Com-

TABLE 4

NUMBER AND PERCENTAGE DISTRIBUTION OF CHRONIC PATIENTS IN
CHRONIC HOSPITALS AND HOMES

| Institutions | Hospitals and homes | | | PATIENTS | | | | | |
| | | | | Number | | | Per cent | | |
	Total	Public	Private	Total	Public	Private	Total	Public	Private
Total	24	8	16	3,781	2,075	1,706	100.0	100.0	100.0
Chronic hospitals . . .	17	8	9	2,988	2,075	913	79.0	100.0	53.5
General	5	4	1	2,139	1,746	393	56.6	84.1	23.0
Cancer	4	2	2	250	192	58	6.6	9.3	3.4
Orthopedic	8	2	6	599	137	462	15.8	6.6	27.1
Homes for incurables .	7	0	7	793	.....	793	21.0	.....	46.5
General	5	0	5	656	.....	656	17.4	.....	38.5
Cancer	2	0	2	137	.....	137	3.6	.....	8.0

forter, 102 per cent of its average occupancy but only 65 per cent of its total capacity. In Table 3 is shown the percentage both of capacity and of occupancy represented by the chronic sick reported in these institutions.

The above table (Table 4) shows the distribution of patients among the chronic hospitals and homes for incurables. Of all the chronic patients in private institutions designed for chronic care, 46 per cent were in homes for incurables without hospital facilities. The patients in these homes represented 14 per cent of all the chronic patients in public and private institutions for the sick.

Orthopedic Hospitals

In the private orthopedic hospitals, the chronic sick patients represented 45 per cent of the total bed capacity. The institution reporting the largest percentage of chronic patients, 85 per cent of total capacity, was the Brooklyn Home for Blind, Crippled and Defective Children, the remaining capacity being occupied probably by blind patients. In the House of St. Giles the Cripple, the patients reported represented 69 per cent of capacity; in the New York Orthopedic Hospital, 45 per cent; in St. Charles Hospital, 43 per cent; and in the Hospital for Joint Diseases and the Hospital for the Ruptured and Crippled, 27 and 24 per cent respectively.

General Hospitals

In the forty-one general and special hospitals studied, one fifth of the total ward capacity was occupied by chronic patients. The application of this percentage to the thirty-six general hospitals omitted from the census, with a capacity of 13,539 ward beds, would give a total of 1,627 chronically ill persons cared for in these hospitals. Including both private and ward beds, the dependent chronic sick represented 12 per cent of the capacity of the general hospitals, and roughly 17 per cent of their average occupancy, based upon the United Hospital Fund's figure for percentage of use in 1928 for its 30 member general hospitals.[19]

The proportion of chronic sick ranged from none in four hospitals to 56 per cent of the ward capacity in one of the special hospitals. Chronic patients occupied a third of the ward capacity in four hospitals ranging in size from 50 to 517 ward beds; and a fifth or more in nine other hospitals, ranging in size from 8 to 333 ward beds. The largest number of hospitals, sixteen, had between 10 and 20 per cent of their ward beds occupied by chronic patients. Seven hospitals had fewer than 10 per cent.

All Private Hospitals

In private hospitals other than general hospitals, 1,706 chronic patients were reported, and 124 were estimated to be in two hospitals not studied, making a total of 3,457 chronically ill patients in all the private hospitals of the city, or 21 per cent of their combined capacity and 32 per cent of their combined ward capacity.

Twenty-seven per cent of the ward beds in all private hospitals are theoretically available for the chronic sick, if, in addition to the capacity of chronic hospitals, 4 per cent of capacity for patients with chronic diseases is considered to be a natural use of general hospitals. In practice, however, the orthopedic and cancer hospitals treat acute as well as chronic conditions. Moreover, the average use of hospital beds that is ordinarily practicable is not over 80 per cent of capacity. Because of these two factors, the actual number of chronic patients who can be cared for at any one time in the private hospitals is considerably less than the number of beds apparently available for them.

Medical Social Service

Less than half of the chronic patients in private hospitals were receiving social service. Of those in hospitals that had a medical social service, three fourths were getting this service. There were fourteen private hospitals without social service that reported chronic patients. A larger proportion of children were known to the social service (85 per cent) than of adults (69 per cent). (See Table 13, p. 72.)

In public hospitals, all of which with one exception have social service, the information as to whether the patient was known to the social service

[19] United Hospital Fund of New York, Fiftieth Year Book, New York, November, 1929; Statistical Report for the year ended December 31, 1928.

was obtained in a much smaller percentage of cases than in private hospitals. One half of those for whom the fact was known were receiving social service.

In chronic hospitals, 91 per cent of the patients were known to the social service, but whether the staff was adequate for full care of these patients is not known. The homes for incurables have no social service. In the general hospitals that had medical social service, 59 per cent of the chronic patients were known to the social service. The census records give no indication of

TABLE 5

CHRONIC PATIENTS IN PRIVATE HOSPITALS CLASSIFIED BY
TYPE OF HOSPITAL, EACH AGE GROUP

| Age group | Total | | TYPE OF HOSPITAL | | | | | |
| | | | Chronic | | Orthopedic | | General | |
	Number	Per cent	Number	Per cent	Number	Per cent	Number	Per cent
Total	2,707	100.0	1,244	100.0	462	100.0	1,001	100.0
Under 16 years . . .	624	23.3	36	3.0	372	80.5	216	21.6
16–39 years	559	20.8	178	14.6	71	15.4	310	31.0
40–59 years	735	27.4	412	33.8	15	3.2	308	30.8
60–69 years	367	13.7	256	21.0	4	0.9	107	10.7
70 years and over . .	396	14.8	337	27.6	0	0.0	59	5.9
Not reported	26	.....	25	.....	0	.....	1	.....

the extent of service rendered to the patients reported as known to the social service, which would be a matter for special study.

The ten general hospitals without social service reported only fifty-six chronic patients in all, and three of them reported none. In three the proportion of ward beds was small, and therefore they might be expected to be less in need of social service than hospitals with more ward beds. The other four, however, had a large proportion of ward beds and two of them were hospitals in Queens serving large population areas with almost no other special facilities.

CHRONIC PATIENTS IN PRIVATE HOSPITALS

Age, Sex, and Race

Contrary to the popular idea that associates chronic illness with old age or the late middle years of life, a complete program for the care of those who suffer from chronic diseases must deal to a large extent with economic and industrial problems resulting from illness in young adults and with problems of child welfare—education, vocational training, and child guidance—for handicapped children. Nearly half of all the chronic sick in the census were under forty years of age and nearly a third were children under sixteen years of age.

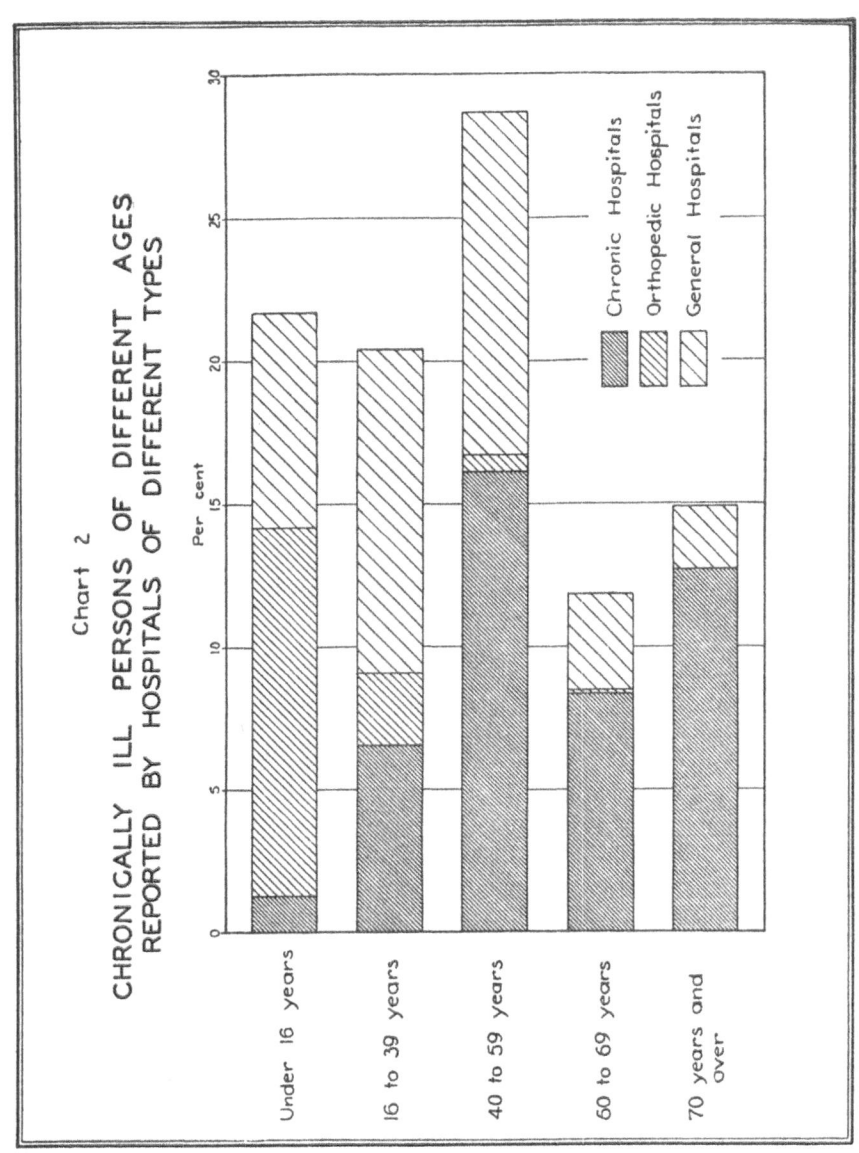

Chart 2

CHRONICALLY ILL PERSONS OF DIFFERENT AGES
REPORTED BY HOSPITALS OF DIFFERENT TYPES

Of all the chronic patients in private hospitals, nearly a fourth were children. In orthopedic hospitals, of which three out of six are institutions entirely for children, four fifths of the patients were under sixteen. In the general hospitals, over a fifth were children. In chronic hospitals, where nearly half of the patients were sixty years of age or over, only thirty-six children were found. Table 5 gives the number of persons of different ages in each type of hospital.

General hospitals, as would be expected, were caring particularly for the younger adult group under forty years of age, who were 31 per cent of their chronic patients and 18 per cent of all the chronically ill in the census. The distribution in different types of hospital for each age is shown in Chart 2. The private hospitals were caring for a younger group of adults than the public hospitals. In private hospitals, 41 per cent and in public hospitals, 57 per cent of the chronic sick were between forty and seventy years of age.

There were more males (52.6 per cent) than females (47.4 per cent) among the patients in general hospitals but the excess of males was slightly less than in the whole census. In the orthopedic and chronic hospitals, females (55.6 per cent) considerably outnumbered males (44.4 per cent).

Of these private hospital patients, 2.2 per cent were Negroes. In the public hospitals, 8 per cent were Negroes. No special hospital facilities have been provided for Negroes through private funds; therefore their care falls mainly upon the public hospitals. In the whole census, the proportion of the chronically ill who were Negores was 5 per cent, which is approximately the percentage of Negroes in the population of the city.[20]

Degree of Disability

In general hospitals, nearly three fourths of the chronic patients were bedridden; in orthopedic hospitals, less than half; and in chronic hospitals, about a fourth. A large proportion of the patients in chronic hospitals, nearly a third, used wheelchairs; and over two fifths were ambulant. Nearly a fourth of the general hospital patients were ambulant. Chart 3 shows the degree of disability among the chronic patients in each type of hospital. The proportion of bedridden patients is largest among the children and younger adults, under forty years of age, and smallest among the aged, seventy years or over.

Diseases

Of the 1,244 patients found in chronic hospitals and "homes for incurables," a sixth were suffering from cancer in some form. Nearly 30 per cent were suffering from diseases of the nervous system; 15 per cent from general diseases other than cancer, of which rheumatism was the most important; 14 per cent from diseases of the circulatory system. The remaining fourth were suffering from a variety of diseases, no one of which was found in large numbers.

[20] Population Bulletin, second series, New York; Composition and Characteristics of the Population, United States Bureau of the Census, 1931, pp. 72–73.

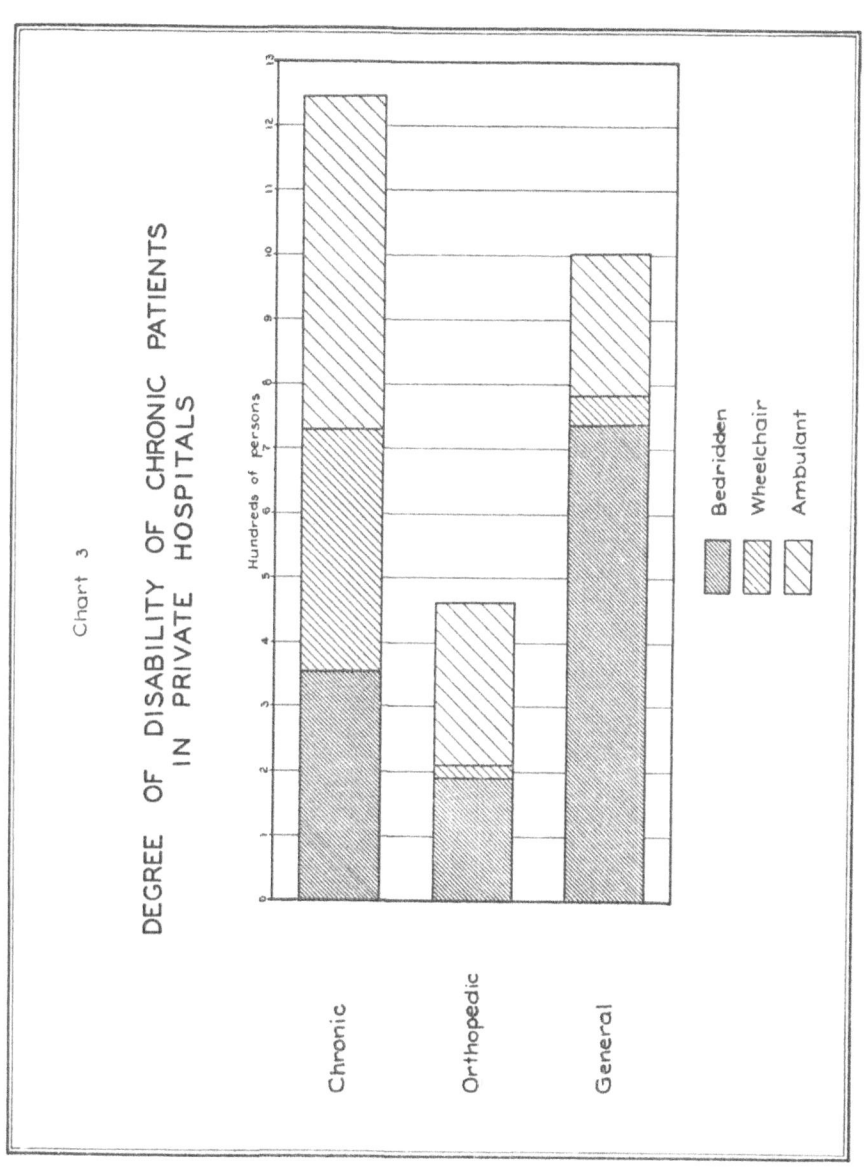

Chart 3

DEGREE OF DISABILITY OF CHRONIC PATIENTS IN PRIVATE HOSPITALS

Of the 462 chronic patients in orthopedic hospitals, the majority of whom were children and nearly all of whom were under forty years of age, the diagnosis of 36 per cent was poliomyelitis. Diseases of the bones and joints, including tuberculosis, came next, with 26 per cent. Tuberculosis of the spinal column and congenital malformations were 7 per cent each; rheumatism and rickets were 6 and 5 per cent respectively.

A fourth of the patients in general hospitals were suffering from diseases classified as "general," among which cancer was chief. Chronic rheumatism

TABLE 6

CHRONIC PATIENTS IN PRIVATE HOSPITALS CLASSIFIED BY
DIAGNOSIS GROUPS, EACH AGE GROUP

Diagnosis group	Total		AGE GROUP				
	Number	Per cent	Under 16	16–39	40–69	70 and over	Not reported
Total persons							
Number	2,707	. . . . .	621	559	1,100	396	26
Per cent	. . . . .	100.0	100.0	100.0	100.0	100.0	. .
Epidemic diseases	368	13.6	39.6	13.2	4.0	0.8	1
General diseases	705	26.1	12.1	23.2	35.9	24.7	7
Diseases of the nervous system . .	499	18.5	9.3	18.8	23.2	18.9	6
Diseases of the circulatory system	363	13.4	7.7	14.5	16.3	12.1	7
Diseases of the respiratory system	66	2.4	2.9	4.3	1.6	1.5	0
Diseases of the digestive system .	89	3.3	0.8	5.4	4.3	1.8	0
Non-venereal diseases of the genito-urinary system	148	5.5	2.1	7.5	5.9	6.8	1
Diseases of the skin	31	1.2	0.3	0.7	1.6	2.0	0
Diseases of the bones	163	6.0	14.0	7.5	2.6	0.8	2
Congenital malformations	50	1.9	6.8	1.1	0.1	0.3	0
Old age	101	3.7	0.0	0.0	0.1	25.3	0
Diseases due to external causes .	107	4.0	4.2	3.4	3.7	5.0	1
Ill-defined diseases	12	0.4	0.2	0.4	0.7	0.0	1
Not reported	5	. . . . .	3	. . . . .	2	. . . . .	0

and diabetes were next. The remainder of the diagnoses were scattered among various diseases. Circulatory diseases were nearly a fifth of all diagnoses, 81 per cent of which were heart diseases. Eleven per cent were suffering from diseases of the nervous system. Another 11 per cent suffered from non-venereal diseases of the genitourinary system, chiefly nephritis.

In Table 6 above, the proportion of the patients in each age group suffering from different forms of disease is shown. In the older middle-aged group between forty and seventy years of age, nearly 60 per cent suffered from general diseases or diseases of the nervous system.

The distribution of different forms of disease among all the chronic patients in private hospitals, as well as in public hospitals and in the total census is shown in Chart 6 of volume I, p. 92. The chief problems of both private and public hospitals are the general diseases and diseases of the nervous system, which together account for 44 per cent of the patients in each group of hospitals. General diseases, which were first in private hospitals and second in public hospitals, were largely cancer, rheumatism, and diabetes. In the total census, epidemic diseases, chiefly poliomyelitis, were most important. Diseases of the circulatory system appeared as the primary diagnosis of about 16 per cent of the patients in public hospitals and also in the total census, and of 13 per cent of those in private hospitals. However, circulatory diseases were present in nearly a fourth of the chronic patients in private hospitals, for nearly 200 persons had a secondary diagnosis of heart disease and most of the 100 persons whose condition was diagnosed as "old age" probably had circulatory disorders.

Mental Abnormality

Although the study was not planned to include patients with mental disorders, the question was asked in regard to each chronic patient whether any mental abnormality had been diagnosed or suspected. As the mental condition of the patient is not ordinarily given special study in hospitals of the types included, this question brought out only the most conspicuous instances of mental abnormality. Emotional disturbances, such as frequently complicate chronic illness without causing marked behavior difficulties, probably would not have been recorded.

Among the private hospitals' chronic patients, some mental abnormality had been noticed in 8 per cent, a somewhat smaller proportion than in the whole census. The same proportion was found also in public hospitals. For about a third, a diagnosis had been made by a physician and for the other two thirds an abnormal mental condition was suspected by a physician or some other person in charge of the patient. The proportion of mental abnormality discovered was over twice as large in chronic hospitals as in the other types of hospital. It was suspected five times as frequently as it was diagnosed in chronic hospitals, twice as often in orthopedic hospitals, and in an equal number of instances in general hospitals.

Home Situation

Most of the children had homes; only 6.6 were reported to have no home of their own. Of the younger adults, nearly a fifth and of the older adults, over a third had no home. Of the aged, seventy years or over, 70 per cent were without homes. In Chart 4, the situation is shown for adults. A somewhat larger proportion of women than men in chronic hospitals were without homes; in general hospitals, the situation was the same for both sexes.

Over half of all patients in the chronic hospitals were reported to have no home. In orthopedic hospitals, the percentage without homes was small since most of the patients were children. In general hospitals, 11.4 per cent were without homes. The percentage in private chronic and general hospitals combined who had no home was 36 per cent, a considerably lower proportion than the 44 per cent of patients reported homeless in public hospitals.

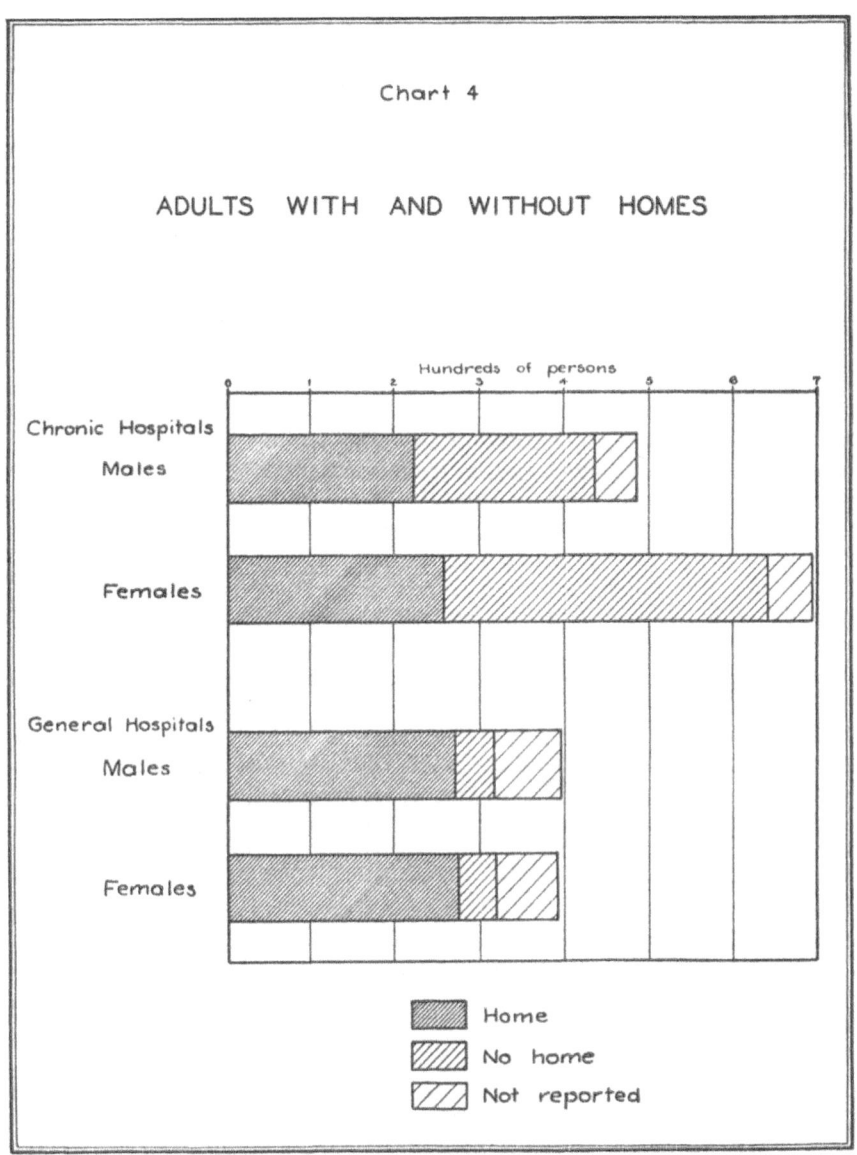

Chart 4

ADULTS WITH AND WITHOUT HOMES

Financial Status

All persons in hospitals were regarded as dependent in the sense that even if they were paying the hospital bill, the hospital was contributing medical care. About 80 per cent of the adults were wholly dependent for both care and maintenance upon resources other than their own, and the remainder were only partly dependent. A fifth of the adults got some assistance from relatives or friends; the rest were assisted either by private agencies alone or by both public and private agencies.

Twenty-seven per cent of all the patients in institutions for the sick were free patients and another 35 per cent were public charges. Less than 40 per cent, therefore, paid anything toward their care. Although the hospitals received some payment, either from the patient and his friends or from the city, for nearly three fourths of their patients, in only two fifths of these instances did it equal the full ward rate. The following table shows the extent of payment by the sources from which payments were received.

TABLE 7

CHRONIC PATIENTS IN PRIVATE HOSPITALS CLASSIFIED BY EXTENT OF PAYMENT FOR HOSPITAL CARE AND SOURCE OF PAYMENT

Source of payment	EXTENT OF PAYMENT		
	Total	Full payment	Part payment
Total payment for hospital care	1,750	39.5	60.5
Public charge	829	32.0	68.0
Patient	274	56.6	43.4
Patient and friend or relative	56	71.4	28.6
Friend or relative of patient	542	37.3	62.7
Other	49	59.2	40.8
No payment	636	....	....
Not reported	321	....	....

The rate allowed by the city for the care of public charges in private hospitals equalled the ward rate of the hospital in less than a third of the instances of city charges. The full ward rate was received more frequently when the patient or his friends and relatives paid the hospital charges than when they were paid by the city.

Length of Care

The patients in private institutions for the sick had been under care an average of two years—3⅓ years in chronic hospitals, 2⅓ years in orthopedic hospitals, and less than three months in general hospitals. Half had been in the institution for less than three months and two thirds for less than a year. About 100 persons had been in the institution ten years or longer. The following table (Table 8) shows the length of time for which the chronic patients in each of the three types of hospital had received care.

In chronic hospitals, more than half of the patients had been under care a year or longer. More than a fifth of them had been under care five years or longer. In orthopedic hospitals, about 40 per cent had been under care a year or longer and 18 per cent, five years or longer. In general hospitals, thirteen patients had been under care as long as a year and 11 per cent, for three months or longer.

In private hospitals, a larger proportion of patients had been under care less than a year than in public hospitals; but the proportion of those under care less than three years was about the same.

TABLE 8

CHRONIC PATIENTS IN PRIVATE HOSPITALS CLASSIFIED BY PERIODS OF
CARE RECEIVED, EACH TYPE OF HOSPITAL

Period of care	Total	TYPE OF HOSPITAL		
		Chronic	Orthopedic	General
Total reporting	2,655	1,226	459	970
Under 3 months	50.1	22.5	41.2	89.2
3 months under 1 year	16.4	21.4	17.6	9.5
1 year under 2 years	8.4	14.2	8.7	0.8
2 years under 3 years	5.0	9.0	5.0	0.0
3 years under 4 years	3.8	6.1	5.7	0.1
4 years under 5 years	2.6	4.3	3.5	0.0
5 years under 10 years	9.6	15.1	14.6	0.2
10 years and over	4.1	7.4	3.7	0.2
Not reported	52	18	3	31

In the whole census, the proportion of children who had been under the care of the agency reporting for long periods was as large as among adults. More of the adults under sixty years of age had been taken under care recently than of the children and older persons, especially those between forty and sixty years.

The number of times the patient had been in an institution because of his chronic illness previous to his admission to the hospital in which the census found him was reported for half of all the patients in private hospitals. Nearly half had been in an institution once before and nearly a sixth, twice. Five or more admissions were recorded for 4.5 per cent. Over a fourth had had no previous admissions.

Chart 5 shows the number of admissions to institutions of the patients in the three hospital groups. In general hospitals, for over half of the patients this was the first time they had been in an institution because of chronic illness. In chronic and orthopedic hospitals, more than half had been in at least one other institution before admission to the hospital and nearly a third had had two or more previous admissions. The age groups varied little in the number of previous institutional admissions reported,

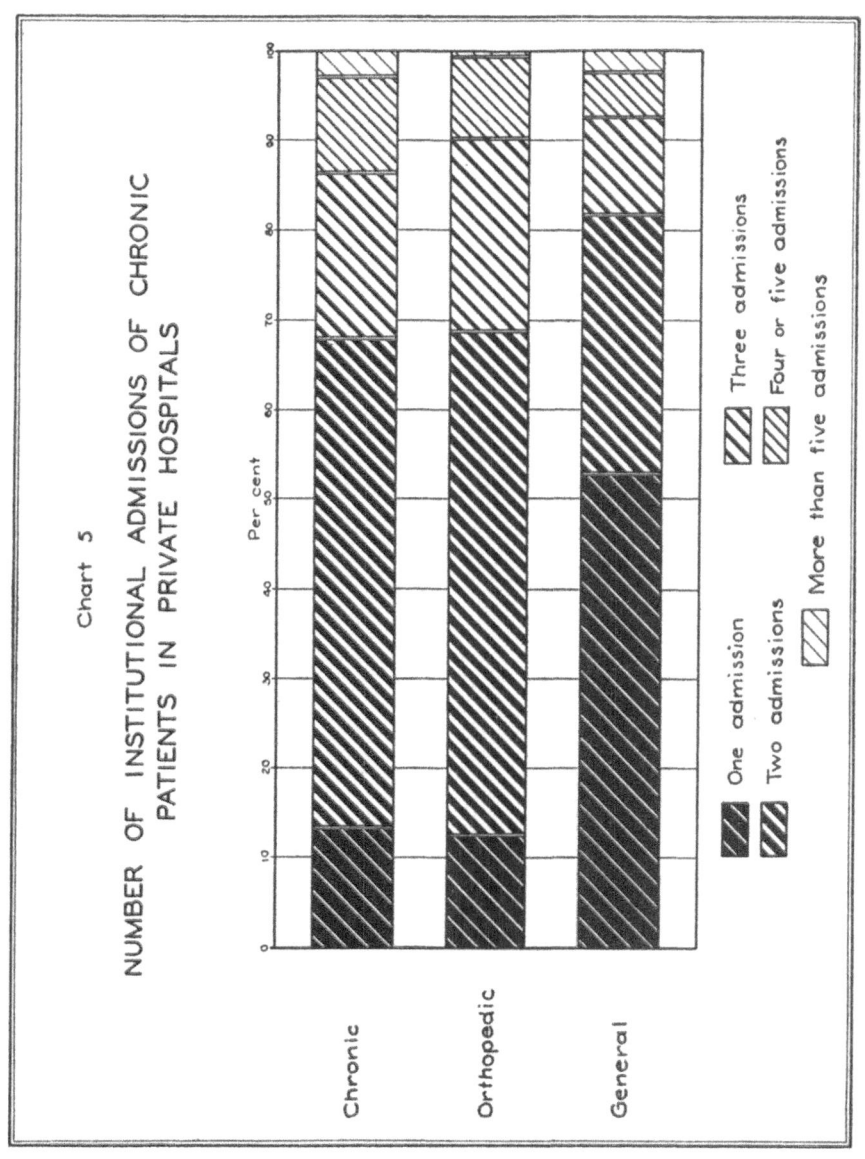

Chart 5

NUMBER OF INSTITUTIONAL ADMISSIONS OF CHRONIC PATIENTS IN PRIVATE HOSPITALS

with the exception of the aged seventy years and over, of whom a much larger proportion had had one previous admission and a smaller proportion two previous admissions.

The length of time since the patient first received institutional care, shown in Table 9 below, reflects the nature of the hospital in which he was at the time. General hospitals for the most part receive the patients who have not suffered long from chronic disease, and over three fourths of their patients had received institutional care for the first time within a year. In chronic hospitals, only about a fourth had received the first institutional

TABLE 9

CHRONIC PATIENTS IN PRIVATE HOSPITALS CLASSIFIED BY TIME SINCE
EARLIEST INSTITUTIONAL CARE, EACH TYPE OF HOSPITAL

Time since earliest institutional care	Total	TYPE OF HOSPITAL		
		Chronic	Orthopedic	General
Total reporting	1,212	448	206	558
Less than 1 year	49.8	26.1	27.7	76.9
1–2 years	12.8	18.5	12.1	8.4
2–3 years	8.0	11.8	12.6	3.2
3–4 years	4.9	7.6	6.8	2.2
4–5 years	4.5	6.3	7.3	2.2
5–10 years	11.8	18.1	19.4	3.9
10–15 years	5.0	5.1	12.1	2.3
15–20 years	1.6	2.9	1.5	0.5
20 years and over	1.6	3.6	0.5	0.4
Not reported	1,495	796	256	443

care less than a year before. In orthopedic hospitals, where most of the patients were children, a little over a fourth had first received institutional care within a year; but for a third, the beginning of institutional care had occurred at least five years earlier.

INADEQUACIES IN PRESENT CARE

Forms of Care Needed and Received

Of nearly 1,400 patients in private institutions for the care of the sick, including the "homes for incurables," who needed hospital care, 92 per cent received it. The remainder were receiving either skilled nursing or attendant care. In public hospitals, 97 per cent of those needing hospital care were receiving it. The smaller proportion in the private institutions is due to the fact that the "homes for incurables" are not equipped for medical care. In the private orthopedic and general hospitals, practically all of the patients who needed medical care received it. In the private chronic institutions, however, only two thirds who needed medical care received it. In the public hospitals, there was little variation on this point in the three types of hospital.

Of the nearly 400 patients for whom clinic medical care would have sufficed, 82 per cent were receiving it but were receiving it in a hospital. Of the remainder, about 1 per cent received skilled nursing care and 17 per cent received only attendant care. More than 100 patients in private hospitals were thought to need "B" care, of whom 72 received it, about 20 received medical care, and a few received attendant care. The private hospitals had 850 patients, or 31.5 per cent of all, who needed only attendant care, of whom nearly a fourth got a more skilled type of care—8.6 per cent, medical care, and 15.4 per cent, nursing care. Over three fourths who needed attendant care in private hospitals, in public hospitals, about half were receiving it.

In Table 10 below the proportion of patients receiving the care they needed in each type of hospital is shown.

TABLE 10

CHRONIC PATIENTS IN PRIVATE HOSPITALS CLASSIFIED BY CARE NEEDED
AND CARE RECEIVED, EACH TYPE OF HOSPITAL

Care needed and type of hospital	Total	CARE RECEIVED					
		Medical		Nursing		Attendant	
		Number	Per cent	Number	Per cent	Number	Per cent
TOTAL							
Total	2,707	1,671	61.7	208	7.7	828	30.6
Medical	1,748	1,576	90.2	5	0.3	167	9.5
Hospital	1,397	1,289	92.3	2	0.1	106	7.6
Clinic	351	287	81.8	3	0.8	61	17.4
Nursing	104	22	21.2	72	69.2	10	9.6
Attendant	851	73	8.6	131	15.4	647	76.0
Not reported . . .	4	0	.....	0	....	4	....
CHRONIC							
Total	1,244	244	19.6	199	16.0	801	64.4
Medical	392	233	59.4	1	0.3	158	40.3
Hospital	309	204	66.0	1	0.3	104	33.7
Clinic	83	29	34.9	0	....	54	65.1
Nursing	83	4	4.8	69	83.1	10	12.1
Attendant	765	7	0.9	129	16.9	629	82.2
Not reported . . .	4	0	.....	0	....	4	....
ORTHOPEDIC							
Total	462	453	98.1	7	1.5	2	0.4
Medical	427	423	99.1	3	0.7	1	0.2
Hospital	196	196	100.0	0	0.0	0	0.0
Clinic	231	227	98.3	3	1.3	1	0.4
Nursing	15	12	.....	3	....	0	0.0
Attendant	20	18	.....	1	....	1	0.0
GENERAL							
Total	1,001	974	97.3	2	0.2	25	2.5
Medical	929	920	99.0	1	0.1	8	0.9
Hospital	892	889	99.7	1	0.1	2	0.2
Clinic	37	31	83.8	0	0.0	6	16.2
Nursing	6	6	.....	0	0.0	0	0.0
Attendant	66	48	72.7	1	1.5	17	25.8

In chronic hospitals, including the "homes for incurables," 40 per cent of those who needed medical care received less skilled care; and nearly one fifth of those who needed attendant care received a more skilled type. In private institutions for the sick, nearly a third of the patients were suitable for custodial care. On the other hand, of those who needed hospital care, 8 per cent did not receive it. Less than three fourths of all the chronic sick in the census in need of hospital care were receiving it; and at the same time 10 per cent of those in need of custodial care were having medical care in hospitals.

The way in which purely social factors operate to modify treatment appears in cases of patients in hospitals whose medical needs could have been cared for in out-patient departments. All three types of hospitals were giving hospital care to a number of patients who needed only clinic care. This was particularly true among children. About 200 children were in an orthopedic hospital, although clinic care would have been sufficient, because they could not be cared for in their own homes.

None of the children and practically none of the younger adults were receiving a less skilled type of care than they needed. A number were getting hospital care although they required only clinic or attendant care. Among those forty years of age or over, a number who needed hospital care got less skilled care; among the aged, nearly a third. Among persons under sixty years of age, more than a third of those who needed attendant care got a more skilled type of care, but among those sixty years of age or over, only 13 per cent.

Among all the chronic patients in both public and private institutions for the sick, 49 per cent were in need of hospital care, 52 per cent in private institutions and 46 per cent in public hospitals. In addition, nearly 5 per cent required skilled nursing care in an institution with hospital facilities. The remainder did not require care in a hospital; 10 per cent needed clinic care and 36 per cent needed care in a custodial institution.

These discrepancies between the type of care best suited to the patients' needs and the type of care they receive indicate that, in addition to the insufficiency and inadequacy of facilities for the chronic sick, there is also considerable misuse of the existing facilities. This haphazard situation in regard to the chronically ill is part of the whole problem of hospital development affecting all classes of the sick. The United Hospital Fund has pointed out that "the need for a community plan for the growth of New York hospital facilities has been recognized for some time,"[21] and has announced its intention to seek funds to undertake a hospital survey with a view to making such a plan. The needs of the chronic sick, so large a group that they occupy a fifth of the capacity of all the general hospitals of the city, should not fail to receive special consideration.

Need for Facilities

It is well known that it is extremely difficult to find a hospital to which a person in New York City in need of a long period of care for a chronic illness

[21] United Hospital Fund of New York, Fifty-Second Year Book, New York, October, 1931, pp. 14, 23.

can be admitted. This is strikingly revealed by the figures brought out in this study. Concrete evidence of it was also found. Montefiore Hospital for chronic diseases, the only hospital in New York equipped for complete medical care of all types of chronic illness, reported that it was necessary to reject many applicants because its facilities were used to capacity. The "homes for incurables" also stated that they are not able to care for all who apply. The social workers in hospitals and family agencies and the visiting nurses all expressed the need for more beds for persons with chronic diseases. For those who need custodial care only, provision can sometimes be made in private nursing homes if the family is able to bear the expense, but the majority of the patients with which this study deals have no such resources.

A similar situation was found also in other cities. The Robert B. Brigham Hospital, in Boston, stated in its 1927 report, "that the free beds have all been occupied throughout the year, but about half of the most highly approved applicants have had to be refused admission for lack of space."[22]

Montefiore Hospital at the time of the census had a list of 149 persons not yet admitted because of the lack of facilities. Forty per cent were to be admitted as free patients, the remainder on a part-pay basis. In 1928, the facilities of this hospital were used to 94 per cent of its total capacity. Beth Abraham Home for Incurables had a waiting list of 181. Three of the other "homes for incurables" had waiting lists ranging from twenty to forty patients. Memorial Hospital, whose function is the treatment of acute phases of cancer, had a waiting list of fifty patients, although it has a rapid turnover of patients; and the need for provision for cancer patients with small means who do not want to be dependent is emphasized particularly by the City Committee for the Control of Cancer.

For older people, the need may be partly met in the future through the recent policy of some private homes for the aged of establishing hospital departments and accepting guests suffering from chronic diseases as well as caring for those who develop such illnesses after admission. Although it has usually been the policy of the homes to refuse to admit anyone with evidences of chronic disease, there were 237 persons found in private homes for the aged who needed medical care, only 64 per cent of whom were receiving that type of care. (See also p. 111.)

It is the middle-aged group, between forty and sixty years, who need hospitalization most frequently. This group constituted 18 per cent of all the persons in the census and 28 per cent of those requiring hospital care. The younger adults under forty years of age were 18 per cent of those in the census and 21 per cent of those requiring hospital care. Those between sixty and seventy years of age were found in equal proportions in the total census and in the group needing hospital care. Children constituted 31 per cent of all persons in the census and 27 per cent of those requiring hospital care. The aged were one fifth of those in the study and 11 per cent of those requiring hospital care.

The general diseases, especially cancer, rheumatism, and diabetes, most

[22] Robert B. Brigham Hospital, Boston, Annual Report for the Year 1927, p. 2.

frequently require hospital care. Nineteen per cent of all persons in the census and 29 per cent of those requiring hospital care were suffering from such diseases. Of the general diseases, cancer is most important, as 65 per cent of the 860 persons suffering from cancer required hospital care. Next in importance are diseases of the circulatory system, largely heart diseases, which constituted 16 per cent of the whole census and 18 per cent of those needing hospital care. Over a fifth of the cardiac patients required hospital care. Diseases of the genitourinary system were twice as frequent among those requiring hospital care as among the whole number in the census.

The two types of illness least often found to be in need of medical care were the infirmities of the aged due to senescence rather than to a chronic disease and diseases of the nervous system. Persons with nervous diseases were 8 per cent of all those requiring hospital care but 14 per cent of all patients.

It was pointed out as early as 1913, in a municipal inquiry into hospitals and city homes, that attempts to make definite provision for the chronic sick in city institutions were made difficult by the demands of the medical staffs for an increase of acute service.[23] The survey of hospitals in New York City made by the Academy of Medicine, in 1924, found the city singularly negligent in its provision for chronic patients.[24] Certain groups of chronic diseases, that is, cancer, orthopedic, cardiac, and neurological diseases, and syphilis, have received some attention from the standpoint of community planning; but no organized effort whatever has been made in this community to provide for the medical needs of a large group of chronic patients suffering from a variety of diseases, who numbered about 8,300 among the 20,700 chronically ill persons in the census. In respect to this particularly neglected group of invalids, medicine has hardly emerged from the era when "the hospital was an institution for the charitable relief of the destitute sick."[25] Although "the idea of going to a hospital because better medical or surgical care can be secured there is now practically universal among the American-born population,"[25] it is frequently only a vain hope for the chronic sufferer.

Additional Institutional Beds Required

There was found to be an actual lack of 1,000 beds, of which three fourths should be in institutions equipped to give full hospital care to chronic patients. In addition, general hospitals were caring for about 1,900 persons who should have been in chronic institutions; and custodial institutions were caring for 2,000 adults without giving them adequate care.

Besides these known deficiencies in institutional provision for the chronic sick, among 1,000 persons at home whose living conditions were not fully reported, many probably needed institutional care of the custodial type.

[23] Wright, Henry C., Report of the Committee on Inquiry into the Departments of Health, Charities, and Bellevue and Allied Hospitals in the City of New York, Board of Estimate and Apportionment, 1913, pp. 763-765.
[24] Corwin, E. H. L., The Hospital Situation in Greater New York. New York, G. P. Putnam's Sons, 1924, pp. 307-310.
[25] Davis, Michael M., Clinics, Hospitals and Health Centers. New York, Harper and Brothers, 1927, pp. 12, 13.

Furthermore, private chronic hospitals were found to be giving unsuitable care to about a third of their patients; and in many instances the institution did not have the equipment to give proper care. These facts brought out by the census, given in more detail in Chapter 2 of volume 1, are represented in Chart 9 in vol. 1, p. 112. They indicate the need for an extensive development of facilities for institutional care of chronic patients. After allowing for all possible readjustments of existing facilities, it is estimated that there is still a need for at least 1,400 new beds for hospital care and probably 2,000 additional beds for custodial care of the chronic sick (see p. 35).

To provide medical care in chronic hospitals for all patients not properly placed, including those found at home, in general hospitals, and in institutions unable to give hospital care, would require at least 2,500 ward beds. More than half, or about 1,350 beds, are needed for adults between sixteen and sixty years of age; about 700 beds, for children; and about 450 beds, for persons sixty years of age or over.

The largest group in the census for whom new hospital facilities are needed are the chronic patients occupying beds in general hospitals. Among the 1,900 chronically ill persons in general hospitals who should have been cared for in chronic institutions were 1,550 in need of hospital care, of whom about 1,130 were in private hospitals and 420 in public hospitals. At the present time, there are no chronic hospitals in which these patients could be given care. They are chiefly adults under sixty years of age. About 950 are adults between sixteen and sixty years of age; and about 350 are children. Only about 250 are persons sixty years of age or over, who might possibly be provided for through an extension of hospital facilities in homes for the aged.

The second group needing hospital care consisted of 800 patients at home, among the 1,000 persons at home who needed to be in an institution of some kind. Of this group, 350 were children; 350 were adults between sixteen and sixty years of age; and 100 were sixty years or older. About 360 were orthopedic patients, largely children and young people. Among the adults, cancer was the most frequent disease. The rest suffered from cardiac and neurological diseases, rheumatism, diabetes, and other chronic conditions.

The third group, patients in institutions without medical facilities, for whom beds in a chronic hospital are needed, numbered approximately 200 persons, the majority of whom were sixty years of age or over.

Over against the need for new hospital provision for those three groups must be set the fact that there were approximately 600 persons receiving hospital care in institutions other than general hospitals although they did not need it, for whom other arrangements would have been more suitable. If there were custodial beds available for these patients, the new provision for hospital beds required would be reduced from 2,500 beds to 1,900 beds. Approximately 500 hospital beds for chronic patients will be provided by institutions opened since the study was made or by various adjustments in present facilities, so that a total number of new beds is actually required for 1,400 persons.

To provide new hospital beds for 1,400 chronic patients, assuming 90 per cent of occupancy to be a maximum standard[26] in chronic hospitals, 1,550 beds in chronic institutions would be needed. Of these 1,550 beds needed, 715 would be in public institutions and 835 in private institutions, if the relative proportion of patients in public and private hospitals intended for chronic diseases continued to be the same as that found in the census. If official responsibility for the chronic sick were fully recognized, an increase in public facilities might be expected to furnish the greater part of these beds.

That the municipal Department of Hospitals could provide additional beds for chronic patients by any means other than new construction is doubtful. Since the time of the study, the municipal provision for cancer has been decreased through the closing of Cumberland Street Hospital's cancer division, but when the new Brooklyn Cancer Institute is completed, late in 1932, the original bed capacity will be restored and the facilities will be greatly improved. Neponsit Beach Hospital, the only municipal orthopedic hospital, was used to 97 per cent of capacity, in 1928, and to 101 per cent of capacity in 1929. Neurological Hospital, the only municipal hospital devoted entirely to general chronic diseases, is continually filled to more than its capacity; and its facilities, moreover, are far below modern hospital standards. The facilities for chronic patients at Kings County Hospital will be improved when the new hospital building is completed; but the three municipal hospitals with chronic services have altogether fewer beds for chronic patients at the present time than at the time of the study. Although Kings County Hospital has about sixty more beds for chronic service, the facilities at City and Metropolitan Hospitals have been reduced by about 100 beds by the demand for acute service and by an increase in the tuberculosis service in Metropolitan Hospital.

To meet the demand for private hospital beds for chronic patients, the Jewish Sanitarium for Incurables, with 250 beds, was opened in 1928. Between 150 and 200 of its patients are hospital cases. It serves largely the Jewish community, which is perhaps already better provided with facilities than the general public. The Sisters of St. Francis are endeavoring to raise a fund to build a new hospital for chronic diseases which will have about 400 beds for all types of care.

For cancer, the chief lack of facilities is not among patients with early or operable cancer but rather among those who, though probably incurable, yet need medical attention such as cannot be given by homes for incurables. The new Kane Pavilion of the Home for Incurables added fifty beds for this purpose. It has medical facilities for ameliorative treatment, including radium and X-ray equipment.

The need for increased orthopedic facilities might be partly met by an extension of the orthopedic service in the Hospital for Joint Diseases, which now uses only about half of its ward beds for orthopedic work. Unwillingness to accept care rather than lack of facilities was probably responsible for

[26] Corwin, E. H. L., The Hospital Situation in Greater New York. New York, G. P. Putnam's Sons, 1924, p. 72.

the fact that 46 per cent of the persons at home needing hospital care were suffering from orthopedic disorders.

Over half of a group of nearly 200 patients already in institutions who should have been in an institution able to give medical care were in homes for incurables. This group of patients might be provided for largely through a reorganization of homes for incurables to include facilities for medical care for some patients and by an extension of hospital facilities in homes for the aged.

To sum up the need for hospital facilities, about 2,500 additional beds in hospitals for chronic diseases were found to be required. Some part of the need for orthopedic beds for children and young persons might be met by an existing hospital; a new institution has provided for 150 to 200 adults; a reorganization of facilities in homes for incurables might provide for perhaps 150 others; and some of the 450 beds for persons of sixty years of age and over might be provided by an extension of medical facilities in homes for the aged. From all of these sources probably not over 500 beds would be provided. Provision of other forms of care for persons receiving hospital care although not in need of it would release 600 beds. It appears then that altogether 1,550 new beds in chronic hospitals are required to care for 1,400 persons, allowing for an average occupancy of 90 per cent.

The need for additional facilities in custodial institutions, which has been discussed elsewhere (see vol. 1, p. 113) may be stated briefly here. Improvements should be made in institutions caring for 2,000 custodial patients without adequate facilities—1,400 in homes for the aged and 600 in correctional institutions. To provide suitably for these 2,000 patients would require various changes in the homes for the aged, particularly the public homes, and the development of a public policy in regard to drug addicts; and it has been estimated that about 600 of the 2,000 persons might be given adequate care merely through improvements in these institutions. Six hundred additional institutional beds are needed for persons found at home or in general hospitals, over a third of which should be in institutions able to provide clinic care. More than 600 custodial beds are required for patients getting hospital care in various institutions outside of general hospitals. Readjustments of existing facilities and facilities created since the study was made would provide over 1,200 of the 3,200 beds needed, so that approximately 2,000 custodial beds remain to be provided through new construction. Among 1,000 patients whose home conditions are not known, there are unquestionably a number for whom custodial care in an institution should be provided, mainly in one with the clinic facilities. To determine the size of this group would require an investigation of each patient's situation. If a fourth should be found to be in need of institutional custodial care, about 250 additional custodial beds might be needed.

The above estimates are based upon facilities actually provided or under construction since the study was made in 1928. Plans for providing some of the additional beds needed for chronic patients are further discussed in

Section B of this chapter, pages 41–42. As all of the plans have not been fully drawn, it is not yet possible to say definitely how far the situation may be relieved in the near future.

SUMMARY

The Need for Chronic Hospitals

Hospital care for chronic diseases is one of the most urgent problems of medical organization.

Chronic patients do not belong in general hospitals. The régime of treatment they require is different from that of the acutely ill; and their presence hampers the hospital in caring for acute patients. Nevertheless, a fifth of the ward beds of private general hospitals are used for the chronic sick.

The lack of institutional facilities for the chronic sick is so great that general hospitals have great difficulty in refusing these patients, although they are not equipped to care for them. Once admitted, it is almost impossible to find a place to which they can be transferred, since the institutions intended for chronic patients have long waiting lists.

Approximately 2,000 chronic patients in public and private general hospitals could have been cared for more suitably in another type of institution.

The modern hospital for chronic diseases is the result both of improvement in medical knowledge and also of a growing public sentiment that the chronic sick are entitled to the benefits of medicine to the same extent as the acutely sick.

Only one such hospital yet exists in New York City; and over 2,500 persons who should have been receiving care in a hospital of this type were found elsewhere.

For the future progress of medicine in its search for the causes of obscure chronic diseases, such hospitals are essential. Only in a hospital devoted to chronic conditions can full opportunity be afforded to physicians and medical students to gain experience in the treatment of these conditions and to carry on research.

Types of Care Required for the Chronically Ill

The chronic sick require three forms of care—(1) medical care, known as "A" care, for those who need active medical study and treatment; (2) nursing, or "B" care, for those who require skilled nursing under medical supervision; and (3) attendant, or "C" care, for those who are disabled and need assistance but cannot be further benefited by medical treatment. Institutional care for the first two groups is given in a hospital, and for the third group in an institution of the custodial type.

Three fifths of the patients in the census of the dependent chronic sick, needed "A" care; 3.5 per cent, "B" care; and over a third, "C" care. As over two thirds of those needing "A" care could have received it outside of an institution, only one fifth of all, or 3,850 persons, needed to be in a hospital for "A" care. As some of those needing "B" care could receive it at home from a visiting nurse, about 600 persons needed "B" care in a hospital. Institutional provision for "C" care was needed by 6,780 persons.

Types of Chronic Patients under Care

Nearly a fourth of the chronic patients in private institutions for the sick were children; 21 per cent adults under forty years of age; 41 per cent, adults between forty and seventy years; and 15 per cent, seventy years of age or over. The proportion of Negroes, 2.2 per cent, was smaller than in the whole census, 5 per cent, and much smaller than in public hospitals, 8 per cent.

The chief diseases found were.the general diseases, mainly cancer, rheumatism, and diabetes, and diseases of the nervous system; and 45 per cent of the chronic patients were found in these two disease groups.

Types of Institutions Caring for the Chronically Ill

The chronic sick were found in different types of institution: (1) "Homes for incurables"—the conception that chronic diseases were always incurable, which prevailed before the days of modern medicine, led to the establishment of these homes usually equipped to give "C" care and sometimes "B" care but without hospital facilities. (2) Homes for the aged—the necessity of caring for guests in private homes for the aged when they become ill has brought about hospital departments in some homes; and in a few homes, the usual policy of not admitting anyone who is chronically ill has been modified so that aged sick persons are sometimes received directly. A home for the aged may be equipped to give "C" and "B" care and to a limited extent "A" care. Many of the private homes and public homes, however, are not equipped to give "C" care adequately. Private homes for the aged had 14 per cent of all the chronic sick, who were nearly half of all their guests; public homes had 8 per cent, or two thirds of all their inmates. (3) Convalescent institutions for children with cardiac and orthopedic diseases which are essentially child-caring institutions, as the children remain for months or years, and should be equipped to provide not only for the child's physical care but also for the development of his personality and normal family relationships. (4) General convalescent homes, which care for some chronically ill persons during recovery from an acute attack of the disease, but also sometimes receive chronic invalids needing custodial permanent care who will not be restored to normal capacity by a period of convalescence. (5) General hospitals for the acutely ill, which are obliged under present conditions to devote a fifth of their ward beds to the chronic sick and care for a third of all those needing hospital care. (6) Special hospitals for the study and care of certain chronic diseases, notably cancer, neurological diseases, and orthopedic diseases. (7) The hospital for general chronic diseases, which is a recent development.

Of 2,707 chronic patients reported by private institutions for the sick, 58 were in two special hospitals for cancer, 393 in one general chronic hospital, 793 in seven "homes for incurables," 462 in six orthopedic hospitals, and 1,001 in thirty-seven general hospitals.

The Cost of Hospital Care

Over 800 chronic patients in the private hospitals studied were "city charges," for whose care the city paid at a fixed rate. The amount paid by the city for two thirds of them, however, was less than the ward rate. In addition, over 600 patients were receiving entirely free care.

The private hospitals received full payment for approximately a fourth of their chronic patients, part payment for over two fifths, and no payment for over a fourth.

Families at the income level of the group covered by this study cannot possibly sustain the expense of prolonged chronic illness. The average period of disability was 5.8 years. The average period of care for the patients in private hospitals was 2 years. Seventy-one per cent of families of five or more persons in the census had a yearly income below the minimum budget for "health and decency" and 92 per cent had an income below the standard budget for a skilled workman's family.

The cost of hospital care for chronic patients is little less than the cost of care for acute patients. In addition to the facilities of a general hospital, the hospital for chronic diseases requires more extensive physiotherapy and occupational services and a larger dietary budget. The need for medical social service is at least as great as in the acute hospital. In institutions where children with chronic diseases, especially orthopedic disorders, are kept for long periods, the standards of child care developed for children's institutions must be maintained and special educational and training facilities added to the equipment.

The expenditure required for hospital care will depend to a great extent upon available facilities for clinic care with social service and nursing service, which make home care possible. Hospital provision without adequate clinic facilities is the most extravagant way to meet the problem.

Inadequacy of the Care Now Given

Of the chronic patients reported by all private institutions for the sick, including the "homes for incurables," nearly a third did not require medical care and could have been cared for in a custodial institution. On the other hand, of those who needed medical care, 8 per cent were not receiving it, owing to a lack of hospital facilities in "homes for incurables."

In the chronic hospitals and homes for incurables, 40 per cent of those who needed medical care were not receiving it; and nearly a fifth of those who needed only attendant care were receiving a more skilled service.

Of all the chronic sick in the census who needed medical care in a hospital, less than three fourths were receiving it. At the same time, 10 per cent of those who needed custodial care were getting medical care in hospitals.

Less than half of all the chronic patients in private hospitals were receiving social service. Fourteen of the fifty-three institutions had no medical social service. In the hospitals with this service, three fourths of the chronic patients were known to the social service. The "homes for incurables" and several of the general hospitals had no social service.

Inadequacy of the Facilities Now Existing

The census of the chronic sick in private hospitals revealed that the existing facilities for their care are insufficient, inadequate, and misused. This situation is part of the need for a community plan for the development of hospitals in New York, which has been generally recognized for some time. The pressing need for provision for the chronic sick makes the necessity for such a plan most urgent.

Official responsibility for the care of the chronically ill, long accepted in regard to tuberculosis and mental diseases, is beginning to be recognized in connection with other chronic diseases, particularly cancer. The resources of private philanthropy, to which the care of the chronic sick has been very largely left in the past, have proved insufficient to make the necessary provision.

A fourth of all the dependent chronically ill in New York City and less than half of those requiring institutional care are under the care of public agencies.

Additional custodial facilities are needed for approximately 2,000 patients among the chronic sick found by the census.

New hospital facilities are needed for 1,400 of the chronic patients found by the census. To provide for this number of persons in hospitals for chronic diseases would require 1,550 ward beds, assuming a maximum average occupancy of 90 per cent of capacity.

If the division of responsibility for the chronic sick between public and private hospitals were to continue as it is, a little over half of these beds might be in private hospitals and the remainder in public hospitals. If, however, the care of the chronic sick is considered to be largely a public responsibility, this lack of 1,550 chronic beds should be provided for the most part through municipal hospital units for chronic diseases.

SECTION B

FACILITIES OF PRIVATE HOSPITALS CARING FOR THE CHRONIC SICK IN NEW YORK CITY

HOSPITAL PROVISION FOR CHRONIC DISEASES IN NEW YORK CITY

Voluntary and Municipal Hospitals

As this study deals with the dependent chronic sick, it is concerned especially with ward patients. At the time of the study, in 1928, there were 4,481 ward beds[27] designed for chronic diseases,[28] almost equally divided between public and private institutions, of which 74 per cent, or 3,324, were in hospitals and 26 per cent, or 1,157, were in "homes for incurables." These institutions, although they have been in the past regarded as institutions for medical care and for convenience are grouped in this study with "chronic hospitals," are usually not equipped as hospitals and are rarely able to give their patients more than custodial care. Of all the 3,324 hospital ward beds provided for chronic patients, 33 per cent were in hospitals under private auspices and 67 per cent were in public hospitals. Proprietary hospitals conducted for profit have not been included in this study, as it deals with the dependent group of chronic invalids.

As it is to be expected that possibly 4 per cent of the ward beds in general hospitals will be occupied at any given time by patients with chronic diseases, 470 of the 11,756 beds in general hospitals might also be said to be available for the chronic sick—319 in private and 151 in public hospitals. In all then, a total of 3,794 hospital ward beds—1,416 in private and 2,378 in public hospitals—were available for the chronic sick at the time of the study.

The total bed capacity of the 142 institutions for the sick of the city in 1931 was 36,537; 24,174 in voluntary and 12,363 in municipal hospitals. The total number of institutional beds designed for the care of the chronic conditions included in this study in that year including private and ward beds, was 5,633, 29 per cent of which were in "homes for incurables."

The changes that have occurred since the census of the chronically ill was made, in 1928,[29] are: the opening of a new institution of 250 beds in Brooklyn, the Jewish Sanitarium for Incurables; the opening of the Hebrew Home for Chronic Invalids, a fifty-bed custodial home; the closing of the Cancer Division of Cumberland Street Hospital; an increase of about sixty beds in the chronic facilities of Kings County Hospital; and an increase of over 100 beds at Montefiore Hospital. The Home for Incurables has rebuilt

---

[27] Allowance has been made for the fact that not more than half of the total ward beds in three orthopedic and one special hospital with a cancer service were occupied by patients with chronic conditions.

[28] The hospitals included among those designed for chronic diseases are:
        Chronic hospitals and homes for incurables, with tuberculosis beds omitted
        Orthopedic hospitals
        Municipal neurological hospital
        Municipal general hospitals with chronic services.

[29] See Appendix Tables 1 and 3 for private and public hospitals included in the census of the chronic sick.

its old plant; and it has about the same number of beds, approximately 300, that it formerly had for general chronic diseases with an additional wing of about fifty beds, the Kane Pavilion, equipped for palliative medical treatment for cancer patients whose condition has been determined to be not amenable to further active treatment. There have been other minor changes in several institutions, amounting to the addition or subtraction of a few beds. Plans for additional facilities are discussed below.

The number of patients found by the census, outside of homes for the aged, who required care in a hospital, was 4,095; and to this number should be added an estimated 630 persons in the care of agencies of the type studied but not included in the census; so that the total number of patients in need of hospital care was approximately 4,725. Allowing for a possible use of 90 to 95 per cent of the 3,794 hospital ward beds available for the chronic sick in 1928, as estimated above, the shortage of hospital beds would appear to be between 1,200 and 1,300. In practice, however, most of the private hospitals in New York City have not been used to that extent. Actually 1,900 patients were found who should have been receiving medical care in a chronic hospital but were either in an institution of a type not suited to their needs or at home; but this 1,900 persons, through possible readjustments of existing facilities and new facilities since created, is reduced to approximately 1,400 persons to be provided for in hospitals for chronic diseases. (For further discussion, see pp. 32–36.)

The city pays for the care of dependent patients in voluntary hospitals at the rate of not more than $3.00 a day.[30] The daily cost per patient in the private institutions is frequently in excess of the amount they receive. Approximately 30 per cent of the chronic patients in the private hospitals were public charges, for whom the city had been requested to make this payment. (See also pp. 10–11.)

Extension of Institutional Facilities Planned

The Memorial Hospital is planning a new building of 300 beds. In the new institution, because of the conditions of a bequest received, there will be fifty beds for advanced cancer patients. The hospital will eventually therefore have about two hundred and fifty beds for patients under diagnosis and treatment. The Beth Abraham Home for Incurables is planning an addition of between 250 and 300 beds, in which one floor of about forty beds will be reserved for acutely ill patients who are now temporarily transferred to general hospitals. The House of Calvary is improving its old build-

[30] Rules of the Department of Finance, City of New York, for payment per day for care of public charges in private charitable institutions, 1931:

Children in general hospitals under the age of five	$1.15
To hospitals for medical and surgical treatment	3.00
To hospitals for consumptive patients	2.00
To hospitals for cancer patients	3.00
For orthopedic treatment of children	1.40
For the chronic, incurable, or infirm	1.15
For maternity service; ten to fifteen days hospital care Per patient	35.00

ing and adding a new building, and its total capacity in both buildings will be 140 beds.

The Lutheran Hospital Association of Brooklyn moved into a new 110-bed general hospital early in 1928. Because it is often under the necessity of accepting chronic patients referred by its affiliated churches, it plans eventually to convert a part of its old dispensary building into a ward for these patients. A similar project is that of St. John's Hospital of the Church Charity Foundation in Brooklyn, which recently moved into a new hospital building and plans to convert its old building into a hospital for chronic patients. The institution eventually will include both a general and a chronic hospital and also a home for the aged.

St. Francis Home for Incurables, a custodial home of 250 beds in a crowded section of the city, has begun a campaign for $3,000,000 to erect a modern 400-bed hospital for chronic diseases. The group of institutions conducted by the Sisters of St. Francis will then include a general hospital, a tuberculosis hospital, a chronic hospital, and a home for the infirm aged.

The municipal Department of Hospitals has under construction a psychiatric division of 600 beds at Bellevue Hospital and a general hospital in the borough of Queens. Plans have been discussed for a new cancer hospital as a unit of Bellevue Hospital to replace the present New York City Cancer Institute and for the reconstruction of the Brooklyn Cancer Institute with 100 beds; additions to Cumberland Street Hospital, which will increase its capacity to nearly 700 beds; and a 500-bed tuberculosis pavilion at Kings County Hospital. When the new 1500-bed building at Kings County Hospital is completed, sections of the old hospital will be used for the chronic service.

HOSPITALS FOR CHRONIC DISEASES AND HOMES FOR INCURABLES

Bed Capacity and Borough Location

The private hospitals for chronic diseases in New York City (exclusive of those serving orthopedic patients, discussed below) consist of three hospitals—Montefiore Hospital, Memorial Hospital, and the New York Skin and Cancer Hospital. The "homes for incurables" were eight in number. The following list shows the number of beds in each of these eleven institutions at the time of the study by borough.

Total	2,010
Manhattan	541
Memorial Hospital	104
New York Skin and Cancer Hospital	98
St. Francis Home	250
St. Rose's Free Home	89
Bronx	1,405
Montefiore Hospital	614
Beth Abraham Home for Incurables	224
Home for Incurables	307
House of Calvary	100

Six of these eleven institutions are in the Bronx; four are in Manhattan; one is in Brooklyn. Excluding the tuberculosis sanatorium of Montefiore Hospital, they had, in 1928, a total capacity of 2,010 beds.

Types of Patients Accepted

Of the three hospitals, Montefiore Hospital serves all types of chronic patients and the other two serve cancer patients who are potentially curable. Of the eight "homes for incurables," two serve cancer patients only; the other six receive all types of chronic disease. Among the eight is included St. Joseph's Hospital for Tuberculosis, in which the top floor has been given over to a ward for women suffering from some form of incurable disease; and this ward, therefore, is subordinate to the main purpose of the hospital.

It is sometimes erroneously reported that Montefiore Hospital, once a "home for incurables," has become a general hospital. This is due to a misunderstanding of its medical policy in regard to admission of patients. As its standards of medical treatment improved, it adopted the policy of selecting for admission chronic patients who might be expected to benefit by medical treatment and ultimately be discharged.

Types of Care Given

Of the eleven institutions, three, Montefiore Hospital, Memorial Hospital, and the New York Skin and Cancer Hospital are organized to care primarily for "A" patients, those needing active medical treatment. With their out-patient departments, they can give patients complete medical care even after discharge from the hospital. Montefiore Hospital is organized to care also for "B" patients, or those needing skilled nursing care under medical supervision, both those admitted as "B" patients and those who have become "B" patients after a period of study and treatment as "A" patients. "C" patients, or those needing only custodial care, are not admitted; but a limited number who become "C" patients while in the hospital are cared for in a special custodial pavilion. The continued care of other custodial patients is arranged for in custodial institutions or in their own homes. None of the other eight institutions were organized to care for "A" patients.

The following table shows the different types of care provided in each of the eleven institutions.

One institution, Beth Abraham Home for Incurables, is organized primarily for "B" care; but it accepts patients for "C" care as well. It is equipped to give adequate care to "B" patients, as far as good medical supervision is concerned; but it is a question whether the nursing staff is

[31] The census was not taken in this institution.

adequate for the care of a considerable number of "B" patients out of its total population. Only 9 per cent of its patients reported in the census were considered to be in need of "B" care.

Two other institutions, St. Francis' Home and St. Joseph's Hospital, care for "B" patients, although they are organized primarily for "C" care. It is believed that "B" patients could be cared for adequately if they were well selected. No such selection is being made at present, since no medical investigation of the patient is made by either of the institutions before admission of the patient.

TABLE II

PRIVATE CHRONIC HOSPITALS AND HOMES CLASSIFIED BY TYPES OF CARE OFFERED

Institution	TYPES OF CARE OFFERED[1]		
	"A"	"B"	"C"
Memorial Hospital	1	. .	. .
Montefiore Hospital	1	2	3
New York Skin and Cancer Hospital . .	1	. .	. .
Beth Abraham Home for Incurables . .	. .	1	2
Faith Home for Incurables	. .	. .	1
Home for Incurables[2]	. .	. .	1
House of Calvary	. .	. .	1
House of the Holy Comforter	. .	. .	1
St. Francis' Home	. .	2	1
St. Joseph's Hospital for Tuberculosis .	. .	2	1
St. Rose's Free Home	. .	. .	1

[1] The numerals indicate the order of importance that each type of care has in the particular hospital.
[2] The new Kane Pavilion of the Home for Incurables is equipped for palliative medical treatment.

The remaining five institutions are organized to give "C" care only. These are: Home for Incurables, House of Calvary, St. Rose's Free Home, Faith Home for Incurables, and House of the Holy Comforter. The selection of their patients is made without adequate medical examination before admission. The first four require that a physician connected with the institution approve the admissions, but no hospital facilities are available for diagnosis. The fifth requires only examination by a graduate nurse before admission.

In the other three institutions that admit "C" patients the practice in regard to medical examination before admission is similar. Beth Abraham Home for Incurables requires a medical examination by one of its doctors before admission, but the diagnostic facilities of the institution are limited. St. Francis' Home[32] makes no medical investigation before admission. St. Joseph's Hospital apparently does not require medical examination, although the services of the medical staff in its tuberculosis division are available for the chronic patients after admission.

[32] For future plans of this institution see p. 42. (see p. 42)

Medical Staff

There were 95 physicians including consultants, at the time this study was made, on the visiting staff of Montefiore Hospital, one of whom was paid. The daily average attendance of visiting men in the hospital was 15. These in addition to the internes and residents, 40 in all, represented one doctor in daily attendance to about every 20 patients.

Memorial Hospital had 2 paid residents, 28 visiting doctors, 7 of whom were salaried, and 4 internes. New York Skin and Cancer Hospital had 37 visiting doctors, of whom 12 were salaried, and 5 internes. These three hospitals each have an out-patient service conducted by the hospital staff. In Montefiore, the out-patient service is comparatively small; but in the other two hospitals it is a very active service.

The Home for Incurables had 3 paid resident physicians, a medical superintendent, and a paid visiting physician who served once a week. It had therefore, 5 doctors for 291 patients, or about one doctor to every 58 .patients. Beth Abraham Home for Incurables had 2 paid visiting physicians and 1 paid resident physician, the proportion of doctors to patients being about one to every 60 patients. In addition there were 32 consultants. The House of the Holy Comforter had 2 visiting physicians, one of whom was paid, for its 66 patients, or one doctor for every 33 patients. Faith Home for Incurables had 1 unpaid visiting doctor for its 64 patients. St. Francis' Home had 1 visiting physician for its 250 patients. St. Joseph's Hospital can call upon its house physician on the tuberculosis service for its 60 chronic patients or upon any of the visiting staff. No physician was assigned special responsibility for these patients. St. Rose's Free Home and the House of Calvary had 1 and 3 visiting physicians respectively.

Nursing Staff

None of these institutions has a nurse's training school except Montefiore Hospital, which at the time of the study had 72 pupil nurses and a graduate staff of 26 nurses.[33] New York Skin and Cancer Hospital had 25 nurses, and Memorial Hospital had 37 graduate nurses and 15 who were not.

In the homes for incurables, the nursing service was performed largely by undergraduate or attendant staff with graduate nurse supervision. The Home for Incurables, with an average daily census of nearly 300 patients, had 4 graduate nurses. Beth Abraham Home for Incurables, with nearly 200 patients on an average, had 2 graduate nurses. The House of the Holy Comforter had 2 graduate nurses, with an average census of 66 patients, and its superintendent was also a registered nurse. Faith Home for Incurables had no graduate nurse, the attendant staff being supervised by a practical nurse. In the Catholic homes, the nursing service is performed by the Sisters of the Order operating the institution, all of whom have usually had training in nursing. In the House of Calvary, there were 7 registered nurses; and in St. Rose's Home for Cancer, 1. In St. Francis Home, the 19

[33] Montefiore Hospital discontinued its school of nursing on March 1, 1932.

nursing Sisters perform the nursing duties; and in the chronic wards of St. Joseph's Hospital, the attendant staff is under the supervision of the nursing staff of the hospital.

Social Service

Social service is provided in only four of these eleven institutions. The homes for incurables studied have no social service. The three hospitals, with a total bed capacity of 816 beds, had 14 social workers. Six of these in Memorial Hospital combined the duties of social service and visiting nurse, giving home nursing care to both bedridden and ambulatory patients. Of the chronic sick patients reported by these three hospitals, 91 per cent were known to the social service.

Medical Records

Memorial Hospital, the New York Skin and Cancer Hospital, and Montefiore Hospital kept medical charts for which the doctors were personally responsible and which were reviewed by active records committees. Beth Abraham Home for Incurables required its doctors to be responsible for keeping the record on medical charts but had no records committee. The nurse here took the responsibility of seeing that the records were completed. Faith Home for Incurables kept no medical records; and medical records were not regularly kept at the Home for Incurables. At the House of the Holy Comforter the medical records were kept up to date by the nurses in the office of the superintendent. St. Francis' Home kept records of its patients on cards or in books and items were recorded by either doctors or nurses. Medical records were not regularly kept for the chronic patients housed by the St. Joseph's Hospital for Tuberculosis. The homes for incurable cancer patients kept no medical records.

Discharges

At Memorial Hospital and the New York Skin and Cancer Hospital, patients are discharged according to a regular hospital discharge procedure. In the homes for incurables, discharges are infrequent because patients are usually accepted for life and discharged only if the patient wishes to return to his home or if his mental condition requires his discharge to a mental hospital. Montefiore Hospital, in addition to its plan of admitting patients for a three-month period and discharging them at the end of the period if they are sufficiently improved, reviews all cases monthly to determine the possibility of discharge. A special committee on discharges meets every six months to pass on difficult cases.

All of the institutions discharge patients with psychopathic conditions to public institutions. One institution discharged 9 patients to public institutions in 1927; another, 10 patients. Patients are discharged to private hospitals for special treatment that the institution cannot provide. All but one institution agreed to take the patients back upon their discharge from the hospital. Beth Abraham Home in 1927 transferred 25 patients for special treatment; the Home for Incurables transferred 3 patients.

Montefiore Hospital discharges a small number of patients to other institutions for custodial care. Fourteen patients were discharged to private institutions for custodial care in 1927. Other patients are discharged to their homes, either cured, improved, or leaving voluntarily with condition unchanged. Montefiore Hospital discharged 784 patients to their homes during 1927; Beth Abraham Home discharged 3; the Home for Incurables discharged 37.

Memorial Hospital does not have occasion to discharge patients to public institutions, since the patients it admits are hopeful cases and as a rule can be cared for in their own homes after discharge. Patients with advanced conditions who are not admitted are sometimes referred to the New York City Cancer Institute after home conditions have been investigated by the social service. This is done in spite of the fact that referral to the Institute has been found to be unsatisfactory because patients so referred have frequently left within a short time. Aside from the Institute, the hospital reported great difficulty in placing those who are refused admission because there seems to be no hope of cure. It finds that facilities for Protestant patients are especially lacking.

Memorial Hospital tries to arrange for the home care of apparently hopeless cancer patients; partly because it is difficult to get them into other institutions and partly because if home care is possible, it is considered more satisfactory to the family and kinder to the patient. The hospital has a visiting nurse service (the Social Service Department is virtually a visiting nurse service), for the home care of such patients.

Costs and Charges

The daily cost per patient was given for six of the institutions, ranging from $2.47 in two of the "homes for incurables" to $8.26 and $9.29 in Memorial Hospital and the New York Skin and Cancer Hospital respectively. It was $3.75 in Beth Abraham Home for Incurables; $2.57 in the House of the Holy Comforter; and $2.47 in the Home for Incurables. In Montefiore Hospital, including both the hospital and the custodial divisions, it was $3.68. It is of interest to compare these figures with $6.32, the average cost per patient of the general hospitals of the United Hospital Fund in 1928.[34]

Five of these eleven institutions provide for private patients, two of which have regular hospital charges; two charge weekly rates of $30.00 and $35.00 to $40.00 respectively; and in the fifth, the rate varies. In four of the institutions, the rates for ward patients are $10.00, $14.00, $15.00, $17.50 respectively; and in four institutions, the rate is $21.00. These eight institutions accept ward patients on a part-pay basis. All have free patients

[34] United Hospital Fund of New York, Fiftieth Year Book, New York, November, 1929; Statistical Report for the year ended December 31, 1928.

but one institution requires an admission fee of $100.00 for burial expenses and also transfer of property. Two of the homes for incurables stated that it was their policy not to receive city charges.

Equipment and Physical Plans

Memorial Hospital, the New York Skin and Cancer Hospital, and Montefiore Hospital have complete hospital equipment. Memorial Hospital is fully equipped for research in cancer problems. It has pathology, chemistry, biophysics, physics, and biology laboratories and radiotherapy, X-ray-therapy, and electrotherapy departments. More than one third of the hospital patients are given treatment in the physiotherapy department of Montefiore Hospital. Beth Abraham Home for Incurables has installed a laboratory, physiotherapy apparatus for mechanotherapy and hydrotherapy, and a dental department and has a pharmacy and an operating room for minor surgery only. The Home for Incurables reported a pharmacy and urinalysis equipment as special facilities. The House of the Holy Comforter reported a dental department for complete dental treatment.

Montefiore Hospital has a separate building for custodial patients. The Home for Incurables reserves an eight-bed infirmary for acutely ill patients. The House of the Holy Comforter houses its patients on two floors, one of which was occupied by sicker patients. The Beth Abraham Home for Incurables reserved one floor for the sicker patients.

It is possible for all the patients to get into the open air in six of the institutions caring for patients over long periods. The buildings, including elevators, all accommodate wheelchairs. All but one institution provide recreation rooms.

Religious Service

Religious service is provided in all the institutions. One of the two Jewish institutions also provides Catholic services. One of the two Episcopal institutions has a resident chaplain. Opportunities "for worship and spiritual consolation are among the first requirements," according to Dr. Boas. "Places of worship and a spiritual head are among the prime necessities."[35]

Recreation

Recreation was provided in eight of the institutions through radio, concerts, and other entertainments. Reading is said to be "by far the favorite form of diversion" and "a good library is indispensable in a hospital for chronic diseases."[36] Movies are given frequently in the various hospitals. Costume parties, programs given by children, and plays or concerts by the patients themselves are favorite forms of entertainment. Memorial Hospital had a singer once a month. At Montefiore Hospital, the patients have a welfare committee that plans various types of recreation and among its activities is the publication of a monthly magazine. Montefiore Hospital

[35] Boas, Ernst P , M.D., and Michelson, Nicholas, M.D., The Challenge of Chronic Diseases. New York, The Macmillan Company, 1929, p. 164.
[36] Ibid., p. 166.

has recently completed extensive improvements in its recreational facilities, including a central radio system and a moving picture hall for sound pictures.

Occupational Therapy

Occupational therapy is provided in three institutions. Montefiore Hospital, with five occupational therapists, has the most highly organized occupational therapy department. There, occupational therapy serves about 30 per cent of the hospital population.

Research

The hospitals in this group all carry on extensive research. Montefiore Hospital has a completely equipped research laboratory, including neuropathological and metabolic laboratories, devoted to the study of chronic diseases. In 1929, the staff of the laboratory division published eleven papers in various medical journals and members of the staff of other departments presented forty scientific papers either at medical conferences or in published form. The New York Skin and Cancer Hospital maintains a research clinic in skin diseases; and seven papers, based on the work of the clinic, were read or published during the year 1930. Memorial Hospital, which is primarily a research institution, and has several endowed funds for research, is the outstanding center in the country for cancer research and education. It is affiliated with the Cornell University Medical College. Extensive work has been done here in developing treatment by radium emanations. In 1930, the medical and technical staff published fifty-six papers as a result of their research work.

ORTHOPEDIC HOSPITALS

Bed Capacity and Borough Location

The orthopedic hospitals are discussed separately, because they treat a form of chronic illness that has become a special branch of medicine and is not usually found in any of the other hospitals or homes for chronic patients, except Montefiore Hospital. There are six orthopedic hospitals in Manhattan and Brooklyn with beds distributed as follows:

Total	1,019[37]
Manhattan	682
New York Orthopedic Hospital	132
Hospital for Ruptured and Crippled	273
Hospital for Joint Diseases	277
Brooklyn	337
House of St. Giles the Cripple	45
St. Charles Hospital	42
Brooklyn Home for Blind, Crippled, and Defective Children[38]	250

[37] A hospital for crippled children in White Plains, with 225 beds, which was not included in the study, has a large percentage of New York City children.

[38] This is the country home of St. Charles Hospital and is designed for the long-time care of patients first treated at the St. Charles Hospital. It houses mental defectives in separate buildings; bed capacity as given here is exclusive of the buildings for mental defectives.

Types of Patient Accepted

The orthopedic hospitals in Manhattan treat both children and adults. Those in Brooklyn accept children only. Four of the six hospitals are designed for the treatment, particularly operative treatment, of acute conditions. They are not intended primarily for long-time post-operative care of orthopedic patients, nor for custodial care of the permanently crippled. One hospital, the House of St. Giles, often cares for children over a period of many years. Its average length of stay was over two months, which was more than three times as long as that of the other hospitals. The sixth hospital, the Brooklyn Home for Blind, Crippled and Defective Children, a branch of St. Charles Hospital, in addition to giving post-operative care, accepts the permanently crippled, gives treatment for the alleviation of their condition, and trains them for whatever vocation they are able to carry on. It cares for many children who need hospital care only because they do not have homes or because their homes cannot be adjusted to the needs of a child who requires special care and training. It often keeps children under care for many years.

Three other hospitals also have country convalescent branches for the care of post-operative cases, which are discussed in Chapter 4, on convalescent homes.

Medical Staff

The New York Orthopedic Hospital had a resident physician, 6 internes and a visiting staff of 18, who made daily visits. The Hospital for Ruptured and Crippled had a visiting staff of 45 and 12 internes. The orthopedic surgeons visited daily. The Hospital for Joint Diseases had a visiting staff of 77 and 13 internes. The House of St. Giles the Cripple had a resident physician and a visiting staff of 18, of whom some visited daily and others were on call.

Nursing Staff

Only one of the orthopedic hospitals gives training to nurses—the New York Orthopedic Hospital, which offers a graduate course for the training of orthopedic nurses. It had, at the time of the study, an average occupancy of 120 patients and a nursing staff of 40 graduate nurses and 10 student nurses. There were also a few ward attendants in the hospital.

The Hospital for Ruptured and Crippled, with an average census of 260 patients, had 28 graduate nurses and 87 trained attendants or practical nurses.

The Hospital for Joint Diseases, with a daily census of about 275 patients, had 42 graduate nurses and 31 attendants or practical nurses.

The House of St. Giles the Cripple, with about 40 patients, had 2 graduate nurses and 8 undergraduates.

In St. Charles Hospital and its Port Jefferson branch for long-time care, the nursing is done by the Sisters, some of whom have had regular nurse's training.

Social Service

All of the hospitals in this group have social service departments, ranging from one worker in St. Charles Hospital to ten in the New York Orthopedic Hospital. In the latter hospital, the social service staff is, strictly speaking, a visiting nurse staff and, as such, is discussed fully in the report of facilities for the care of the chronic sick in nursing services in Chapter 6. Of the chronically ill patients reported by these hospitals, 90 per cent were known to the social service.

Among the duties of the social service department in some of these hospitals is the investigation before admission of all persons unable to pay full ward rates and the responsibility for adjusting charges to such patients.

Medical Records

All of these hospitals keep complete medical records, for the items of which the physicians are personally responsible. In the Hospital for Joint Diseases, the New York Orthopedic Hospital, and the Hospital for Ruptured and Crippled, there is an active records committee. Records are freely available to the medical staff for study immediately after the discharge of the patient.

Discharges

The fact that all of these hospitals except the Hospital for Ruptured and Crippled have country branches simplifies their discharge problems. The House of St. Giles the Cripple and the New York Orthopedic Hospital discharge all patients needing care beyond the hospital stage to the convalescent homes, where they may remain for many months or in the case of the former institution, for years. The latter institution does not receive Negro adults in its country branch and finds great difficulty in placing them for prolonged post-hospital care.

The Hospital for Joint Diseases discharges tuberculous bone and joint cases to its country branch; but it finds a shortage of facilities for other patients who need from three to six months of further care, particularly patients in plaster casts. Since many of them must convalesce at home, the hospital provides ambulance service both for taking them home and for returning them to the hospital when the casts need to be removed. The hospital doctor visits once a month, and in addition, the patient is often referred to the Henry Street Visiting Nurse Service. Even then the hospital does not consider this a proper solution, because the patient's home usually cannot furnish sufficient care, light, and air. Discharge to Welfare Island also has not been satisfactory, because a change in the treatment plan has often defeated the work of the surgeon. The hospital superintendent suggested that visits to the homes of these patients by masseuses would be helpful.

This hospital also finds difficulty in discharging the less hopeful cases that need only custodial care, such as hemiplegia in adults or birth palsy in children. Before any patients are discharged to their homes, a home investigation is made either by the social service or, in the case of children, by the Association for the Aid of Crippled Children.

The Hospital for the Ruptured and Crippled has no convalescent home but uses other resources for convalescent care. Of 360 placements made by the social service in 1928, 49 per cent were sent to orthopedic convalescent homes or to summer homes giving three or four months' care to orthopedic patients; 30 per cent, to vacation homes for orthopedic patients; and 19 per cent, to general convalescent homes. With the exception of twelve children sent to Neponsit Beach Hospital, these post-hospital placements were not for patients needing care for months or years, such as those sent to the Country Branch of the New York Orthopedic Hospital, where the average stay in 1928 was 130 days.

Among the chief discharge problems of the Hospital for Ruptured and Crippled are the adults in plaster casts who, for lack of other facilities, must often be kept in the hospital for months, at times overcrowding it. Other difficulties in placement are the number of chronic patients who are admitted for ameliorative treatment but need continuous supervision, such as patients with arthritis or with various forms of paralysis. For all patients, home conditions are investigated before discharge and facilities for further treatment made available.

Since St. Charles Hospital keeps children, either in the Brooklyn Hospital or the Port Jefferson Home, until they reach sixteen years of age whenever necessary, it has few of the ordinary discharge problems. Home investigation is always made before the child reaches the age for discharge. Care in a boarding home is often arranged, when the home conditions are unsatisfactory. For badly handicapped children, an attempt is made to secure institutional jobs in order to solve the problem of transportation to and from work.

Costs and Charges

The daily cost per patient of operating the hospital was given for four of these institutions in 1928 as follows:[39]

Hospital for Joint Diseases $6.36
Hospital for Ruptured and Crippled 5.94
House of St. Giles the Cripple 2.85
New York Orthopedic Hospital 4.92

In the last two, the cost includes the convalescent branches. The average cost per patient of these four institutions was $5.39 or nearly one dollar less than the daily cost per patient in general hospitals of the Fund for the same year. In 1929, the costs per patient in the same hospitals, not including their convalescent branches, were $6.17, $6.36, $3.05, and $5.25, or an average per patient of $6.31. The cost per patient for general hospitals for the same year was $6.79.[40]

[39] United Hospital Fund of New York, Fiftieth Year Book, New York, November, 1929; Statistical Report for the year ended December 31, 1928.
[40] United Hospital Fund of New York, Fifty-First Year Book, New York City, October, 1930; Statistical sheet for the year ended December 31, 1929.

In the hospitals, the full ward rates vary from $21.00 a week in the House of St. Giles, the Hospital for Joint Diseases, and St. Charles Hospital to $28.00 in the New York Orthopedic Hospital. In the Hospital for Ruptured and Crippled, the rate for adults is $23.00 and for children, $12.00. In the Brooklyn Home for Blind, Crippled, and Defective Children, the rate is $10.50. All of these institutions accept patients for part payment in accordance with the patient's ability to pay.

Equipment

In addition to complete hospital equipment, all of the orthopedic hospitals have physiotherapy departments. The Hospital for Ruptured and Crippled probably has the most complete equipment. In 1928, it gave nearly 63,000 treatments, 70 per cent of which were given to clinic patients, 14 per cent to ward patients, and 16 per cent almost equally divided between private patients and workmen's compensation patients.

All of the hospitals have laboratories, X-ray departments, special provision for dietetic care, and complete dental service. The Port Jefferson Home of St. Charles Hospital had a swimming pool for muscle reëducation. At the time when the study was made, the home had as patients five children suffering from spastic paralysis, sent from the State Orthopedic Hospital[41] for the swimming treatment, with the expectation that if it were successful it would be adopted in the state plan of treatment. The Hospital for Ruptured and Crippled and the House of St. Giles the Cripple have installed pools since the study was made. All of the hospitals are well adapted to the use of wheelchairs and are so arranged that all patients can get into the open. The House of St. Giles the Cripple has vita glass windows on the sun side in all wards.

Recreation

A fairly extensive program of recreation is carried on in all of these hospitals, with the exception of the New York Orthopedic Hospital. In the House of St. Giles the Cripple, it is closely tied up with the educational program through the household science work, the gymnasium activities and the work of the music and dramatic departments. This hospital seems to have combined the aims of education, physical therapy, and recreational therapy effectively in many of its activities. The Hospital for Joint Diseases has a number of auxiliary groups that provide entertainment for the patients in various ways. The recreational aspect of the occupational work taught in the hospital is stressed more than its therapeutic values. Nearly all of the hospitals have radio and movie equipment. Some have libraries.

Religious Service

All of these hospitals with the exception of the New York Orthopedic Hospital make provision for religious services for the patients.

[41] Now known as the State Reconstruction Home.

Occupational Therapy

The Hospital for Joint Diseases and the Hospital for Ruptured and Crippled each have two trained occupational therapists on the staff. In the latter hospital, in 1928, a total of 426 patients were served by this department—from 80 to 105 each month. The hours of work done by the patients averaged about forty-six hours for each patient. The New York Orthopedic Hospital has given up its occupational work, since patients are sent to its country branch as soon as possible and while in the hospital are not in a condition to be benefited by occupational therapy. The House of St. Giles the Cripple had no occupational therapy department but had the services of a volunteer once a week. In the country branch of St. Charles Hospital, the vocational work is planned for its therapeutic value as well.

Educational Service

The Brooklyn Home for Blind, Crippled, and Defective Children, because it keeps children for many years, is equipped to give complete grammar school work. In addition children are taught music, painting, dancing, and acting whenever they show aptitude in any of these directions. Two years of commercial training are given to those who have completed the work of the grades. All girls are taught sewing and allied arts.

The Hospital for the Ruptured and Crippled had during 1928 an average of about 90 children at one time and a total of 450 children in its school classes. The House of St. Giles the Cripple had, in addition to the regular teachers furnished by the Board of Education, departments of household arts and science, music, dramatics, and physical education, each with a director. The hospital has a band, and it has produced with patients as performers both musical and dramatic programs.

Research

Three of the hospitals, the Hospital for Joint Diseases, the New York Orthopedic Hospital, and the Hospital for Ruptured and Crippled are equipped for research and teaching. The last-named hospital is doing extensive research in the causes and treatment of arthritis. The New York Orthopedic Hospital, since 1927, has had a full-time research surgeon studying the end results of surgical treatment given to patients in previous years. In 1928, a study of the effects of the sun treatment was in progress. During 1928, the laboratory staff of the Hospital for Joint Diseases were engaged in twelve scientific problems of research and prepared eight scientific papers for medical journals.

GENERAL AND OTHER SPECIAL HOSPITALS

Sample of General Hospitals Included

All of the special and chronic hospitals were included in the study; but a sample of private general hospitals was selected, and 32 of the total of 68 private general hospitals in the city were included.

In selecting these 32 hospitals, an effort was made to get a representative sample of the general hospitals, so that the proportion of chronic sick found in those studied might be applied to the remainder. First, the 56 non-Catholic hospitals were arrayed in descending order of average stay of patients in 1926. The first 14 were selected, but two of these later were omitted because of difficulties in obtaining data from them. Then another 11 hospitals were selected at random by using every fourth one in the array according to average stay.

This selection was further modified to exclude all hospitals with less than 25 beds and to be representative in such factors as borough location, total bed capacity, percentage of occupancy, proportion of hospital beds to number of staff physicians, affiliation with a medical school, affiliation with racial and religious groups, and ward rates. The sample was then increased by 9 Catholic hospitals in which a census had been taken, 7 in the boroughs of Brooklyn and Queens and 2 in the New York Diocese. The other 3 in the New York Diocese were discarded at the request of the Catholic Charities on the ground that they had not reported all of their chronic patients. The original plan had been to make a census in all of the 12 Catholic hospitals.

In addition to the 32 general hospitals studied, 9 of the so-called special hospitals are treated with the group of general hospitals, as previously stated, 6 of them because their function is identical with that of general hospitals except that they serve only children or only women and children. Three others, Neurological Institute, Reconstruction Hospital,[42] and Rockefeller Institute were included in this group, because, although special in function, they are treating acute conditions or acute manifestations of chronic diseases rather than chronic conditions. These 9 hospitals had a bed capacity of 1,058, 69 per cent of which were ward beds.

Slightly over half of the general hospitals in the city were studied, having nearly 60 per cent of the total bed capacity of the city and nearly two thirds of the total ward capacity. Since the study is concerned only with those chronic patients who are, at least in part, dependent for their care upon public or private social resources, only patients using ward facilities were included in the census.

Bed Capacity and Borough Location

The 77 general hospitals in the city, including the 9 special hospitals that are treated with this group, and the 41 general hospitals included in the study are analyzed by their borough location and the number of their beds in Appendix Table 2.

Nearly half of the hospitals studied, more than half of the beds, and nearly 60 per cent of the ward beds were in Manhattan. The hospitals in Manhattan are larger than in the other boroughs and have a larger percentage of ward beds.

[42] On January 1, 1930, this hospital was merged with the New York Post-Graduate Medical School and Hospital, and it is now known as the Reconstruction Hospital Unit of that institution. Since 1929, the United Hospital Fund of New York has classified it as an orthopedic hospital.

Policy in Regard to Admission of Chronic Patients

The general hospital is intended for the treatment of acute medical and surgical cases; and patients suffering from contagious, mental, or chronic diseases are generally excluded. The policy of every hospital from which information was gathered is not to accept chronic patients. "We avoid chronic patients, and it is understood that patients must be removed if they become chronic" was the usual statement of this policy.

The fact that the census found chronic patients occupying ward beds in different hospitals is proof that it is not possible to live up to this policy under the present condition of insufficient facilities for the chronically ill. Only 4 of the 41 general hospitals studied reported that they had no chronic patients at the time. (See also p. 17.)

With few exceptions, all the hospitals from which information was obtained reported that they were frequently called upon to admit chronic patients, some specifying "daily," "almost daily," or "every week." The exceptions were small hospitals with no out-patient departments, where patients are admitted chiefly through the staff physicians who are not interested in treating chronic patients in the hospital. The greatest demand is made upon the large hospitals with active out-patient departments and upon hospitals supported by religious, national, or racial groups who expect their hospital to admit all sick persons of the group. The lack of facilities elsewhere was given as the chief reason for the demand upon the general hospitals.

One Jewish hospital states that its patients, who are orthodox Jewish, are unwilling to go to the city institutions, because Kosher food is not provided, and that Montefiore Hospital is often inaccessible or overcrowded. This demand for admission of chronic patients, the superintendent said "is an unnecessary and avoidable hardship for us."

Eight hospitals gave reasons for making occasional exceptions to their policy of not admitting chronic patients. These exceptions are as follows:

Beth Israel Hospital admits some chronic patients who may be improved by hospital treatment.

At Knickerbocker Hospital, the superintendent said, "We have made occasional exceptions of patients who live in the neighborhood and for whom we feel sorry."

Mt. Sinai Hospital accepts chronic patients who present obscure conditions requiring prolonged and intensive scientific investigation.

At New York Hospital, certain chronic patients referred from the out-patient department were accepted for teaching purposes.

The Norwegian Lutheran Hospital had six beds regularly reserved for chronic patients. Patients suffering from tuberculosis or cancer were accepted and alcoholics, if non-transient, living in the neighborhood, and not too disturbing. When the six beds were occupied, others could not be admitted.

The Lutheran Hospital of Brooklyn accepts chronic patients sent by churches affiliated with the hospital. It plans, in the future, to convert part of its old dispensary building into quarters that can be used for chronic patients.

The Presbyterian Hospital accepts chronic patients who present acute symptoms that in the opinion of the attending physician or surgeon are capable of being relieved.

St. John's Hospital, supported by the Church Charity Foundation of Long Island, is compelled to take a few chronic patients referred to it by affiliated churches of the diocese. Because of the pressure of the demand for caring for chronic patients, the hospital plans as a part of a future building program to convert to this purpose its old hospital, which was recently abandoned for a new 200-bed institution.

New York Infirmary for Women and Children. Chronic patients are admitted if the doctor or the social service recommends them for admission and they are wanted at the time for teaching purposes.

St. Mary's Free Hospital for Children. Although this hospital accepts children suffering from chronic diseases as well as those with acute conditions, it reported no chronic sick at the time of the census, and the superintendent reported that chronic patients were very infrequent in the hospital.

Neurological Institute. This hospital does not accept neurological patients for custodial care but accepts for diagnosis and temporary treatment many patients whose condition is of a chronic and long standing nature. Facilities for their further care are often lacking after the two months usually allowed by the hospital as a maximum stay are over.

Reconstruction Hospital. Since this hospital is for the purpose of rehabilitating persons suffering from occupational and traumatic diseases, it often cares temporarily for chronic patients; but it does not accept for treatment those whose disability is permanent and for whom there is little hope of rehabilitation.

Rockefeller Institute. At the time of the census, among the conditions being accepted by this institution for study were the following chronic diseases: Bright's disease, rheumatic fever, and chronic heart disease.

A record of the number of patients refused admission and the reasons for refusal was kept by only four of the general hospitals from which information was obtained. These were Beth Israel Hospital, Mt. Sinai Hospital, St. Luke's Hospital, and the Bronx Hospital. About 150 chronic patients were rejected by Beth Israel Hospital in 1927; 192 by Mt. Sinai Hospital; and 97 by St. Luke's Hospital. The total figures for 1927 were not available at the Bronx Hospital. Other hospitals gave such estimates as "4 or 5 a week"; "365 in the year"; "1 or 2 daily." Almost all of the other hospitals refused chronic patients admission during 1927, but kept no record of rejections.

Two hospitals reported that no chronic patients were rejected in 1927. These were the Norwegian Lutheran Hospital and Staten Island Hospital. The former had six beds for chronic patients; the latter always had plenty of room since its bed capacity was 265 and its average occupancy only 152.

At the Staten Island Hospital, all chronic patients were admitted if only for twenty-four hours and then transferred to Bellevue Hospital for disposition elsewhere.

The applications of chronic patients for admission are usually troublesome to general hospitals. There are exceptions to the general rule in different hospitals, and the degree to which the restriction against chronic patients is enforced depends upon many variable factors, such as the extent to which the hospital facilities are used, the requirements for teaching material, and the medical interests of the staff physicians. It, therefore, comes to be generally known that some hospitals accept chronic patients more readily than others although the reasons for these variations may not be understood.

One hospital requires that all applications for admission be accompanied by a certificate of the physician stating the nature and probable duration of the disease, and patients with definitely acute symptoms are given preference. The superintendent of another hospital, by way of illustrating the difficulty of maintaining a policy of always rejecting chronic patients, told of a case he had dealt with recently. A woman tried to have her father, suffering from a chronic disease, admitted to the hospital; but the superintendent did not yield, although a city official and later a member of the executive committee of the hospital interceded in the patient's behalf.

The problem would be less difficult for the general hospital if there were adequate facilities elsewhere, to which patients refused admission could be referred. Because adequate facilities are lacking or because the hospital lacks the social service personnel to take the responsibility, few hospitals assume the medical guidance of chronic patients refused admission. A majority of the hospitals frankly admit that they take no responsibility for guiding patients elsewhere. Two hospitals say that the staff doctors interested in securing admission advise the patients. Seven hospitals simply give names and addresses of other hospitals to which patients may make application. One hospital makes recommendations through its admitting room, which arranges for placement in urgent cases. The social services of four other hospitals make arrangements for placement of urgent cases refused admission, especially those referred by the doctors in their outpatient departments. The Babies Hospital, which refused admission to 450 patients in 1927, assumes responsibility for the medical guidance of patients refused and refers them to the proper hospital or agency for assistance.

Waiting lists were kept in fourteen of the hospitals for which information was gathered. In eighteen of the hospitals, no waiting list was kept, except, in a few hospitals, for maternity cases. Chronic patients were not generally put on the waiting list in those hospitals that occasionally accepted them.

Policy in Regard to Discharge of Chronic Patients

Three hospitals reported that they never discharged patients to public institutions; one hospital reported that it rarely did so and that in 1927 no patient had been discharged to a public institution. The remaining hospitals discharge to public institutions as the need arises. In the case of patients whose condition and circumstances indicate that they will eventually have to go to one of the city institutions on Welfare Island, some hospitals transfer them there directly and others transfer them to Bellevue Hospital or Kings County Hospital. Some of the factors that determine how the transfer shall be made are: the distance of Welfare Island from the transferring hospital, the willingness of the patient to go to Welfare Island, and the willingness of the transferring hospital to accept responsibility for explaining the patient's chronic condition to him.

Twenty-two of the 38 hospitals that discharge to public institutions reported a total of nearly 500 patients sent to the city institutions in 1927. The Staten Island Hospital discharged 90 patients to public institutions, more than any other hospital that reported. This is probably due to the fact that, since there is no municipal hospital on Staten Island, many patients are accepted who would otherwise be referred to a public hospital in the first instance. Knickerbocker Hospital discharged 72 patients to public institutions; New York Hospital, 70; St. John's of Long Island City, 56; and St. Vincent's Hospital, nearly 50. Other hospitals reporting discharged from 1 to 35 patients to public institutions.

Besides discharging chronic patients to public institutions, some of the general hospitals make other arrangements for their further care. Patients who can live at home and go to a clinic are referred to the out-patient department of the hospital or to another out-patient department or clinic. For patients needing continued institutional care, the hospitals are sometimes able to secure a bed in a private institution for chronic patients. For other patients, the hospitals sometimes request the services of visiting nurses or social agencies. Occasionally a patient able to pay a low rate of board is referred to a nursing or boarding home.

Five hospitals report that they make no arrangements for further care of chronic patients except to send them to public institutions. Seven hospitals do not refer patients to out-patient clinics, because they have no out-patient departments of their own. Nine hospitals say they do not try to secure beds for discharged chronic patients in other institutions, nor do they call upon social agencies and visiting nurses to help patients after discharge.

Institutional care is not always necessary in order to meet the problem adequately. By ingenious arrangements, social workers sometimes succeed in making suitable provision for patients even under inauspicious conditions in their own homes. One social worker tells of an afflicted wife of a street cleaner for whom the Department of Street Cleaning, at the suggestion of the social worker, arranged that he be transferred to his own neighborhood, so that he could give his wife the few minutes care that she needed at various times during the day. In this way the couple were kept together and the chronic patient got all the special attention that was required.

The hospitals that make no effort to assist chronic patients to secure further care needed after discharge are hospitals, in most instances, that do not have a social service. Three hospitals, however, without social service departments do endeavor to secure further care for a discharged patient when needed through referring him to social agencies or other private institutions or clinics.

Costs and Charges

The daily costs per patient of general hospitals at the time of the census are best indicated by the cost figures of the United Hospital Fund. During the year 1928, the thirty general hospitals belonging to the Fund had an average daily cost per patient of $5.56 for ward patients, of $7.69 for private patients, and of $6.34 for all patients. On this basis the 1,000 chronic patients under the care of private general hospitals were costing those hospitals about $5,600 a day and, on the basis of the average time under care of the chronic patients reported by general hospitals, had already cost the hospitals approximately $475,000.

The ward charges in 39 of the 41 hospitals studied ranged from $14.00 to $28.00 a week. Two hospitals, St. Mary's for Children and Rockefeller Institute, made no charge. The most usual charge was $21.00, the rate in 21 hospitals. The rate in 12 hospitals was either $24.50 or $28.00; in 6 hospitals, less than $21.00.

Medical Social Service

Of the 41 hospitals, 10, with a total of 1,186 beds, had no social service. These 10 hospitals had 15 per cent of all the beds and 13 per cent of all the ward beds in the hospitals studied. Three of them reported no chronic sick and the remaining 7 reported less than 6 per cent of the chronic sick found in private general hospitals.

The other 31 hospitals had a total of 152 social workers, an average of nearly 5 per hospital. Twelve hospitals had one each, 9 had from 2 to 5, 3 had from 5 to 10, and 7 had 10 or more, one of which had 26 and another 15.

Of the 945 patients reported by the 31 hospitals with social service, 59 per cent were known to the social service. Seventy per cent of the children were known to the social service; but the percentage was smaller in the other age groups.

Research

Research in some form is carried on in nearly all of these general and special hospitals. Rockefeller Institute is entirely a research institution selecting patients primarily for the research interest of their malady. At the time of the study, this institution was carrying on research in acute rheumatic fever, chronic cardiac disease, pneumonia, and other acute respiratory infections, chickenpox, measles, and Bright's disease. The Neurological Institute, since it moved to the New York Hospital-Cornell University Medical Center, has had a special Committee on Research and Publication, which by the end of 1931 had already subsidized seven major research projects and had begun the publication of the quarterly *Bulletin of the Neurological Institute.* Its first issue contained eight original articles. The Matheson Commission on Encephalitis was carrying on a research program in this hospital.

Examples of some of the chief research activities announced in the annual reports of the hospitals may be mentioned to indicate the extent and importance of research work in the program of a general hospital. The New York Hospital, an outstanding research institution, was studying especially asthma, urology, and heart disease. Its professional staff published about forty papers in 1929. In its new quarters in the New York Hospital-Cornell University Medical Center, its research program will be enlarged. The New York Post-Graduate Medical School and Hospital has a number of funds for research in asthma, pyelitis, nutrition, eye conditions, mental deficiency, paralysis agitans, and pellagra, besides general research. The Presbyterian Hospital in the city of New York also has many research funds, the chief of which is the $500,000 Harkness Research Fund, the income of which is used for laboratory research. In addition, there are special funds for research in arthritis, physical diagnosis, Bright's disease, common colds, the nervous system, and other special problems. Long Island College Hospital is a teaching and research hospital and is making a special study of arthritis.

Lenox Hill Hospital has several research funds and its staff is carrying on research in eye diseases, metabolism in children, colitis, etiology of arteriosclerosis, etiology of Hodgkin's disease, and other subjects. Its staff published forty-two scientific papers or textbooks in 1930. Woman's Hospital also has an active research program, chief among which has been a study of results in the treatment of cancer covering a period of eleven years. Beekman Street Hospital, since it has a large workmen's compensation service, specializes in research in traumatic surgery. Its staff has in the last four years presented fifteen scientific papers in this field.

Mt. Sinai Hospital has many special funds for research. Among the studies conducted in 1930 were researches in thrombo-angiitis, heart diseases, peritonitis, allergy and radiation, typhoid, gastroenterology, electrocardiography, and otology. The Jewish Hospital of Brooklyn carries on extensive research. Its medical staff published sixty-four scientific papers during the year 1930. Beth Israel Hospital's most extensive research is in the field of diabetes.

SUMMARY

The private institutions for the sick in New York City in which the chronically ill were receiving care, at the time of this study in 1928, consisted of: (1) 11 institutions for chronic patients, of which 8 are "homes for incurables" without hospital equipment; one, a cancer hospital; one, a hospital with a special cancer service; and one, a hospital for all chronic diseases; (2) 6 orthopedic hospitals, of which 3 are primarily for operative or other short-time care and the other three, for children, give long-time care; and (3) general hospitals, which make no intentional provision for chronic patients but are obliged to receive them owing to the lack of special provision for chronic diseases.

The public institutions providing hospital care for the chronic sick included in 1928: (1) 11 general hospitals, three of which had chronic services; (2) 2 cancer hospitals; (3) 1 chronic hospital; (4) 1 orthopedic hospital and provision for bone and joint tuberculosis in a tuberculosis hospital; and (5) 4 contagious hospitals, in which chronic diseases are treated when there is an element of contagion.

Public care is also provided to some extent through the agency or private institutions to which the city may pay not over $3.00 a day for the care of a dependent patient.

Some changes have occurred in institutional provision for chronic patients since 1928. Several private homes for incurables have increased their bed capacity or are planning to do so, and two new homes of this type have been opened, one of which has hospital facilities. Montefiore Hospital's bed capacity has been enlarged. One of the municipal cancer hospitals has been closed, but is to be rebuilt. The number of beds in the chronic services of municipal general hospitals has been decreased.

The total ward capacity of all private institutions in the city intended to care for chronic patients of the class with which the study deals, including hospitals and homes for incurables, was approximately 2,200 beds. In addition, an estimated 4 per cent of beds in general hospitals may legitimately be used for temporary care of chronic patients.

The total bed capacity for the chronic sick in municipal hospitals was approximately 2,200 beds.

Of all the ward beds provided for the chronic sick by private agencies, 51 per cent were in homes for incurables not equipped for hospital care. Twenty-six per cent were in orthopedic hospitals and 23 per cent in chronic hospitals.

The lack of hospital facilities for the chronic sick was estimated to be provision for about 1,900 persons. In this estimate allowance was made for the use of a small percentage of general hospital beds.

Through new facilities created since the time of this study and through various adjustments of present facilities, this deficiency may be reduced to a lack of provision for 1,400 chronic patients, requiring at an average rate of occupancy of 90 per cent, 1,550 hospital ward beds, of which 650 should be in children's wards.

CHAPTER 2

Medical Social Service in Relation to the Care of the Chronic Sick

FUNCTIONS OF MEDICAL SOCIAL WORK IN RELATION TO CHRONIC PATIENTS

A CHRONIC disease, whether it results in prolonged illness and incapacity or merely in a limitation of ordinary activities, necessarily creates social problems. Frequently the family as well as the patient are involved in the necessary readjustments. Questions of financial support, change of occupation, altered living conditions, or provision for the care of children may be as fundamental to a patient's welfare as his medical treatment. His state of mind and attitude toward his illness, upon which his readiness to cooperate to his treatment depends, are affected by his ability to deal with such difficulties. The attitudes of different members of his family toward his illness and its consequences must also be taken into account in making plans for a chronic patient.

The chronic sick demand much more of the time of medical social workers than the acutely ill, not only because a larger proportion require assistance in becoming adjusted to their disabilities but also because chronic conditions are as a rule more difficult to diagnose and often cannot be understood without the information in regard to social situations and psychological attitudes that constitutes a social examination. In a hospital with a well-developed social service, the greater part of the social workers' time is undoubtedly devoted to the chronic patients. Among a thousand social service cases analyzed to show the functions of hospital social workers, which were selected to represent the practice of various departments throughout the country, approximately half were cases of chronic disease such as this study deals with and the rest were for the most part other forms of chronic disease not included in this study and obstetrical cases.[1]

There seems to be little general recognition, however, of the fact that medical social service is one of the chief agents of treatment for chronic patients. Writing of the importance of the social service in a hospital for chronic diseases, Dr. Boas says: "Happily the time is past when arguments must be marshaled for the justification of social service departments in general hospitals. They have long been accepted as representing an essential phase of hospital activity. But it still seems necessary to insist on the importance of social work in the care of subjects of chronic diseases, whether within or without an institution. This can be due only to lack of interest and inattention, for it is evident, as has been set forth in previous chapters, that the chronicity of disease brings in its train innumerable social and

---

[1] The Functions of Hospital Social Service: A Report of the Committee on Functions. American Association of Hospital Social Workers, Monograph No. 1, June, 1930, p. 60.

economic complications."[2] He points out that the "problems that arise are most difficult of solution," and he believes that "the social worker will find that she must do more intensive case work than she would in a general hospital; her cases will be of much longer duration, and she will have to maintain very close contact with many of her families for prolonged periods of time."[3]

There is no statistical basis at present for estimating the proportion of patients with chronic diseases as defined in this study among all the patients in hospitals and clinics who need medical social service. The percentage will naturally vary in hospitals of different types and in clinics for different diseases. It has been found that 20 per cent of the patients discharged from one general hospital have no need of social service. (See p. 81.) It is assumed, however, that dependent chronic patients in hospitals, the group under discussion in this report, with few if any exceptions have social problems requiring some attention from the social service and that their situation should be reviewed by a social worker in order to discover their social needs.

In the prevention of severe illness and serious disability due to chronic disease, the medical social worker has as important a part as in the care and treatment of incapacitated patients. The preventive aspects of their work were stressed by the medical social workers organized by the Section on Medical Social Service of the Welfare Council in a statement of the problem of the chronic patient as it presents itself to them, in which they urged the need for the present study, as follows: "(1) Chronic patients are frequently readmitted to general hospitals for treatment of recurrent acute phases of the disease. They are commonly referred to the medical social service on each discharge. They are a recurrent problem; for social workers consider from their experience that there is not sufficient visiting nursing service to which to refer these patients for home care and that facilities for institutional care of those who for medical or social reasons cannot be cared for at home are not sufficient. (2) Certain chronic patients can be kept in condition adequate to a productive life by regular clinic supervision and treatment; and for many others, more serious incapacity and institutionalization can be prevented by such care. How can medical social service be adequately staffed so that contact may be made with each patient in order to find those who need social care and so that adequate follow-up may be maintained?"

The indifference often found among physicians in general hospitals toward the treatment of chronic diseases is no doubt largely due to their inability to carry out a successful plan of treatment because of a lack of assistance from the social service in making the necessary economic and social adjustments. The physician may realize that his efforts to cure or improve the chronic patient are likely to be futile without continuous oversight of such factors; but he does not always realize that such service can be

[2] Boas, Ernst P., M.D., and Michelson, Nicholas, M.D., The Challenge of Chronic Diseases. New York, The Macmillan Company, 1929, p. 140.
[3] Ibid., pp. 141–142.

obtained nor recognize the hospital's obligation to provide it. Too often the physicians think of the social service only as a means of removing from the wards chronic patients for whom they feel no further responsibility.

The social service encounters great obstacles in the care of chronic patients due not only to the lack of community resources but also to the inability or unwillingness of patients to carry out a long course of treatment. Part of the skill of the trained medical social worker, however, is the ability to influence patients to take a constructive attitude toward their illness and to help them to find and use their individual resources to the best advantage, and at the same time to make the hospital's experience contribute to the development of new resources in the community.

The data on medical social service obtained for this study include a survey of the facilities of fifty-five social service departments and an item on the schedule used in taking the census of the chronic sick in hospitals to indicate whether the social service was in touch with the patient. A census of all patients known to the social service departments of the city was not attempted, for most of the departments keep no classification of problems presented or services rendered, a patient whose ability to pay his hospital bill is investigated being classed with one for whom an elaborate plan of social treatment is carried out; so that the figures obtained by a census would have covered too great a range of services to be significant. Clinic patients, who make up the greater part of the case load of the departments, are not included in the study, as it was not found practicable to take the census in clinics. A study of the functions of medical social service departments in relation to the care of the chronic sick, which must necessarily be based upon individual case studies, was outside the scope of the survey.

However, although the data concerning medical social work obtained in the course of the study are limited, there is a good deal of information available to throw light on the practices and standards in this field in New York City and elsewhere. Since medical social service is one of the most important and least understood factors in a community program for control and care of chronic diseases, it has seemed desirable to gather together in this report some of the available information indicating its functions and development in general and the extent to which it is utilized in New York City.

The treatment of cardiac diseases was one of the first medical fields in which medical social work was recognized as essential; and in New York there has been a further development of social service for cardiac patients than for any other group of the chronic sick. In the standards for cardiac clinics,[4] it is specified that a social worker must be part of a cardiac unit. The patient with heart disease must follow a prescribed régime and to this end, he frequently needs continuous personal instruction and help in effecting changes in his way of living. Nevertheless, the staff of many cardiac

[4] Standard Requirements for a Cardiac Clinic. Prepared by the Committee on Cardiac Clinics of the Heart Committee of the New York Tuberculosis and Health Association, Inc., October, 1931.

clinics in New York is still insufficient for adequate service. The superintendent of a children's hospital speaking of children with cardiac disorders said: "What are the vital problems in children's cardiac clinics? Any doctor will tell you that what he can do for these children in the clinic is little beside what can be done for them in their homes. He will tell you that in the search for a cure for this baffling disease, his hands are tied without the knowledge and patient follow-up of the trained social worker."[5] A general hospital superintendent speaking of the necessity for medical social service said: "No amount of surgical skill or expert judgment can bridge the gap between the patient and his life situation without the aid of the medical social worker. If patients suffering from medical complications, particularly cardiac and diabetic conditions are readmitted again and again to our hospitals—is this not frequently due to improper instructions to the patient and his family at the time of discharge—or a lack of information regarding the home into which he is being sent?"[6]

The treatment of diabetes is particularly a medical social problem. The adult patient who must change his mode of life and follow a strict dietary régime needs personal education and encouragement and frequently also assistance in making the necessary changes in his mode of living. For the child with diabetes, the stamina required to follow his régime, is as important as medical treatment. As medical social service is most needed at the beginning of treatment, when the patient first learns about his condition, a diabetic clinic should have a social service adequate for contact with every patient. But many of the diabetic clinics in the city have no social service and others refer only an occasional patient to the general social service department. About half of the hospital patients with diabetes in the census of the chronic sick were not known to a social worker. This subject has been discussed more fully in another section of the report.[7] Among twenty-three diabetic clinics of the city, in which inquiry was made, a great variety was found in the arrangements for providing social service. One clinic had no social work. Half of the remainder had the services of a social worker, sometimes for half or three quarters of her time, and in eight clinics, the social worker was present during all sessions of the clinics. The other half referred special problems to the general social service department.

The need for increase and improvement in social service for patients with cancer has been discussed in the section dealing with that disease.[8] Of nearly 500 cancer patients in hospitals in the census, about 60 per cent were not receiving any attention from a social worker. The municipal cancer hospital has a well-organized social service department and the Director of the Division of Cancer in the Hospital Department has expressed his belief that "in no other branch of health service is the social worker more

[5] Social Service and Preventive Medicine, discussed by John R. Howard, Jr., and Michael M. Davis. *Bulletin of The Welfare Council of New York City*, vol. 5, No. 4, April, 1931, p. 5.
[6] Address by William B. Seltzer, Minutes of the Meeting of the Medical Social Service Section of The Welfare Council of New York City, March 11, 1931, p. 2.
[7] See also vol. 1, Chapter 3, The Special Problems of Some Main Groups of Chronic Diseases, p. 206.
[8] *Ibid.*, pp. 185; 186.

essential" than in the treatment of cancer.[9] One of the objects of the Brooklyn Cancer Welfare Service, a recently organized committee of Brooklyn women, is to promote medical social service for patients with cancer where it is needed. The New York City Cancer Committee has directed attention to the need for an increase of social service for cancer.

All orthopedic hospitals and clinics in the study have some form of home service, but it is frequently limited to a nursing service for follow-up and does not attempt intensive social case work. The necessity for the latter service was emphasized in the report of the Massachusetts survey of the care of crippled children, in 1931. In regard to nearly a thousand children who needed treatment and were not receiving it, the report states: "The difficulty seems to lie with the lack of adjustment of the families, in which there are crippled children, to the complete system of treatment which exists. Lack of adjustment can be remedied by the establishment of specialized social service for crippled children. Medical social service has developed to a certain standard in the adjustment of the patient to the hospital, and the proper follow-up of the patient on leaving the hospital. This service for crippled children has not been sufficiently developed. It calls for a special technical knowledge of the possibilities of treatment, and particularly an appreciation gained from experience with the attitudes of parents and children toward treatment."[10]

The value of medical social service in the treatment of arthritis has been demonstrated at the Robert B. Brigham Hospital in Boston, which is one of the few modern chronic hospitals in the country and is devoted particularly to arthritis. It has a staff of two trained social workers for approximately 350 patients a year under care in both wards and out-patient department.[11] At the end of the year 1929, there were ninety-six patients receiving intensive social service to keep them "at their best levels—as far as possible from needing any return of chronic hospital care." It is clear that this type of social work is impossible with the facilities reported by a number of New York arthritis clinics in which inquiry was made. In some of them, special problems were referred to the general social service department; in one hospital, a social worker gave half time to the clinic which sometimes had as many as 150 arthritis patients at a session; in another hospital, one social worker covered other clinics in addition to the arthritis clinic.

The treatment of drug addiction, after the first withdrawal of the drug under medical supervision, depends upon psychiatric and social service. The Mayor's Committee recommended a staff of social workers as essential in an institution for the rehabilitation of narcotic users.[12]

[9] Kaplan, Ira I., M.D., The Social Service Worker's Responsibility in Cancer Work. *Hospital Social Service*, vol. 25, No. 3, September, 1931, pp. 195, 196.

[10] Final Report of the Department of Public Welfare Relative to the Number and Care of Crippled Children, House Document No. 401, Commonwealth of Massachusetts, Boston, December, 1931, pp. 47, 49.

[11] The Robert B. Brigham Hospital, Annual Report, Boston, 1929, p. 22.

[12] Report of the Mayor's Committee on Drug Addiction to the Hon. Richard C. Patterson, Jr., Commissioner of Correction, New York City. Reprinted from the *American Journal of Psychiatry*, vol. 10, No. 3, November, 1930, pp. 446–447.

The trend of modern medicine is more and more toward the conception that the physician treats not merely a diseased section of the body but the whole person. The director of the study made by the Commission on Medical Education pointed out that "the content and scope of medical training are in the process of undergoing significant changes. . . . Greater emphasis is being placed in some of the schools in study of the patient as a whole, in which factors of emotional life, conditions of employment, habits of living, family life, and other human factors are considered in arriving at a diagnosis or in outlining treatment."[13]

In agreement with this conclusion is the following statement by the director of the new medical center of the New York Hospital-Cornell Medical College Association: "If the medical student is to gain in interest and enthusiasm for the broader social opportunities that surround the doctor, he must be brought in contact with hospital social work practised by professional and scientific methods. It is essential that he should not only be brought in contact with it, but should participate in its performance in order that his social and human development may take place beside his technical and scientific training . . . the doctor must view man as body and mind inseparable and must know him in his human surroundings as well as in his physical world if he is to render service of the highest type. It is here that social service has a rôle to play in medical education. It may be an important factor in shaping the destinies of our doctors of the future."[14]

It follows that social factors should be dealt with as definitely and systematically as medical factors. A major function of the social service therefore is to take part in the original study of the patient. To quote from a report of the American Association for Hospital Social Workers: "Such inquiry is not the chance discovery of episodes in the patient's past life or of his present needs and desires. It is a deliberate, methodical undertaking, directed to specific ends. It takes place by direct observation on the part of the inquirer, and by the securing of testimony from the patient himself and from others associated with him. It should reveal all the facts essential to a knowledge of the meaning of his sickness and the means he has, or lacks, for meeting his disability. It may be brief or extended. Even a brief inquiry, planned and carried out with enough precision to give facts which make the main issues clear will save much waste motion for patient and for hospital."[15]

The social factors that may affect the health of patients have been classified in the report on the functions of a hospital social worker quoted above, as follows:

"1. Social conditions which bear directly on the health of the patient, either inducing susceptibility to ill-health, or helping or hindering the securing and completing of medical care.

[13] Rappleye, W. C., M.D., Current Problems of Medical Education. The *Journal of the American Medical Association*, vol. 94, No. 13, March 29, 1930, pp. 915–917.

[14] Robinson, G. Canby, M.D., An insert in *Better Times*, The Welfare Council of New York City, vol. 14, No. 6, November 7, 1932, p. 15.

[15] The Functions of Hospital Social Service: A Report of the Committee on Functions. American Association of Hospital Social Workers, Monograph No. 1, June, 1930, p. 60.

"2. Social distress caused to others by the illness of patients; such as, loss of income, neglect of children, etc.

"3. Social problems not having direct cause-and-effect relation to the health condition, but collateral to it. Such problems would exist independently of the sickness." It is pointed out that "these factors exist in many possible combinations."[16]

It is clearly the function of the hospital social service to deal with factors of the first group in direct service to the patient. As a rule factors of the second and third groups in a well-organized community are primarily the function of specialized agencies and are dealt with through coöperative relations with these other agencies. Frequently a combination of these direct and indirect services is required for the same patient. Also in problems of the first group other agencies must often be called upon for special services. In any case, it is the responsibility of the medical social worker to see that the patient's social problems are handled in a way to promote his medical care; and therefore, she must learn from the physician the exact nature of the disease process and its possible consequences; and if different parts of the body are affected, she must learn how the various disease processes are interrelated. It has been aptly said: "It is the part of good medicine to synthesize as well as to analyze the patient, and the social worker must ask no less of the physician."[17]

When the treatment of the patient's social problems is carried on through a coöperative relationship with another agency, the medical social worker must not only be able to give practical and intelligible information about the patient's physical condition to the agency but must also have enough detailed knowledge of the functions and facilities of the agency to judge whether the application is well placed. To make two or more agencies work together for the good of a patient requires not only knowledge of all factors in the situation but also considerable skill. It is generally recognized that policies for such coöperative work should be worked out by the hospital social service departments and the social agencies of different types based upon fundamental principles of social organization. The Medical Social Service Section and Family Service Section of the Welfare Council through a joint committee have agreed upon policies to be tried experimentally.[18] In Cleveland, similar efforts have been made to formulate policies for children's agencies coöperating with hospitals.[19] The Children's Hospital in Boston has successfully developed foster home care for convalescent and chronically ill children through its agreements with certain children's agencies. In New York, the Heart Committee is studying the possibilities of foster home care for cardiac children.

[16] *Ibid.*, p. 59.

[17] Cannon, Mary Antoinette, Approach to Social Case Work in the Hospital. *Hospital Social Service*, vol. 10, No. 4, October, 1924, p. 172.

[18] Byington, Margaret F., On Division of Labor. *Better Times*, The Welfare Council of New York City, vol. 13, No. 18, February 1, 1932, p. 15.

[19] Peck, Gracil Green, The Inter-Relationship of the Medical Social Worker and the Children's Workers of the Non-Medical Agency. *Bulletin of the American Association of Hospital Social Workers*, vol. 5, No. 1, January, 1932, p. 10.

Among other types of agency with which hospital social service departments must frequently coöperate are convalescent homes, visiting nurse services, sheltered workshops, and employment centers for the handicapped. In most instances, the social service department attempts to conform to the policies of the other agency without further effort to arrive at an agreement by which both agencies working together may accomplish the best result for the patient. For example, the Employment Center for the Handicapped furnishes other agencies with a clear and comprehensive statement of the types of handicapped persons it serves; and the social service departments refer such patients to the center. A well-defined coöperative relationship here would show the need for some knowledge of vocational guidance for the handicapped on the part of the medical social worker, not in order to give vocational advice or make the placement but to help the patient to adjust himself to his disability and to prepare him for placement. She needs to know the requirements of different occupations and processes in industry in order to judge how the patient's special skill and experience may be conserved and adapted to a new job.

Whether the service given by the hospital social worker involves intensive medical social treatment, a coöperative relationship with another social agency, or some special bit of advice or assistance, the characteristic that gives it professional value is that it should be done in the light of the patient's total welfare. This has been well put by Miss M. A. Cannon: "The giving of a single service, piece of information, explanation or recommendation is of value in proportion as it rests upon a truthful analysis of some person's need, and so applies the individual or case method to an individual. Case workers in the hospital can save waste that comes from routine, therefore indiscriminate, handling of individual patients. By application of case method even the smallest piece of work may be made to fit into place in a complete plan of treatment."[20]

As social work has come to be recognized as essential in medical diagnosis and treatment, it naturally follows that one function of a social service department is to contribute to medical research. This subject is discussed further on in connection with the facilities for medical social service in this city. The College of Surgeons in recommending follow-up for certain chronic conditions—cancer, cardiac and renal disorders, tuberculosis, arteriosclerosis—in order to "enrich scientific knowledge as to diagnosis and treatment and promote the prevention of disease" pointed out that "such follow-up and desirable results cannot be successfully assured without a well organized social service department."[21]

So far, medical social work has been identified almost entirely with medical institutions and has extended only in rare instances into public health agencies. Massachusetts for a number of years has been developing social service in the State Department of Public Health, first in its venereal disease program and later in connection with the control of cancer and

[20] Cannon, Mary Antoinette, Approach to Social Case Work in the Hospital. *Hospital Social Service*, vol. 10, No. 4, October, 1924, pp. 172–173.
[21] American College of Surgeons, Hospital Standardization Report for the Year 1931, Chicago, p. 31.

tuberculosis, and has given consideration to the place of social work in relation to the control of other chronic diseases.[22]

The rôle of the medical social worker in public health has not yet been evolved. Although much thought and discussion have been given to coöperative relations and differentiation of functions between public health nurses and medical social workers, and effective working relations have been developed in many local situations, the principles and policies differentiating the responsibilities of these two groups are not yet clearly defined. This issue has been briefly stated as follows: "It is of course obvious that at many points these fields overlap and that either worker may have a considerable degree of knowledge and experience in the field of the other. The important point is that a major responsibility should be assumed by either worker in the field in which her training and experience give her the right to speak with some degree of authority. It is in the region in which both groups recognize an interest and some degree of responsibility that the necessity for clarification becomes necessary."[23] The White House Conference report states that "leaders in both public health nursing and medical social work agree that this problem should receive more thoughtful study" and finds that "there is a serious need for thought and discussion on this subject."[24]

CHRONIC PATIENTS RECEIVING SOCIAL SERVICE IN THE HOSPITALS STUDIED

In the census of the chronic patients in hospitals made for this study, the question was asked: "Is the patient under care of the medical social service?" The nature and extent of the service rendered are questions beyond the scope of the study. Special case studies would be necessary for such an evaluation of the service. The information obtained in the census therefore indicates that the patient was known to a social worker in the hospital but does not show the extent of this knowledge or the quality of the care given. The service given may range from an interview with a relative concerning the patient's care or a report of his condition to another social agency to intensive case work in studying a patient's situation and carrying out over a period of months a plan for his future care or occupational rehabilitation.

There were 96 private hospitals and 21 public hospitals in the city, exclusive of special hospitals for the types of illness not covered by this study, that is, tuberculosis, mental diseases, and diseases of the eye and the ear. Thirty-eight of the 96 private hospitals and 1 of the 21 public hospitals had no social service.

Eighteen of the 77 public and private hospitals in which the census of the

[22] Kelly, Eleanor E., The Social Worker in Adult Hygiene. *The Commonhealth*, Quarterly Bulletin of the Massachusetts Department of Public Health, vol. 16, No. 4, December, 1929, pp. 129–133.

[23] Byington, Margaret F., Team Work Between the Nurse and Social Worker. *Public Health Nursing*, vol. 24, No. 1, January, 1932, p. 14.

[24] Hospitals and Child Health; Report of the Sub-Committee on Medical Social Service, by Ida M. Cannon, Chairman. White House Conference on Child Health and Protection called by President Hoover, New York, The Century Company, 1932, pp. 188–189.

chronic sick was taken had no social service, including 1 public orthopedic hospital with 2 per cent, 7 private chronic hospitals with 14 per cent, and 10 private general hospitals with 1 per cent of all the chronic patients in hospitals. The records of 29 per cent of the chronic patients in hospitals with social service did not contain the information as to whether or not the

TABLE 12

PER CENT OF CHRONIC PATIENTS KNOWN TO THE SOCIAL SERVICE IN PUBLIC AND PRIVATE HOSPITALS OF EACH TYPE

Hospitals	Per cent reporting	Known to social service	Not known to social service
Total	70.8	63.1	36.9
Public	56.0	49.9	50.1
General	45.0	68.4	31.6
Special	58.6	100.0	0.0
Chronic	99.8	0.8	99.2
Private	92.7	74.9	25.1
General	89.3	58.6	41.4
Orthopedic	97.4	90.0	10.0
Chronic	94.9	90.9	9.1

patient was known to the social service. This information was obtained for a much larger proportion of patients in private hospitals, 93 per cent, than in public hospitals, 56 per cent. It is believed, however, that the records of chronic patients in public hospitals for whom this information was reported,

TABLE 13

PER CENT OF CHRONIC PATIENTS KNOWN TO THE SOCIAL SERVICE IN PUBLIC AND PRIVATE HOSPITALS, EACH AGE GROUP

Age group	Total		Public			Private		
	Known to social service	Not known to social service	Per cent reporting	Known to social service	Not known to social service	Per cent reporting	Known to social service	Not known to social service
Total	63.1	36.9	56.0	49.9	50.1	92.7	74.9	25.1
Under 16 years .	85.0	15.0	38.3	80.0	20.0	95.5	85.6	14.4
16–39 years . .	63.6	36.4	55.5	50.2	49.8	91.7	70.8	29.2
40–59 years . .	58.6	41.4	57.3	47.8	52.2	92.8	71.3	28.7
60–69 years . .	50.4	49.6	55.5	47.9	52.1	89.0	56.6	43.4
70 years and over	52.8	47.2	60.4	48.4	51.6	84.5	71.8	28.2

although less than three fifths of the whole number, fairly represent the whole situation in regard to the extent to which chronic patients are receiving social service in the municipal hospitals.

The 59 hospitals with social service reported 4,595 patients, of whom 63 per cent were said to be under the care of the social service department. Although a chronic disease almost invariably constitutes a social problem, 37 per cent of these patients were not even known to a social worker in the hospital. In Table 12, the proportion known to the social service in different types of hospitals is shown, together with the percentage of all the chronic patients for which the item was reported. All or nearly all of the chronic patients were known to the social service in 5 hospitals, which included a

TABLE 14

NUMBER AND PER CENT OF CHRONIC PATIENTS WITH CERTAIN DISEASES KNOWN
TO THE SOCIAL SERVICE IN PUBLIC AND PRIVATE HOSPITALS

	Children			Adults		
Type of disease	Total	Known to social service		Total	Known to social service	
		Number	Per cent[1]		Number	Per cent[1]
Orthopedic disorders	551	351	63.7	245	103	42.0
Poliomyelitis	165	152	92.1	32	22	68.8
Rickets	33	29	87.9	0	0	....
Congenital malformations	53	33	62.3	14	5	35.7
Diseases of bones and organs of locomotion	115	64	55.7	143	47	32.9
Tuberculosis of spine or joints . .	185	73	39.5	56	29	51.8
Diabetes	6	5	83.3	104	42	40.4
Cancer	6	1	16.7	485	201	41.4
Diseases of digestive system	6	3	50.0	136	54	39.7
Diseases of skin	8	4	50.0	134	48	35.8
Heart disease	86	50	58.1	558	186	33.3
Arthritis or rheumatism	37	29	78.4	426	126	29.6
Fractures	31	12	38.7	177	69	39.0
Nephritis	16	8	50.0	105	29	27.6
Neurological diseases	66	47	71.2	1,113	292	26.2
Old age	0	0	....	248	51	20.6

[1] Based upon the total number with the given diagnosis reported by hospitals.

cancer hospital, a contagious hospital reporting 5 chronic patients, 2 public general hospitals with chronic services, and a private general hospital.

In the private hospitals less than half of all the chronic patients were known to the social service. There was no social service in 17 of the 57 private medical institutions covered by the census. In institutions in which there was a social service department, three fourths of all the chronic patients were known to a social worker. Ninety per cent in chronic and orthopedic hospitals and less than 60 per cent in general hospitals were known to the social service.

In public hospitals, 48 per cent of the adults and 80 per cent of the children were known to the social service. All for whom the item was reported were known to the social service in the special hospitals; practically all in the chronic hospitals; and 68 per cent in the general hospitals.

The percentage of children, 85 per cent, known to the social service was much larger than the percentage of adults, 69 per cent. The proportion of patients in different age groups known to the social service in both public and private hospitals is shown in Table 13.

The proportion of chronic patients not known to the social service increases almost consistently with each age group in both public and private hospitals.

TABLE 15

CHRONIC PATIENTS KNOWN TO THE SOCIAL SERVICE IN PUBLIC AND PRIVATE HOSPITALS CLASSIFIED BY CARE NEEDED, EACH AGE GROUP

Care needed	AGE GROUP						
	Total	Under 16	16–39	40–59	60–69	70 and over	Not reported
Total	2,053	564	432	599	250	197	11
Medical	1,406	515	321	376	125	67	2
Hospital	1,080	296	281	334	103	64	2
Clinic	326	17	40	42	22	3	0
Nursing	122	32	29	42	22	12	0
Attendant	516	0	81	180	97	118	8
Not reported	9	0	1	1	6	0	1

The extent to which hospital patients with different forms of chronic disease were receiving social service, is shown in Table 14.

Less than half of the adults in each disease group were known to be receiving social service with the exception of those suffering from the results of poliomyelitis and non-pulmonary tuberculosis. In nearly every group, children received attention from the social service more frequently than adults.

Table 15 shows the types of care needed for the chronic patients known to the social service department; that is, whether their condition called for medical study and treatment, nursing care by a trained nurse, or attendant care by a skillful but not necessarily trained person.

The large majority were patients needing medical care, which could be given in clinics for nearly a fifth, mainly children. Nearly a fourth of the whole number needed attendant care and a small proportion nursing care.

Three fourths of these social service patients were receiving the type of medical or nursing care suitable for their condition and were being cared for under satisfactory conditions at the time of the census, as shown below in Table 16. A fourth were not receiving satisfactory care, of whom nearly half were children requiring clinic care.

MEDICAL SOCIAL SERVICE FACILITIES IN NEW YORK CITY

Since there is no differentiation in the records of medical social service departments between work in behalf of the acutely ill and of the chronically ill, the social service facilities of hospitals have been treated as a whole in the discussion that follows. It is probably true that patients with chronic conditions, including both clinic and ward patients, demand the greater part of these facilities; but no estimates of the division of service between chronic and acute patients are available and the situation would naturally vary according to the nature of the hospital's medical work. The object of this discussion of medical social service facilities is to present available information showing the amount and character of the medical social work

TABLE 16

CHRONIC PATIENTS KNOWN TO THE SOCIAL SERVICE IN PUBLIC AND PRIVATE
HOSPITALS CLASSIFIED BY PRESENT SITUATION, EACH AGE GROUP

| | AGE GROUP | | | | | | |
Present situation	Total	Under 16	16–39	40–59	60–69	70 and over	Not reported
Total	2,053	564	432	599	250	197	11
Suitable care	1,535	318	358	519	202	129	9
Unsuitable care . . .	508	246	73	79	42	67	1
Not reported	10	0	1	1	6	1	1

done in the hospitals of New York, since it is assumed that these are factors of fundamental importance in the community's care of the chronic sick both in relation to the prevention of illness and disability and also in relation to the provision of economical and kindly care for chronic invalids.

No general survey of hospital social service departments, such as was made recently in Philadelphia,[25] has been made in New York City. The present study of these facilities included fifty-five departments, mainly those in hospitals in which the census of the chronic sick was taken, and covered items related especially to the care of chronic patients. (See pp. 92 to 96.) The annual reports of the social service departments indicate that there is great variation in the proportion of patients served and in the character of the services rendered. Two departments with about the same number of social workers report respectively about 1,900 and 7,000 patients. Three other much larger departments with comparable staffs report approximately 650, 5,000, and 7,000 patients. One of the latter group reports 3,000 home visits and another 245 home visits. Most of the reports make no attempt to interpret or evaluate the quality or usefulness of the service.

It may be assumed that most of it comes within the category usually defined in statistics of medical social work as "slight service"; for an examination of the records in the Social Service Exchange of the number of cases registered by six social service departments selected at random, during the year 1930–1931, indicates that each had registered a small proportion of its patients. All of these departments together report nearly 23,000 patients

[25] Social Service in Hospitals and Dispensaries: Chapter 18 of Philadelphia Hospital and Health Survey, 1929, by Haven Emerson, M.D., Sol Pincus, and Anna C. Phillips. Published by the Philadelphia Hospital and Health Survey Committee, 1930.

dealt with in the course of a year; and yet in the year cited all six registered only 2,230 patients. It may not be practicable to clear all clinic cases in the Social Service Exchange; but no definite or uniform principle seems to have been established for selection of the cases to be cleared. The report of the Exchange for the year 1930–1931 showed "wide variations in the number of clearings made by medical social service departments of different types of hospitals. Illustrative of this, one large special hospital with a medical social service staff, cleared 5 cases during the year. Another special hospital with similar facilities cleared 3 cases. A third cleared 2,730. One of the largest general hospitals in the city cleared 2,042 cases, while another general hospital with a smaller bed capacity but about the same number of social workers, cleared 1,098 cases."[26]

Standards and Coördination

Agencies Engaged. The agency for standardization and development of medical social work in New York City is the local branch of the national professional organization of medical social workers, the North Atlantic District of the American Association of Hospital Social Workers. The agency for coördination in this field is the Medical Social Service Section of the Welfare Council, representing ninety-six social service departments. Another local organization, the Hospital Social Service Association, composed of member agencies represented by both social workers and lay committee members was organized in 1912 to stimulate the growth of social work in hospitals and dispensaries and to standardize such work. It publishes a monthly magazine, *Hospital Social Service,* which has a national circulation. As other local and coördinating agencies in the field of social service have developed, its local activities have diminished and it is now known chiefly for its publication of the outstanding magazine in the field of medical social work. The New York Tuberculosis and Health Association also brings together social workers in different medical fields in conferences for educational purposes. The Associated Out-Patient Clinics Committee of this organization had a subcommittee on medical social service which united with the corresponding section of the Welfare Council when the latter was organized.

The North Atlantic District of the American Association of Hospital Social Workers, with headquarters in New York, covers the eastern half of New York State, all of Connecticut, and the northern half of New Jersey. Its object is to work toward improvement and development of standards of social work among its membership in the hospitals and within its territory. For the past two years, it has conducted institutes for its members, consisting of conferences under the direction of a leader.

The Associated Out-Patient Clinics of the City of New York was organized in 1912; and, at the instance of the Public Health, Hospital and Budget Committee of the New York Academy of Medicine, its statement of purpose

[26] McDermott, Valeria D., The Uses Made of the Social Service Exchange by Medical Social Workers. Reprinted from *Hospital Social Service,* vol. 26, No. 5, November, 1932, p. 358.

in promoting proper standards of treatment provided for "the study of the relative need of home visiting and of social service in the different departments of a general dispensary, with a view to the encouragement of development of such work along the lines of greatest immediate need and benefit."[27] Although the Medical Social Service Section of the Associated Out-Patient Clinics was not organized until 1921, in the standards set up for each of the medical sections there was always a recommendation that the clinics be equipped with social service, preferably by having social workers a part of each clinic's personnel, or that service should at least be available from a general social service department in the hospital. Early in 1926, this association, which had been merged in 1920 with the Committee on Dispensary Development of the United Hospital Fund, became the Associated Out-Patient Clinics Committee of the New York Tuberculosis and Health Association. In 1927, its Medical Social Service Committee became the Executive Committee of the Medical Social Service Section in the Health Division of the Welfare Council.

This Section of the Welfare Council, in which 99 agencies are represented,[28] meets about six times a year. The requirements for agency membership in the Section are: (1) a responsible and active governing body, (2) a legitimate purpose concerned with medical social service, (3) reasonable efficiency, and (4) a willingness to coöperate with other members in preventing duplication of work and in promoting other essential objectives of the Welfare Council. The Section has committees on the division of labor between family and medical social agencies, the development of social service in eye clinics, the use of the Social Service Exchange, problems of venereal diseases, extension of medical social service to meet the needs of the chronic sick, and relief problems in hospitals; and it has recently organized a lay committee composed of members of auxiliaries and advisory committees of medical social service departments.

Standards of Organization. The American Association of Hospital Social Workers adopted in 1928 a statement defining the minimum standards to be met by social service departments in hospitals. It is assumed that a hospital organizing a social service department under that name is under an obligation to meet certain accepted standards. The fundamental requirements are: (1) that since the primary purpose is "to further the medical-social case study and treatment," "the major activity of the department should be medical-social case work"; and (2) that since "it is important to the hospital that its medical and social work be closely integrated in function and organization," the department should function "as an integral part of the institution."[29] These minimum standards were embodied in full

---

[27] The Associated Out-Patient Clinics of the City of New York, First Annual Report, 1913, p. 9.

[28] These 99 agencies include 96 medical social service departments, 1 medical research institute, the Central Council of Social Service Auxiliaries, and the Hospital Social Service Association of New York City.

[29] A Statement of the American Association of Hospital Social Workers which Defines the Minimum Standards to Be Met by Hospital Social Service Departments, Adopted May, 1928. *Bulletin of The American Association of Hospital Social Workers*, July, 1928, pp. 1-2.

in the Hospital Standardization Report, 1930, of the American College of Physicians and Surgeons.

A more detailed outline of standards of social work in hospitals together with suggestions for putting them into practice had previously been prepared, in 1926, by a Committee of the Social Service Section of the Associated Out-Patient Clinics of New York City and published in pamphlet form under the title "Technique of Hospital Social Service." The Committee offered this statement "not as a final word on the subject, but as a convenient basis for further discussion and experiment which may eventually lead to constructive and comprehensive standards of hospital social service practice."[30] Six years later, however, few of the 96 social service departments of the city have been able even to approximate either the standards here outlined or the minimum standards adopted by the American Association of Hospital Social Workers.

As mentioned above, the cardiac clinics have come nearer to a general standard of social work than any other medical unit, in that the standards outlined by the Committee on Cardiac Clinics[31] and accepted by a majority of the clinics require that there shall be a social worker in each clinic whose duties and responsibilities are defined.

Professional Training. The national organization, the American Association of Hospital Social Workers, has sought to influence standards for personnel. It has continually endeavored to raise its requirements for membership; but these requirements are still very broad. Graduation from a recognized school of social work with special experience in medical social work is accepted as the standard for membership. However, five years of experience in social work is accepted as a substitute for regular training; and for those who have had nursing training only three and a half years of experience in social work is required. These membership requirements embrace a wide range of personnel. The medical social worker who has graduated from a school of social work may have been through college and received two years of postgraduate education in the theory and practice of medical social case work. At the other extreme is the social worker or nurse without special education in medical social work, who may not have received as much as a high-school education and who qualifies for membership only through practical experience acquired in many instances under a supervisor who is also without training in social work. As the association has no means of evaluating this experience, the membership is greatly diversified in regard to background and ability.

No common standards of training for medical social workers are generally accepted in New York City. In the selection of social workers for hospitals and clinics, there is no general recognition of the qualifications required for

[30] Technique of Hospital Social Service. Prepared by a Committee of the Social Service Section, The Associated Out-Patient Clinics of the City of New York, February, 1926, p. 4.
[31] Standard Requirements for a Cardiac Clinic. Prepared by the Committee on Cardiac Clinics of the Heart Committee of the New York Tuberculosis and Health Association, Inc., October, 1931, pp. 7–8.

membership in the American Association of Social Workers. Some of the workers in the social service departments do not meet even the widely inclusive membership requirements of the American Association of Hospital Social Workers. Only a few of the private hospitals will appoint a social worker without nurse's training, but very few require recognized social work training. The development of hospital social work in New York was initiated by the nursing group, in contrast to other communities where it grew out of social work. Nursing education, therefore, was assumed to be the primary requisite for hospital social work; and social workers were considered ineligible regardless of the extent of their medical social training. It is only within the last ten years that workers other than nurses have been accepted in any of the social service departments of New York hospitals. In the municipal hospitals, it is still an invariable requirement that the staff of the social service departments shall be nurses and the requirements for experience in social work are poorly defined. The Presbyterian Medical Center requires medical social training without regard to whether the social worker has or has not had nurse's training. Mt. Sinai Hospital also gives preference to persons who have had special training in medical social case work.

"In 66 or one-sixth of the 430 social service departments listed by the American Association of Hospital Social Workers in 1924, the head worker bears after her name upon the list the letters R.N. ('Registered Nurse'). In the remaining 364 she has had no such designation, and if she has had nurse's training probably considers it less important than the social training which she has also received. Thirty of the 66 registered nurses just referred to belong to hospitals within New York City, in which, following the example of Bellevue Hospital, it has until recently been the custom to consider that the training of a nurse was in itself nearly or quite sufficient to qualify one for social work. This point of view, however, has never been held in other parts of the country and is beginning to be abandoned even in New York."[32]

The first training course in medical social work was organized in 1912; but for the first ten years or so, the growth of such courses was slow and there was little coördination with the field of practice. The American Association of Hospital Social Workers formed its Education Committee in 1925 for the purpose of fostering relations between the schools of social work and the practitioners. "Of the 28 schools now belonging to the Association of Schools of Professional Social Work, 10 offer training for medical social work and in another plans are going forward for such training. . . . In most of the schools an undergraduate degree is required for admission. Where the degree is not obligatory, at least two college years, or its equivalent, is required, and in addition evidence of other education more or less formal in character. Completion of medical social training in most of the schools gives academic recognition to the degrees of A.M. or M.S. The

[32] Cabot, Richard C., M.D., Hospital and Dispensary Social Work. *Hospital Social Service*, vol. 18, No. 4, October, 1928, pp. 308–309.

fact that medical social training is classified in all schools as graduate work means that standards in all parts of the training plan must meet requirements for graduate work in universities."[33]

It is well known that in many hospitals in New York and elsewhere little consideration is given to professional education for medical social work in the selection of the social service staff. Although it is now ten years since the American Hospital Association appointed a committee of eighteen representative physicians, nursing educators, hospital social workers, and educators in general social service to study the subject of training for hospital social service and to make recommendations, which were adopted and published,[34] many hospital administrators and boards have not yet given consideration to the standards of education for social workers recommended in the Committee's report.[35]

Probably this indifference to special preparation for medical social work by many hospital authorities is due to their failure to realize exactly the nature of the duties and responsibilities of the social worker, as Robert M. MacIver has suggested in a remarkably lucid account of the nature of a social worker's functions. He says: "I have dwelt on the magnitude of his function, because until it is realized more generally he cannot gain the status necessary for its performance. The old ideas still linger in the public mind though the old order has passed. Even in the minds of many social workers it still lingers, in the minds of those, for example, who think that apprenticeship is an all-sufficient training for the work they have to perform. Do they not know that in every other sphere of worthwhile endeavor —except perhaps, and unfortunately, politics—the day when apprenticeship suffices is past? Important, even necessary as it was and is, it provides only the foreground of the social worker's training."[36]

A number of reasons may be given for the fact that many physicians still do not have the conception of medical social work as a service requiring trained professional skill. The term "medical social worker" is used loosely to apply to persons differing widely in education and ability. The salaries paid are frequently too low to attract professionally trained persons; for example, in Philadelphia 75 per cent of the social workers in hospitals in 1929 were receiving less than $1,800 a year and 90 per cent less than $2,100 a year.[37] In many hospitals because of too small a staff, the trained social workers are obliged to perform a variety of duties which are not medical social work but rather assistance in administration. Under these conditions,

[33] Hospitals and Child Health; Report of the Sub-committee on Medical Social Service, by Ida M. Cannon, Chairman. White House Conference on Child Health and Protection called by President Hoover, New York, The Century Company, 1932, pp. 197–198.

[34] Report of the Committee on Training for Hospital Social Work Appointed by the American Hospital Association, Inc., Bulletin No. 55. Chicago, American Hospital Association, Inc., 1923.

[35] See Appendix II for a brief outline of the standard course recommended for medical social workers by this committee of the American Hospital Association, Inc.

[36] MacIver, Robert M., The Contribution of Sociology to Social Work. Publications of the New York School of Social Work, 1931, p. 80.

[37] Philadelphia Hospital and Health Survey, 1929, Conducted under the Auspices of a Citizens' Survey Committee, by Haven Emerson, M.D., Sol Pincus, and Anna C. Phillips, p. 801.

it is natural that convincing demonstrations of the value of medical social work as a professional service are still confined to a comparatively limited number of centers throughout the country.

Staff Required. No satisfactory estimate of the number of social workers needed in relation to the number of admissions has yet been made that is generally applicable. The proportion of patients requiring social attention and also the amount of attention required per patient vary in different types of illness. Other factors such as administrative duties, teaching, contributions to research, also affect the size of the staff. The proportion of children in the hospital's clientele and to some extent the economic level of its patients are other factors to be taken into account. Therefore, general estimates of staff in relation to admissions will show wide variation; and for practical purposes, the percentage of patients who may be expected to have social needs must be estimated for the individual hospital and for each separate service.

The conclusion reached by an officer of the American College of Surgeons, after a survey of over one thousand hospitals, was that "there should be one social worker for every 150 to two hundred patients in a mixed hospital caring for free, part-pay, and pay patients."[38] In the Philadelphia Hospital and Health Survey, the desirable minimum for social service as indicated by the usual practice in the best equipped hospitals was found to be one social worker to every 2,000 annual admissions to hospital or clinics.[39]

At the time of this study, in 1928, there were 47 social workers in the 42 cardiac clinics represented in the Committee on Cardiac Clinics or one social worker to 250 patients under treatment. The variation in different clinics was from one social worker to 36 patients to one social worker to 680 patients.

A study by the staff of the Social Service Department of the Presbyterian Hospital, New York, of 300 cases consecutively discharged from the hospital in 1930, indicates that 20 per cent, in the opinion of the workers, had no need of social service; 50 per cent were of the "self-directing" group who need instruction or interpretation and guidance; 30 per cent presented social problems that had to be met in order to have the patient benefit fully from the medical care.[40]

The ratio between the social staff and the annual admissions in 29 New York hospitals, according to figures published in their annual reports, is shown in Table 17. As the footnotes on the table indicate, there are points in which these figures are not strictly comparable; but they serve to indicate roughly the very great disparity that exists in the relation of social service staff to number of patients in hospitals of various sizes.

[38] MacEachern, Malcolm T., Ratio of Hospital Personnel to Patients. *Bulletin of the American Hospital Association, Inc.*, vol. 4, No. 10, October, 1930, p. 16.

[39] Philadelphia Hospital and Health Survey, 1929, Conducted under the Auspices of a Citizens' Survey Committee, by Haven Emerson, M.D., Sol Pincus, and Anna C. Phillips, p. 805.

[40] The Presbyterian Hospital in the City of New York, Annual Report, 1930, p. 62.

Half of these 29 hospitals had a ratio of 1 social worker to 4,000 admissions or over; and more than a third had a ratio of 1 social worker to 5,000 admissions or over. There were only 2 hospitals with 10,000 or more annual admissions that had a ratio of 1 social worker to 2,000 admissions or less. Only 6 hospitals in all had 1 social worker to 2,000 admissions or less. The ratio was one to less than 1,000 in 3 of the smaller hospitals and in one with over 10,000 admissions.

TABLE 17

HOSPITAL AND CLINIC ADMISSIONS PER SOCIAL WORKER IN RELATION TO
TOTAL ADMISSIONS[1] IN 29 PRIVATE HOSPITALS[2] OF NEW YORK CITY, 1928[3]

Admissions per social worker	Total	ADMISSIONS						
		Under 5,000 admissions	5,000– 10,000	10,000– 15,000	15,000– 20,000	20,000– 30,000	30,000– 40,000	50,000 or more
Total	29	5	3	6	4	4	5	2
Under 1,000 . . .	4	3[4]	..	1	0	0	0	0
1,000–2,000 . . .	2	1	..	..	..	1	0	0
2,000–3,000 . . .	6	..	3	..	..	1	1	1
3,000–4,000 . . .	2	..	..	1	..	..	1	0
4,000–5,000 . . .	4	1	..	2	1	0	0	0
5,000–10,000 . . .	4	..	..	..	1	..	2	1
10,000–15,000 . .	3	..	..	2	..	..	1	0
15,000–20,000 . .	2	..	..	..	2	0	0	0
20,000 or more . .	2	..	..	..	..	2	0	0

[1] Total hospital and clinic admissions as shown in annual reports were used. These figures in many cases do not allow for duplication between admissions in various departments of the clinic or between admissions to the hospital and the clinic.
[2] Selected on the basis of information available in annual reports. Includes 2 chronic, 3 orthopedic, and 24 general hospitals.
[3] In five instances, 1926, 1927, or 1929 figures were used because 1928 figures were not available.
[4] One of these has no clinic service.

Although all of the public hospitals except one have some provision for social service, the staff of social workers on the whole is not large enough to care for the needs of chronic patients. It may be assumed that every dependent chronic patient admitted to a public hospital should receive the benefit of an inquiry into his social needs at the time of admission; but 52 per cent of the adults and 20 per cent of the children in our census in public hospitals were not known to the social service. The distribution of this service is very uneven. In one large hospital, 98 per cent of the chronic patients reported were known to the social service, and in another, only 7 per cent were known to the social service. One hospital had a staff of 13 workers and another with nearly as large a bed capacity had only 4 workers in the social service. The municipal hospital for children with tuberculosis of the bones, glands, and joints had no social service department, although it is generally recognized that such an institution, where children may remain for years, should be conducted according to the standards of a child-caring agency with ample provision for social service. In the city homes for the infirm and aged, the provision for social service is deplorably inadequate. (For details see vol. 1, Chapter 4, dealing with the municipal institutions.)

Forms of Organization

Various forms of organization were found in the fifty-five social service departments studied. The department is sometimes financed and administered wholly by an auxiliary group that is only loosely responsible to the hospital administration. In other instances, the hospital budget provides for a social service department but allows so little that the greater part of the department's budget is raised by an auxiliary group, who to a greater or lesser extent affect its administration. There are a few hospitals in which the social service is a part of the organization just as the nursing service is and in which the hospital accepts full responsibility for raising the social service budget. This last type of organization does not preclude volunteer committees or workers, who may give important assistance either in raising money or in other capacities. Most of the hospitals have a committee of lay persons with an interest in social service.

As pointed out in the report on medical social work prepared for the White House Conference, "a department of social work should be an integral part of the institution it serves. In a survey made by the American Hospital Association in 1920, 50 per cent of the departments were found to be controlled and financed by the medical institution as a definite department. In our present survey this figure has risen to 89 per cent. . . . Many social service departments have been inaugurated by auxiliary groups and not by those intimately concerned with hospital administration, such as hospital executives or trustees. These groups have been more or less familiar with other fields of social work and have become aware of the need for social service in a hospital. They undoubtedly have made possible in many cities earlier attention to the social problems inherent in the institutional practice of medicine than would otherwise have occurred. . . . Departments thus established have not always had well defined policies regarding working relationships with hospital executives, medical staff and departments of nursing. . . . This type of organization has the advantage of the backing and financial support of a group of people vitally interested in the development of medical social service, but it has the disadvantage of so separating the social service department from the affairs of the hospital that it may be unable to interpret its functions adequately to administrative and medical staffs and to absorb thoroughly the hospitals' traditions."[41]

The study of medical social work conducted a few years ago under the auspices of the American Association of Social Workers in hospitals throughout the country found the prevailing form of organization to be as follows: "In the majority of hospitals the social service department is now under the administrative direction of the medical director or superintendent. The

[41] Hospitals and Child Health; Report of the Sub-committee on Medical Social Service, by Ida M. Cannon, Chairman. White House Conference on Child Health and Protection called by President Hoover, New York, The Century Company, 1932, pp. 193–194.

board of trustees frequently appoints a social service committee, composed of persons from its own membership or outsiders, to serve in an advisory capacity to the department. It assists in interpreting the needs of the social service department to the board of directors, raising additional funds, interpreting to the community the work of the department, and stimulating outside interest in health education and social needs. But its function is advisory, both to the board and to the director of the department."[42]

There seems to be a trend toward the development of another type of auxiliary committee for medical social service departments dealing not with the administration or development of the department as a whole but rather with a special problem, such as tuberculosis or cardiac diseases in children; that is, a committee representing various interests in the community concerned not with the internal problems of the hospital but with the relation of the hospital to community problems. An auxiliary committee of this type may serve as a central committee for a number of hospitals. The Central Social Service Committee for the Municipal Hospitals of Brooklyn is forming a number of divisions to deal with special aspects of disease, including a division on the chronic sick for the development of services for chronic patients in the medical social departments of city hospitals.

The minimum standards adopted by the American Association of Hospital Social Workers, referred to above (pp. 77–78), contain the following statement in regard to the most effective form of organization: "It is important to the hospital that its medical and social work be closely integrated in function and organization. The Social Service Department, therefore, should function as an integral part of the institution. . . . The head of the Social Service Department should be a member of conferences called by the director of the hospital, or by the chief of any department, to discuss or to formulate policies pertaining to the social care of the patient and to the community relationships of the hospital."[43]

The Jewish Communal Survey of Greater New York, in 1928, reported that the Jewish hospitals of this city with one exception lacked this approved form of organization of social service: "A serious defect in the organization of social service in nearly all of the Jewish hospitals is the lack of direct participation by the medical staffs, through representation on the advisory or policy-determining committee. Hospital social service should exist primarily as an aid in the medical care of the patient. If it is really to aid in this way, it must be guided closely by the professional staff in charge of patients, as an essential diagnostic and therapeutic aid in certain cases. The existing type of organization of social service at most of the hospitals seems to reflect a conception of it as an half-extraneous service of humanitarian or financial rather than of medical value. Mt. Sinai Hospital is the one exception in the Jewish group. There the medical social workers often make bedside reports in a case to the physician, and members of the medical staff

[42] Odencrantz, Louise C., The Social Worker; Chapter 9, Medical Social Work. New York, Harper and Brothers, 1929, p. 152.
[43] Bulletin of the American Association of Hospital Social Workers, July, 1928, pp. 1; 2.

may and do attend meetings of the Auxiliary when problems come up about medical care of patients."[44]

At the request of the lay delegates in the Medical Social Service Section of the Welfare Council who expressed the need for a central forum for discussion of their common problems as distinguished from the problems of the social worker in the hospital, a Lay Committee was organized in 1932. The first action of the committee has been to seek definite information by the questionnaire method concerning the functions and practices of all the medical social service auxiliaries of the city.

The degree to which the social service is integrated in practice with the medical work of the hospital varies in the fifty-five hospitals included in the study. In some institutions, the social service is a separate department to which doctors refer social problems as they discover them in the course of their treatment of patients. In others, the social worker is a member of the hospital or clinic personnel and social diagnosis and treatment are considered a definite part of the hospital's provision for the care of the patient. The social factors bearing on the medical situation are then regarded as part of the patient's history with which the doctor is equipped, and the social worker may initiate social treatment without waiting for the doctor to discover the existence of a social problem.

An interesting method of bringing the social service into close working relations with the medical work of a general hospital has been in operation at the Beth Israel Hospital in Boston for over two years. The social worker responsible for the service accompanies a resident physician and the senior house officer on weekly ward rounds. Each patient is discussed in turn on the ward. The senior house officer having received an outline of facts relating to the patient's background and environment, emotional factors, and considerations for after-care prepared by the social service, presents additional data, such as a statement of the specific problem and the diagnosis, the patient's physical and mental condition, the prognosis, the probable duration of hospitalization, recommendations for after-care, and a statement of the patient's ability to resume activity and the need for limitation of activity if indicated. Following the rounds, the doctor and social worker review the cases together and select those problems that indicate the greatest need for medical study and treatment. These ward rounds establish the correlation of medical and social treatment and enable the patient to understand and carry through his treatment in an effective way. The hospital benefits by a shorter period of hospitalization, because the patient is referred early and the medical social plan is made promptly so that the patient is discharged as soon as practicable.[45]

Social service in the municipal hospitals of New York is under the supervision of a General Director of Social Service in the Department of Hospitals responsible to the Commissioner of Hospitals; and the director of

[44] The Jewish Communal Survey of Greater New York, Health Section, Chapter IV, Hospital Social Service, The Bureau of Jewish Social Research, 1928, pp. 9–10, MS.

[45] Cohen, Ethel, An Integrated Medical and Social Service. Reprinted from *Hospital Social Service*, vol. 25, No. 3, March, 1932, p. 223.

social service at Bellevue Hospital serves also as her first assistant. There are still great differences among the departments in different hospitals both in regard to standards of work and size of staff. The development of social work in these hospitals has been promoted by the efforts of the New York City Visiting Committee of the State Charities Aid Association. Auxiliary committees have organized social service at the request of the hospital authorities in many of the city hospitals. Other special auxiliaries exist for the purpose of assisting the social work in special departments of hospital service. A Central Council of delegates from the social service auxiliaries of the different hospitals, meeting three times a year, has advisory powers in all municipal hospitals. Several other agencies also provide various helpful services to patients through the social service. The Social Service Committee of the Free Synagogue and other Jewish societies maintain Jewish workers in the social service departments of seven city institutions. An account of the social service of the city hospitals is given in the section of the report dealing with municipal institutions.[46]

The smaller private hospitals in New York often have no social service. This was found to be the case among the thousand hospitals studied by the American College of Surgeons mentioned above. The Hospital Standardization Report of this Association, for 1930, points out that: "It is not occurring to the management of smaller hospitals that they too have problems of a social nature which must be met by a person well trained for the work."[47]

When social service is regarded as a necessary and integral part of the work of a hospital or clinic, the first question to be faced is what proportion of the whole hospital budget should be devoted to this purpose. As expressed by the President of the Presbyterian Hospital: "Any service directly contributing to the medical diagnosis or treatment of the case should be provided as a charge against hospital general funds. Professional nursing is such a service and at least equally is social service. And so the hospital trustee is or should be prepared to budget social service against general hospital income as a necessary expense chargeable to professional care of patients."[48] Five per cent of the whole budget for ward and clinic expense was considered the highest ratio possible in this hospital "without endangering other departments."[48]

The total amount spent for medical social service in New York City is at present a wholly unknown figure. The private hospitals do not as a rule segregate in their accounting the expense of social service. In many hospitals, the amounts raised by auxiliary committees for this purpose do not appear in the institution's books; and such auxiliary funds often constitute the greater part of the budget of the social service department. The public hospitals segregate and publish their expenditures for social service, but here also the contributions of the auxiliaries are not included and such funds represent a substantial part of the total expense for social service in the city

[46] See also vol. 1, Chapter 4, The Care of the Chronic Sick in Municipal Institutions, pp. 236–239.
[47] American College of Surgeons, Hospital Standardization Report, 1930, p. 47.
[48] Medical Social Service from the Viewpoint of the Hospital Trustee, by Dean Sage, address at a meeting of the Medical Social Service Section of the Welfare Council, January 30, 1931.

hospitals. It is to be hoped that in the study of income and expenditures of hospitals that has been undertaken by the Research Bureau of the Welfare Council, it will be possible to collect these figures in both public and private hospitals for at least one year and to show how much is being expended annually for medical social service.

The United Hospital Fund in a study of the cost of out-patient service attempted to differentiate the cost of social service but found that "outside auxiliaries, in a large percentage of cases finance and administer the social service departments. Since these funds do not pass through the accounting divisions of the hospitals, there is an inaccurate knowledge of the cost on the part of both the hospital administration and the auxiliary." It was also noted that "hospitals fail to take into consideration the floor space occupied and the light, heat, lunches and other maintenance expenses required by the social service department."[49]

The report on medical social service at the White House Conference stresses the importance of budgeting the cost of the social service as a part of the whole hospital budget: "Support by groups other than hospital authorities may allow for more rapid expansion than hospital budgets would permit, but it may tend to isolate the department rather than to foster well defined working relationships with other departments of the hospital organization. . . . It is essential for the members of the social service department to have a sense of financial security in regard to tenure of office, provided their practice is acceptable. A director should also have some assurance that additional workers can be secured at a reasonable rate of growth upon adequate demonstration of need. Budgets depending upon voluntary subscriptions from auxiliary groups may not furnish this sense of security. Hospital budgeting may limit rapid expansion of the work, but will probably stabilize the financing of the social service department. With proper demonstration of need, hospital administrators and trustees should see that social service for their patients is adequately staffed as are their medical and nursing services."[50]

Records and Statistics

It is an axiom of social case work that good records and good work go together. The importance of the record of social history and treatment has been generally recognized by medical social workers, but less frequently by the hospital administration. Good recording is expensive and the expense must be justified "in terms of records that are really useful. The art of writing a record depends primarily on the recognition that records are to be read, not merely filed away."[51] The social records must be good in order to be of use to the medical staff, they must have time and money expended

[49] Babbitt, Henrietta D., Social Service—A Large Item in O. P. D. Expense. Reprinted from *The Modern Hospital*, October, 1930, pp. 10, 11.

[50] Hospitals and Child Health; Report of the Sub-committee on Medical Social Service, by Ida M. Cannon, Chairman. White House Conference on Child Health and Protection called by President Hoover, New York, The Century Company, 1932, pp. 197–198.

[51] Hamilton, Gordon, Notes on Current Practices in Medical Social Case Recording. Reprinted from *The Family*, May, 1931, p. 67.

on them in order to be good, and before this support is obtained the hospital administration must be convinced that they are of value; so that a vicious circle is formed until an opportunity arises to demonstrate the usefulness of good social records in some particular part of the medical work of the hospital.

A few years ago a committee of the American Association of Hospital Social Workers drafted a medical social record form which was recommended as meeting a minimum standard.[52] The main features of this form of record are that it states the medical social problem, the tentative plan of treatment, summarizes the medical social treatment, and when the record is closed gives the reasons for discontinuing treatment and a statement of the situation at the time. There are few social service departments in New York City that have approached this standard. Evidence of this is found in the report of a survey of social service departments made by Dr. Corwin in 1925: "What most of the records needed very badly was a topical arrangement of information under several general headings and the segregation of data in such a way that the details of the investigation would be separated from the main facts about the physical condition of the patient and his economic and social difficulties. Above all there was an apparant need of similarity in recording the facts and also in assigning precise meanings to the terms used."[53] Since that time several departments have improved their methods.

The Presbyterian Hospital introduced in 1916 what is known as "the unit history system" of records, in which all information concerning a patient is kept in one place and the history obtained by the social service appears chronologically in the medical record. This type of record serves a two-fold purpose—it keeps the medical problem clearly before the social worker and the social factors pertinent to the medical case are made readily available to the physician, which "must inevitably result in a closer working relationship between the doctor and the social worker and a definite fusion of objectives."[54]

"A Medical Social Terminology"[55] now in use in many hospitals of the country has been issued by the social service department of this hospital as a guide to enable medical social workers to classify the social situations and behavior of patients and as a guide to the precise use of terms.

A discussion of the relation of the social information to the medical record appears below in connection with a description of facilities in the fifty-five social service departments included in this study. (See p. 94.)

Recording of statistics of the amount of service given in the social service department is necessary in every hospital, but as each department does it according to a method of its own, the volume of work in different depart-

[52] *Ibid.*, p. 72.

[53] Corwin, E. H. L., The Desirability of a Uniform Record Card for Hospital Social Service Work. Reprinted from *Hospital Social Service*, vol. 12, No. 4, October, 1925, p. 185.

[54] Hall, Beatrice, The Social Service Record in the Unit Medical History. Reprinted from *Hospital Social Service*, vol. 20, No. 1, July, 1929, p. 26.

[55] Hamilton, Gordon, A Medical Social Terminology. Published by The Social Service Department of The Presbyterian Hospital in the City of New York, 1930.

ments cannot be compared and the total volume of this service in a given community cannot be appraised. A few years ago, efforts were begun to develop a method for recording uniform statistics of medical social work on a national scale. In 1928, a Committee on the Registration of Social Statistics, working at the University of Chicago, invited the American Association of Hospital Social Workers to take part in its project. Two years later, in July, 1930, the work of this committee was taken over by the United States Children's Bureau. The care with which the work has been done is reflected in these excerpts from a handbook issued by the Bureau:

"It has been the aim of the joint committee to formulate a method of statistical recording in the field of medical social work, a method which will enable those who use it to express numerically the volume of medical social work done. The system which is described and defined in this handbook is the result of the efforts of the Committee to evolve a method which is based on the essential character of medical social work and which makes possible its quantitative expression in terms of service rendered in behalf of patients.

"Any method of statistical recording must be adapted to the processes it is intended to measure, and must change as they change. It is evident, therefore, that the problem of evolving a method of statistical recording in medical social work is a continuous one, and that this is only the first of a series of handbooks. Medical social work, as one of the special fields of social case work, is still emerging, with certain functions crystallized and others not yet clear. However, social case workers have used statistical reports as a service-accounting device ever since social agencies saw the light of day; and community funds and welfare federations have gathered service statistics from an increasing number of agencies and cities in the last ten or twelve years. As these figures are being used for the purposes of inter-agency and inter-city comparisons of the amount of service rendered and its cost, it is imperative that earnest effort be made to develop a method of statistical recording which while it does not measure the qualitative factors and the accepted standards of work, nevertheless takes these factors into account. Since statistics are already being gathered over a wide geographical area, it is necessary to attempt to formulate a method of statistical recording which will yield figures as fundamentally sound and as comparable as possible.

"Statistics in the field of medical social work should be of value in:

"1. Keeping account of the volume of service rendered to patients by medical social service throughout the country.

"2. Showing change in volume of service from time to time; i. e., month to month, and year to year.

"3. Securing facts of value in making comparisons, such as among social service departments, and of medical social work with other fields of case work.

"4. Yielding facts of value in making decisions within the social service department, and by the hospital administration.

"5. Furnishing one means of interpreting the work to those who support it."[56]

This plan for statistics of medical social service is now being used experimentally in a number of hospitals elsewhere but not in New York City. Grasslands Hospital in Westchester County is using it.

The North Atlantic District of the American Association of Hospital Social Workers, in coöperation with the Department of Statistics of the Russell Sage Foundation, for several years carried on a project for central reporting of medical social service statistics. When it was begun in January, 1929, twenty-eight New York City clinics undertook to become a part of the reporting system. As the standardization of reporting proceeded, however, the number of clinics taking part decreased until by the end of 1931 only fifteen clinics were reporting their monthly social service statistics. It became increasingly evident, moreover, that these statistics did not constitute a measure of medical social case work, in view of the varying meanings with which the same terms were used in different hospitals, so that the project was discontinued.

The Section on Medical Social Service of the Welfare Council, through its Committee on the Development of Social Service in Eye Clinics, is attempting to develop a very simple form of monthly reporting that will show the fundamental facts in the clinic treatment of patients afflicted with the major eye diseases, which without proper medical treatment and supervision may result in blindness. The purpose is to measure the clinic activities, to serve as a stimulus in raising standards of practice, and to make possible comparisons between clinics that have been heretofore impossible. A plan for central reporting of statistics of mental hygiene clinics, including a few items in regard to the social work of the clinics, was developed by the Mental Hygiene Section and the Research Bureau of the Council, and has been in operation since January, 1932, with twenty-nine clinics participating.

Research

When social service became available in hospitals, it was natural that doctors carrying on medical research should seek the assistance of the social workers in obtaining facts and observations concerning the patients in their social relationships. It was also natural that the social workers should obtain the help of the doctors in studying the problems arising out of their work. The practice of collaboration between the medical staff and the social service in the study of medical social problems has now become so general that in plans for a modern medical social service department, provision is usually made for research as a major activity. In some instances, trained research workers have been added to the staff.

It is peculiarly the responsibility of the medical social service to find out what can be done for patients disabled by chronic disease to save them from

[56] A Tentative Plan for Statistics in the Field of Medical Social Service. Prepared by a Joint Committee of the American Association of Hospital Social Workers and the Advisory Committee on Social Statistics of the United States Children's Bureau, June 2, 1931, pp. iv, v.

chronic invalidism. Quoting from the annual report of the social service of the Presbyterian Hospital, 1929, "we are only at the beginning of learning what we can do in such cases. It is, we believe, a great field for preventive social work." This responsibility was pointed out many years ago by Ida M. Cannon: "That the treatment of chronic diseases has been distinctly promoted by the assistance of hospital social service departments is without question. The future holds further opportunities for them to contribute to the study of chronic disease in its social incidence and cost, in its loss of working capacity and its frustration of satisfactory living."[57]

The facilities for social service in most of the hospitals in New York City are inadequate for any direct contributions to research. But the annual reports of some of the hospitals give evidence of a trend toward collaboration between the medical service and the social service in research projects. The Presbyterian Hospital has been conducting a study of the significance of social factors in the medical situation. The medical service appointed a representative to take part and the auxiliary of the social service department provided the funds. Referring to this joint project, the director of the Department says: "We believe that a measure of clarification must result from the mere display and enumeration of the many lets and hindrances to medical care which are found in the social relationships of an unselected series of hospital cases. Also a number of questions are emerging from the study of these cases as to the influence of discovered deprivations, strains, and shocks in engendering states of ill health."[58]

The social service department of Mt. Sinai Hospital has participated in two medical social studies recently, one dealing with treatment of children suffering from asthma and the other with the course of the disease in a thousand children with rheumatic fever.

The research program of the cardiac clinics of this city is an example of the dependence of medical investigation upon social service. A number of "Statistical Studies Bearing on Problems in the Classification of Heart Diseases"[59] have been published, since 1926, by The Heart Committee of the New York Tuberculosis and Health Association, which would not have been possible without the assistance of social service in following up patients and keeping them under treatment. So far, this research has been confined to medical data and the attempt has not yet been made to collect and analyze social data, since the available social service facilities in the cardiac clinics have not been adequate for the task of defining the problems for study, standardizing the terminology, and establishing the necessary criteria for observing and recording facts.

[57] Cannon, Ida M., Social Work in Hospitals: A Contribution to Progressive Medicine. New York, Russell Sage Foundation, March, 1923, p. 77.

[58] The Presbyterian Hospital of the City of New York, Annual Report, 1930, p. 67.

[59] Statistical Studies Bearing on Problems in the Classification of Heart Diseases: I. Introduction by Alfred E. Cohn, M.D.; II. Etiology in Organic Heart Disease by John Wyckoff, M.D., and Claire Lingg; III. Heart Disease in Children by May G. Wilson, Claire Lingg, and Geneva Croxford; IV. Tonsillectomy in Its Relation to the Prevention of Rheumatic Heart Disease by May G. Wilson, Claire Lingg, and Geneva Croxford. Distributed by The Heart Committee of the New York Tuberculosis and Health Association, New York City.

Survey of Fifty-five Social Service Departments

The purpose of the survey of social service departments in hospitals made for this study was to find out to what extend medical social service is available for chronic patients. However, since the social work of the hospitals is not organized separately for chronic and acute services, these facilities were studied as a whole and as far as possible related to the data on the chronic patients in hospitals who were reported in the census of the chronic sick as being under the care of the social service. Probably the greater part of the social service required for the chronic sick is needed for the rehabilitation of the large number of clinic patients rather than for hospital patients who are fewer in number and as a rule more seriously disabled; but since the study did not include a census of clinic patients, the medical social service facilities for clinic patients are only incidentally discussed in this report.

The directors of the social service departments in fifty-five hospitals were interviewed and information gathered concerning the number of workers in each department and their functions and procedures. In Appendix III, hospitals included in the study are listed.

As stated above (p. 71), there are nearly 100 private hospitals and twenty-one public hospitals in New York that care for patients coming within the definition of the chronic sick as used in this study, exclusive of special hospitals for tuberculosis, mental diseases, eye and ear disorders, and maternity service. Two fifths of the private hospitals have no social service. All of the public hospitals except one have social service. The fifty-five hospitals selected for study include all public hospitals of the types studied and about 70 per cent of the private hospitals with social service of the types studied.

Three hospitals with departments for home care that give visiting nurse service rather than social service are not included in this section of the report; and the work of these departments is considered in the section dealing with nursing services. (See Chapter 6, p. 216.) They are Memorial Hospital, the New York Orthopedic Hospital, and the Norwegian Lutheran Deaconesses' Hospital. However, in the census of the chronic sick, the patients in these three hospitals who were receiving visiting nurse service were counted among those receiving social service, since the actual service is similar to that given in some medical social service departments.

Contact with Patients. Knowledge of a patient's social situation is frequently necessary for a complete understanding of his medical condition and is usually of great assistance in carrying out wise treatment. Although the practice is still somewhat rare, it is considered advisable by many physicians and social workers that a social worker should interview both ward and clinic patients, or the persons responsible for them, either upon admission or shortly afterwards. The social worker should meet the patient naturally in the course of hospital procedure, and if necessary keep in touch with him during treatment. For chronic patients, who almost invariably have problems of social as well as of medical care, this is especially important. It is particularly desirable to learn as early as possible what the social problems of the chronic patient are, so that plans for social adjustment and continued treatment can be completed before his discharge.

Less than half of the hospital social service departments studied had any provision for including all ward patients in their service. Of the 55 departments, 26 reported that each ward patient was regularly interviewed and 29 that they were not. Of the latter 29, 26 gave service to ward patients only when requested by the doctor or someone else interested in the patient. The remaining three departments regularly interview certain groups of patients; one, the prenatal and gynecological patients before admission to the hospital; one, the orthopedic, congenital lues, and cardiac patients before admission to the hospital; and one, the cardiac and rheumatic fever patients just before discharge, mainly for research purposes.

Contact with every clinic patient is even more infrequent. Only 5 of the 53 social service departments in institutions with clinics reported that each clinic patient was regularly interviewed by a social worker. These were the social service department of the House of St. Giles, Lenox Hill Hospital, Brooklyn Hospital, New York City Cancer Institute, and New York Nursery and Child's Hospital. Thirty-one departments interviewed only patients referred to them by the doctors. The remaining 17 departments interviewed every patient among certain groups. Of the 17, 12 served all cardiac patients, both adults and children, 1 served all cardiac children; all obstetrical patients were seen by 5 departments; and all children in the pediatric clinics, diabetics, and syphilitics, were seen by 3 departments. Other groups in which contact was made with every patient by one or two departments were: mental hygiene; tonsils and adenoids; surgical follow-up; dental; orthopedic; infant hygiene; asthma; tuberculosis; neurological; and nose and throat.

Among the chronic sick, cardiac patients are evidently the group that most frequently receive complete service. Among any of the other groups receiving special attention from the social service, there may be chronic patients; and some of these groups represent chronic diseases; but the majority of the chronic sick are likely to be in the large group of patients who pass through the clinic unnoticed by the social service.

An administrative procedure, followed in some hospitals, that gives the social service department a natural contact with all patients is to have a medical social worker on the social service staff as the clinic executive. In the 55 hospitals studied, 21 had social workers as clinic executives in one or more clinics, but only three had this organization throughout the entire out-patient department. Unless the staff of social workers is adequate for all functions, there is danger in this system that the social service will not be able to perform its essential functions of social diagnosis and treatment.

Follow-up. By "follow-up" is meant the effort made by the clinic or hospital to keep patients in attendance at the clinic as long as the doctor considers it necessary. The term is loosely used in hospital statistics, as mentioned above, so that it is impossible to tell whether it involves a card asking the patient to return or an educational visit to enlist the interest of the patient or his family in coöperating with the clinic in his care. In the hospitals studied, this was sometimes a function of the social service and sometimes it was done as a clerical routine. Home visits were in some cases made by the social service when follow-up letters met with no response, or the service in some institutions was limited to letters. When the social service becomes acquainted with the patient and his social situation upon his first visit to the clinic or upon his admission into the hospital, this continued contact is more readily maintained and incomplete treatment is more likely to be avoided. This "follow through" system has proved superior to the follow-after or follow-up system.[60]

Fifty of the 55 social service departments reported that they did follow-up work and 5 that they did not. Of the 55, only 6 departments follow up all of their patients. Forty-four departments did follow-up work only for referred patients or for certain diagnostic groups. Of these, 13 departments did follow-up for referred patients only; 9 for social service patients only. Others followed up one or more of the following groups: cardiacs, congenital luetics, diabetics, prenatal or postpartum patients, patients in the neurological, rheumatic fever, tuberculous, venereal, pneumonia, orthopedic, surgical, mental hygiene, infant hygiene, nose and throat, pediatric, or medical services, and patients discharged from the hospital and referred to the out-patient department.

In nearly all the hospitals, follow-up is the responsibility of the social service; but in six hospitals, the responsibility was given to clerical workers rather than to social workers. In three of these hospitals, the clerical workers were responsible to the head of the social service and in three they were responsible to the hospital administration. Where clerical follow-up is done under the direction of the hospital administration, patients are referred to the social service when follow-up letters produce no results. It may be a more economical division of labor to have clerks for the routine follow-up procedures and to leave social workers free for the functions of social diagnosis and treatment as a part of the whole process of rehabilitating the patient. This arrangement is considered to be best particularly when the follow-up is merely to determine end results, as in post-operative cases. The simplest routine worked out for follow-up on all patients is the system whereby the doctor indicates on the medical record of the patient at each visit the date on which he should return. If the patient does not return, the doctor then indicates whether he should be followed up.

Relation of Medical and Social Records. Various methods are used to bring to the doctor the social information concerning his patient. It is agreed that to depend on conferences alone is not sufficient. Neither isolated items of social information included in the medical record nor periodic summaries of the social service record have been found altogether satis-

[60] Davis, Michael, Clinics, Hospitals and Health Centers. New York, Harper and Brothers, 1927, p. 485.

factory. The filing of the social record with the medical record is still an experiment; but it seems reasonable to believe that, since social service is coming more and more to be regarded as an integral part of the complete care offered to patients by a clinic or hospital with its many special services, the social record will eventually be treated as an integral part of the medical record. At the Presbyterian Hospital, where the social service was carrying on studies for the purpose of developing higher standards of hospital social work, the social record was filed with the medical record.

TABLE 18

HOSPITALS GROUPED BY NUMBER OF SOCIAL WORKERS IN THE
SOCIAL SERVICE DEPARTMENT

Number of social workers in the department	Number of hospitals	Total number of social workers
Total	55	290
One worker	15	15
Two workers	6	12
Three workers	9	27
Four workers	7	28
Five workers	4	20
Six workers	1	6
Eight workers	2	16
Nine workers	1	9
Ten workers	3	30
Eleven workers	1	11
Twelve workers	1	12
Fourteen workers	1	14
Fifteen workers	1	15
Sixteen workers	1	16
Twenty-seven workers	1	27
Thirty-two workers	1	32

Information showing how the doctor obtains social information regarding the patient was secured for 53 departments. In 5 hospitals, the social information in full is filed with the medical record—Presbyterian Hospital, Beth David Hospital, Jewish Hospital of Brooklyn, Brooklyn Hospital, and Montefiore Hospital. The last two mentioned had just begun this system at the time of the survey. In all of the other 48 departments, interviews between doctor and social worker were chiefly relied upon for integrating medical and social care. The doctor might ask for such social information as he cared to have; or the social worker might bring to the doctor such information as she considered of value to him in making a diagnosis or a plan of medical treatment. In the larger clinics, it is practically impossible for the doctors to find the time to receive this information verbally from the social workers.

In 3 of these 48 hospitals in which the social information is filed separately, an exception is made for certain diagnostic groups and it is filed with the medical record. In one hospital, this is done for cardiac, tuberculous, and syphilitic patients; in one for cardiac, mental hygiene, and infant hygiene patients; and in one for cardiac, syphilitic, and mental hygiene patients.

Four departments file a summary of the social information with the medical record for all patients under the care of social service. Six others file a summary with the medical record only in certain groups. In one, it is done for ward patients only; in another, for ward patients when the doctor requests it. In two departments, a summary is filed with the medical record for a patient in whose care the social worker thinks it would be of value to the doctor. A fifth department files summaries with the medical records of all pediatric and cardiac patients, and a sixth, of all asthmatic, syphilitic, tuberculous, and cardiac patients.

All but six of the institutions in which the social service was studied had central medical records. Unless a unit system of filing has been installed, the social record may as well be filed separately. Three of the six institutions without a central medical record were planning a reorganization of their filing system.

Distribution of Social Workers. The 55 social service departments studied had staffs ranging from 1 to 32 social workers, with a total of 290 social workers. The average number for a department was about 5. Three fourths of the departments had a staff of 5 or less. Table 18 groups the hospitals by the number of social workers in the department.

The predominance of the small department is indicated by the fact that, although the average number of social workers is over five, two thirds of the hospitals had less than five.

SUMMARY

Since medical social service is one of the most important and on the whole least recognized agencies for the prevention and care of chronic illness, in addition to the data obtained for this study, other available information has been assembled in order to throw as much light as possible upon standards and practices in this field in New York City. No general survey of medical social service departments has been made in this city, such as was recently made in Philadelphia.

Of 117 public and private institutions for the sick in New York City that receive chronic patients of the types included in this study, 39 have no social service department.

Considerably more than a third of the chronically ill patients in hospitals with a social service department had received no attention from a social worker. Among those reported as known to the social service, the service given ranged from a single interview to intensive study and treatment.

Functions of Medical Social Service in Relation to Chronic Patients

Chronic illness is always a medical social problem; and, therefore, it may be assumed that chronic patients as a rule require attention to their social needs and very frequently require social service as well as medical care.

Chronically ill patients require medical social service more frequently than the acutely ill. It follows that the major part of the work of the social service department of a hospital has to do with the chronic sick.

In the prevention of chronic illness and incapacity, medical social service is as important as medical or nursing service.

Successful medical treatment in hospitals and clinics is not possible for some chronic conditions without social service. This has been demonstrated particularly in regard to heart disease and diabetes.

In certain cases of chronic disability, after the condition has once been diagnosed, responsibility for the patient's care rests chiefly upon the social service.

Medical social workers in hospitals meet insurmountable difficulties in caring for chronic patients because of lack of facilities for their care in the community and lack of staff for adequate service.

The service given by medical social workers in hospitals may involve intensive medical social treatment, assistance or advice in regard to a special problem, or coöperation with another social agency.

Research in medical institutions depends increasingly upon a well-organized social service, as the emotional and social factors in chronic illness are becoming better understood. The medical social worker contributes data in connection with the study of the disease and the plan for treatment, supervises the care and treatment of the patient at home, and follows up the results of the treatment.

The rôle of the social worker in public health work is still undefined and should receive the joint consideration of physicians, public health nurses, and medical social workers.

Facilities for Medical Social Service in New York City

Organization. Few of the social service departments of New York City have attained even approximately the minimum standards adopted by the American Association of Hospital Social Workers, in 1928, and embodied in the standards of the American College of Surgeons.

The report on medical social work prepared for the White House Conference on Child Health and Protection, in 1931, is a comprehensive summary of the functions and practices of medical social workers; which should be a valuable guide in the organization of social service departments.

In many of the hospitals in this city, the organization of the social service is not in accordance with the accepted standard, that is, that the department should be an integral part of the institution and that its work should be integrated with the medical work and the other departments. In some instances, the department is administered almost entirely by an auxiliary group; and in other instances, so little allowance for its support is made in the hospital budget that its policies are controlled by the auxiliary group which provides the main support.

There is need for a clearer understanding of the functions of auxiliary committees and for the development of standard policies for their guidance.

What proportion of the hospital budget should be expended for social service is a question that hospital boards and administrators are beginning to consider. It will of course vary in different types of hospital according to the nature of the patients served and of the services undertaken. Hospital administrators who recognize the values contributed to the hospital's work by the social service endeavor to secure for this service as adequate a staff as for the medical and nursing services.

Personnel. Professional education for medical social work is now offered in ten educational institutions as a graduate course, usually recognized by the degree of A.M. or M.S.; but no standards of professional education for medical social workers are generally accepted in New York City. In many hospitals, little consideration is given to special training in the selection of personnel for social service. The salaries paid to social workers in most hospitals are not high enough to attract professionally trained persons.

In this city, medical social service was initiated by nurses in contrast to other communities where it has grown out of social work. This led to the tradition that nursing education was essential for hospital social work, which still persists in the requirement that all social workers in municipal hospitals shall be nurses without the requirement of recognized social training.

The 55 social service departments surveyed, with staffs of from 1 to 32 persons, had a total number of 290 persons. Three fourths of the departments had a staff of 5 or less. Only 7 departments had 10 or more.

The ratio between number of patients served and social service staff in different hospitals reflects the fact that the social service department is rarely planned in relation to the hospital's needs. The range is from one or two social workers for less than 2,000 annual admissions to one social worker for over 20,000 annual admissions.

The distribution of social service in the municipal hospitals is very uneven. A large part of the service is supported by voluntary auxiliaries, which are more active in some hospitals than in others.

The facilities of most of the social service departments are inadequate for direct contributions to research. A few hospitals give evidence of a trend toward collaboration of the medical staff with the social service in medical social research.

Records. The value of a good record system in improving the quality of the social service and increasing its contribution to the medical work has been demonstrated; but except in a few hospitals the records of New York City social service departments are far below the accepted standards.

In the recording of statistics, nearly every department follows its own method. The United States Children's Bureau is attempting to collect statistics of hospital social service departments, along with other types of social agency, according to a carefully developed plan; but no department in this city has followed it so far.

CHAPTER 3

The Care of the Chronic Sick in Private Homes for the Aged

SECTION A

THE CHRONICALLY ILL PERSONS FOUND BY A CENSUS IN PRIVATE HOMES FOR THE AGED

NUMBER OF CHRONICALLY ILL GUESTS

In Proportion to All Chronically Ill Persons in the Census

IT is commonly assumed that homes for the aged are institutions for the able-bodied aged and should not be expected to receive the sick. With few exceptions, the homes under voluntary auspices refuse admission to an applicant who is ill or suffering from a chronic disease that is likely to incapacitate him. Nevertheless, 13 per cent of the chronically ill persons of all ages in the census were in private homes for the aged. The number of chronically ill guests reported by these homes, 2,822 persons, was as large as the number of chronic patients reported by any group of agencies except nursing services. It is evident that the private homes for the aged have already assumed a large part of the community's responsibility for the care of the chronic sick, although it has not as a rule been their policy to do so.

The census of the chronically ill included all sick persons receiving care from the medical and social agencies of the city who were incapacitated through chronic illness lasting at least three months and likely to last indefinitely, with the exception of persons suffering from tuberculosis or mental diseases, the blind, and the deaf. The total number of chronically ill persons found under the care of agencies of all types was 20,754. A third of the whole number were in the later years of life, sixty years and over; and nearly a third were children. Half of the remainder were between sixteen and forty years of age; and the other half were between forty and sixty years of age.

In the chart that follows (Chart 6) it will be seen that the private homes for the aged are caring for as many of the chronic sick as either the private or the public hospitals and for more than the public homes for the aged.

Homes for the aged are particularly concerned with persons of sixty years and over. Only about 2 per cent of their chronically ill guests were found to be under the age of sixty years. Nearly two fifths of all the chronically ill sixty years of age and over found by the census were in private homes for the aged. Of those of this age who needed only custodial care, without medical treatment or nursing, nearly half were in the homes for the aged. More than half of all who were seventy years of age and over were found in these homes.

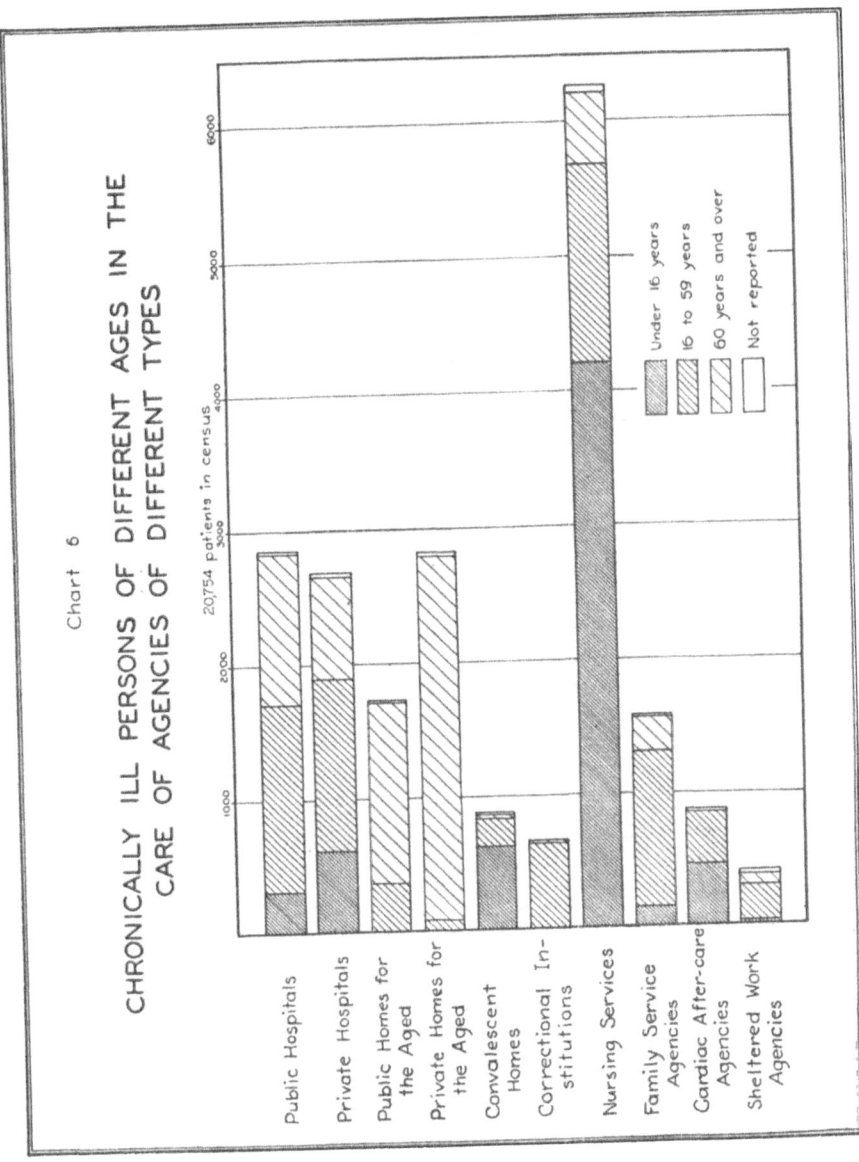

Chart 6

CHRONICALLY ILL PERSONS OF DIFFERENT AGES IN THE
CARE OF AGENCIES OF DIFFERENT TYPES

The chart that follows (Chart 7) shows that the private homes for the aged were caring for twice as many of the chronic sick of sixty years of age and over as any other group of agencies.

Two thirds of the chronically ill in the homes were foreign-born, a proportion slightly higher than among persons sixty years and over in the whole census. All but 4 per cent of the foreign-born had been in the United States ten years or longer.

The borough distribution of the residence of the chronically ill is about the same among guests in homes for the aged as among older persons reported by other agencies. Residence at the time of admission to the home was reported for two thirds of the chronically ill guests. Of these, 9 per cent lived outside of New York City. Of those in the city, nearly one half were Manhattan residents; one third, Brooklyn; 15 per cent, Bronx; and 4 and 2 per cent, Queens and Richmond respectively. The percentage of Manhattan residents is higher than Manhattan's percentage of the city population in 1928. The percentage of residents of other boroughs is lower than the percentage of the population in these boroughs. The difference is largest for Queens, which had 14 per cent of the city's 1928 population.

In Proportion to All the Guests in the Homes

Although most of the homes require that a guest shall be free from incapacitating disease, that he shall be ambulant and able to care for himself when admitted, nearly half (48 per cent) of all the guests in the sixty homes included were found to be chronically ill. Moreover, one tenth were bed-ridden and another 6 per cent were confined to wheelchairs, so that 16 per cent of those who were ill, or 7 per cent of all the guests, were not able to walk about. (See Chart 8.)

In view of the practice of the homes, as a rule, to admit only the able-bodied aged, it might be expected that the illness, in most instances at least, would occur after the guest had been in the home for some time. On the contrary, as the following table (Table 19) shows, the large majority of the chronically ill guests had been receiving care for their illness during practically their entire residence in the home. This was true both of those in the home for many years and of those recently admitted.

A number of the larger homes maintain a hospital department, that is a part of the institution equipped for medical care of the sick with a resident physician and a nursing staff. As these homes do not refuse admission to an applicant suffering from a chronic disease, it is natural that a very large proportion of their guests were reported among the chronically ill. Some homes provide infirmary beds for their sick guests, that is special rooms set aside for the sick with medical care from a visiting physician. Other homes make no special provision for the care of the sick. Even in homes that had an infirmary, there were sometimes two or three times as many sick guests as infirmary beds. Some who occupied infirmary beds may of course have been suffering from acute or temporary illnesses. In the homes with no beds provided for sickness, a larger proportion of chronic patients were found

TABLE 19

CHRONICALLY ILL GUESTS IN PRIVATE HOMES FOR THE AGED CLASSIFIED
BY TIME IN THE INSTITUTION AND PERIODS OF CARE RECEIVED

Time in institution	Persons	PERIOD OF CARE RECEIVED									
		Less than 3 months	3 months under 1 year	1 year under 2 years	2 years under 3 years	3 years under 4 years	4 years under 5 years	5 years under 10 years	10 years under 15 years	15 years and over	Not reported
Total	2,488	5.8	17.7	17.9	13.1	10.6	7.2	15.3	7.7	4.7	327
Less than 3 months	128	100.0	...	...	...	...	...	...	...	...	0
3 months under 1 year	396	0.5	99.5	...	...	...	...	...	...	...	6
1 year under 2 years	413	0.2	3.2	96.6	...	...	...	...	...	...	17
2 years under 3 years	297	1.0	2.7	3.0	93.3	...	...	...	...	...	28
3 years under 4 years	240	...	1.7	2.9	2.5	92.9	...	...	...	...	32
4 years under 5 years	183	...	2.2	4.4	4.4	3.2	85.8	...	...	...	38
5 years under 10 years	461	1.3	2.6	3.9	5.9	5.4	3.0	77.9	...	...	92
10 years under 15 years	225	0.9	1.8	0.9	2.7	3.1	1.3	7.5	81.8	...	53
15 years and over	145	0.7	1.4	1.4	2.1	2.1	3.4	2.8	5.5	80.7	37
Not reported	31	1	1	1	1	1	2	...	...	...	24

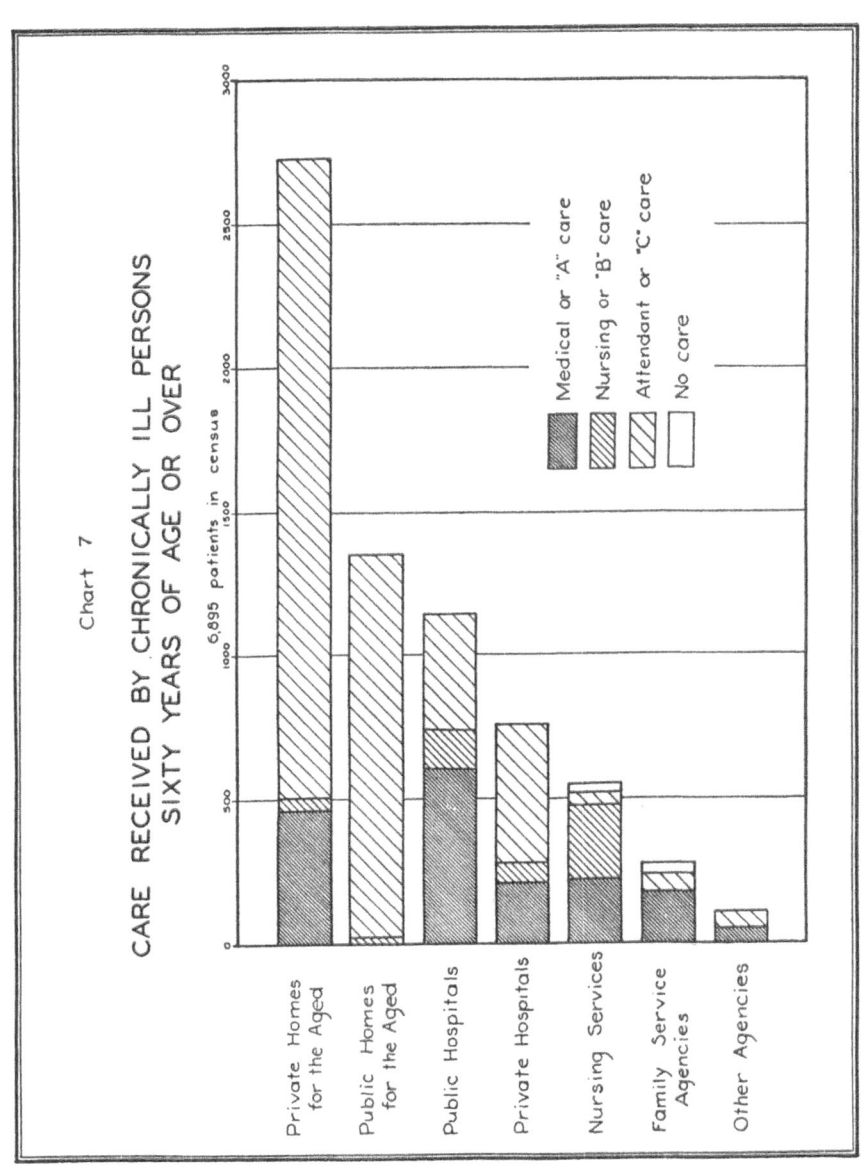

Chart 7

CARE RECEIVED BY CHRONICALLY ILL PERSONS
SIXTY YEARS OF AGE OR OVER

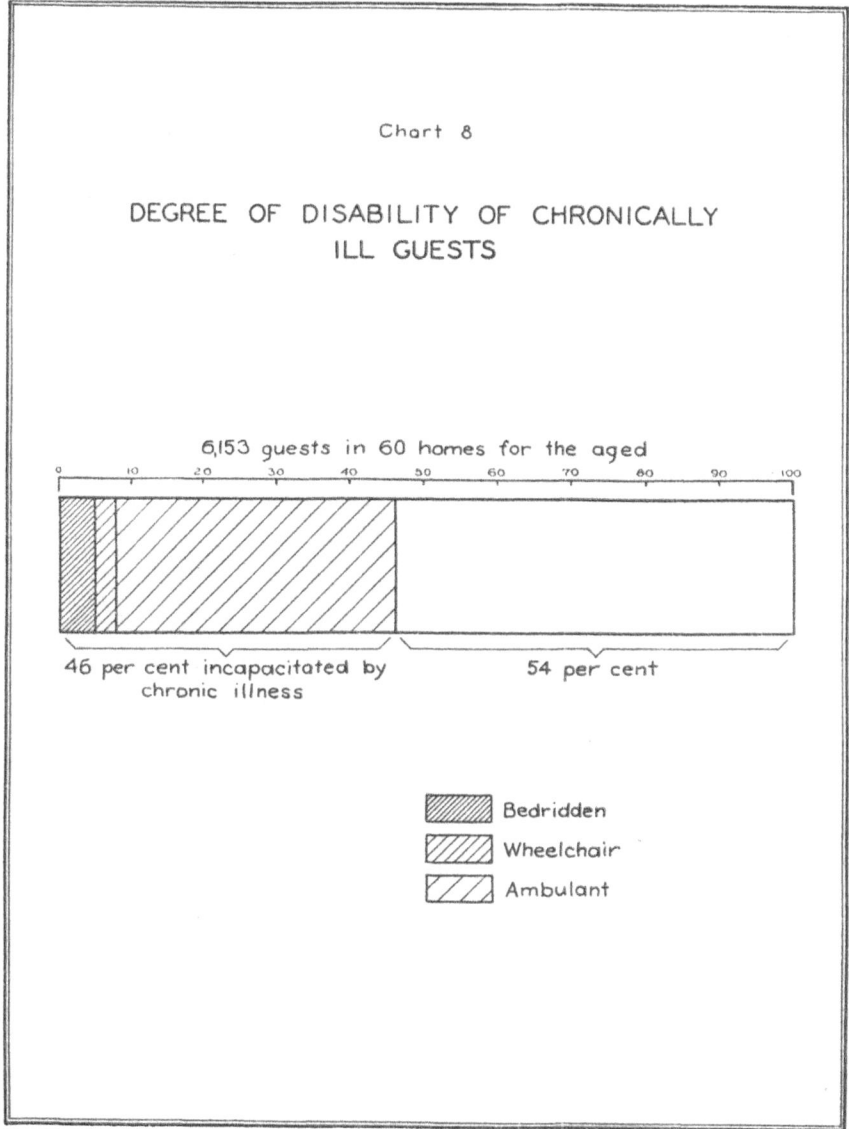

Chart 8

DEGREE OF DISABILITY OF CHRONICALLY
ILL GUESTS

6,153 guests in 60 homes for the aged

46 per cent incapacitated by
chronic illness

54 per cent

Bedridden
Wheelchair
Ambulant

than in the homes with infirmary beds, as seen in Chart 9, showing that the homes that have not made any special provision for the sick have to deal with at least as large a problem of chronic illness as the homes that have found it necessary to provide special facilities for the care of the sick.

A large proportion of chronically ill guests was found in both the largest and the smallest homes. The homes of intermediate size, between 100 and 300 beds, reported a smaller proportion. The distribution of chronically ill

TABLE 20

CHRONICALLY ILL GUESTS IN PRIVATE HOMES FOR THE AGED CLASSIFIED
BY AGE, SEX, AND MARITAL STATUS

| Age and sex | Total | MARITAL STATUS | | | | Not reported |
| | | Married | | Single, widowed, or divorced | | |
		Number	Per cent[1]	Number	Per cent	
Total						
Total	2,822[2]	366	13.2	2,414[2]	86.8	42
40–59 years	65[3]	10[3]	15.4	55	84.6	0
60–69 years	642	103	16.2	531	83.8	8
70 years and over	2,090[2]	252	12.2	1,806[2]	87.8	32
Not reported	25	1	....	22	....	2
Male						
Total	1,491	244	16.6	1,223	83.4	24
40–59 years	58[3]	9[3]	15.5	49	84.5	0
60–69 years	407	69	17.1	334	82.9	4
70 years and over . . .	1,016	165	16.5	832	83.5	19
Not reported	10	1	....	8	....	1
Female						
Total	1,329	122	9.3	1,189	90.7	18
40–59 years	7	1	....	6	....	0
60–69 years	235	34	14.7	197	85.3	4
70 years and over . . .	1,072	87	8.2	972	91.8	13
Not reported	15	0	....	14	....	1

[1] Percentages are not shown for units of less than fifty.
[2] Includes two persons whose sex was not reported.
[3] Includes one person thirty-four years of age.

guests among homes of different capacities appears in Chart 10. The largest homes, those of 300 beds or more, have shown a tendency to provide medical facilities for the permanent care of guests with chronic disease through hospital departments. At the time of the census, nine of the smaller homes, with the exception of one with 100 beds, were planning provision for the care of chronic patients by increasing their infirmary beds; and three other small homes were adding infirmary beds for the first time.

Three fourths of the chronically ill guests were in the later years, seventy years and over. Of the rest, more than one fourth were between sixty and sixty-five years of age and nearly two thirds between sixty-five and seventy

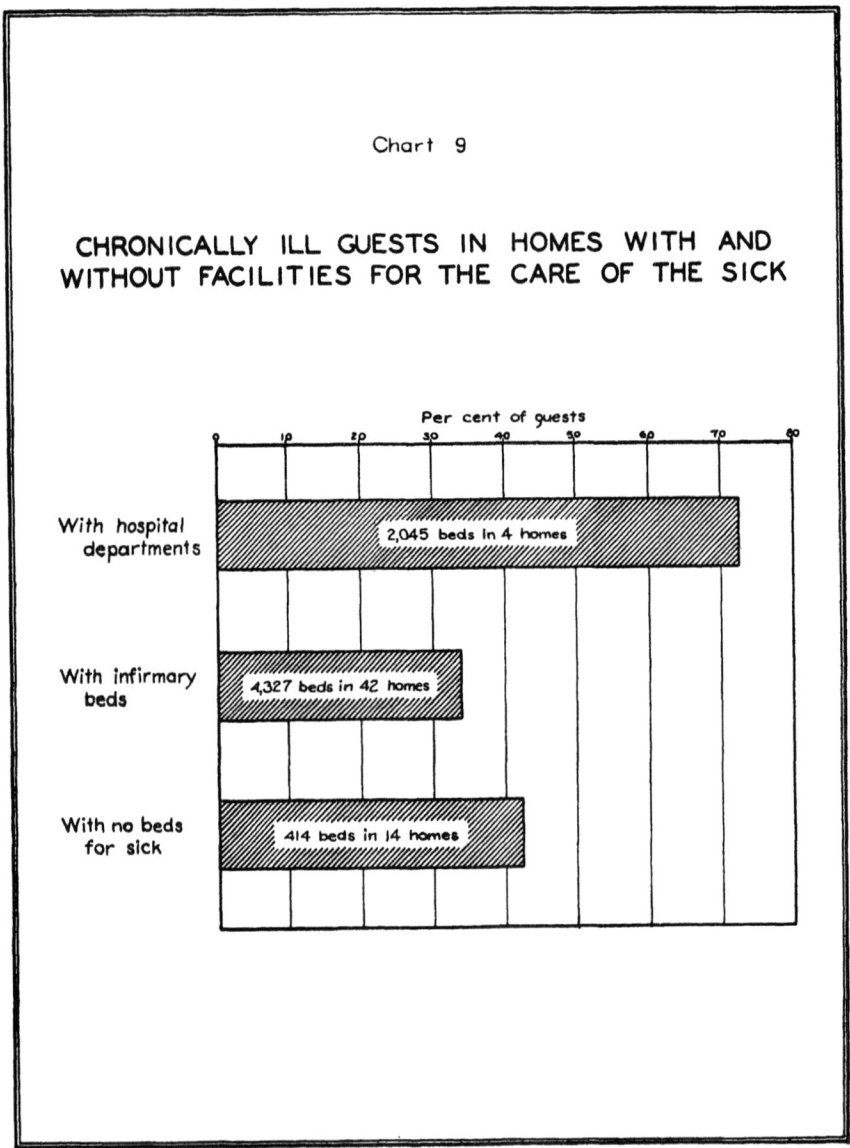

Chart 9

CHRONICALLY ILL GUESTS IN HOMES WITH AND
WITHOUT FACILITIES FOR THE CARE OF THE SICK

years. A small number (2.3 per cent) were under sixty years of age. One person under forty years of age, a cripple, was reported. It is significant that even this small number of persons younger than those ordinarily classi-fied as "aged" should be found, for it seems to indicate a tendency to admit some who have become infirm through chronic disease at an early age. The proportion of all the guests in the homes who are under sixty years is not known at present. Of all the applicants to the Central Information Bureau for the Care of the Aged, which receives applicants for private homes for the aged, in 1928, 6.3 per cent were under sixty years of age.

The ages of guests with chronic illness together with their marital status is shown in Table 20. A larger proportion of the men (16.6 per cent) than of the women (9.3 per cent), were married and had a spouse living. The proportion of those who were single, widowed, or divorced was larger among the women. A similar preponderance of married men was found in a study of aged dependents at home, in this city, in which 66.8 per cent of the men and 26.2 per cent of the women were married.[1]

FORMS OF ILLNESS

The most frequent cause of illness was general physical deterioration connected with senescence, classified as "old age," from which 30 per cent of the chronically ill guests, with few exceptions persons seventy years of age or over, were suffering. Circulatory diseases came next as the chief cause of illness of 22 per cent. Of all the patients with heart disease in the census, 15 per cent were in the private homes for the aged. An equal num-ber, 13 per cent, were suffering from diseases of the nervous system and gen-eral diseases. Almost every form of chronic illness was found among the remaining 22 per cent. The diseases found most frequently among guests of different ages may be seen in Appendix Table 4.

There was no medical diagnosis recorded in the homes for 16 per cent of the guests who were chronically ill. Information in regard to the nature of the diseases from which these guests were suffering was obtained from a nurse, social worker, or other officer in charge, who was able to describe the obvious symptoms or to remember that a medical diagnosis had once been made. For the bedridden patients a physician's diagnosis was usually on record. When the guest is helpless or his complaint is noticeable, he usually receives medical attention. A guest, however, may be equally in need of medical supervision although his symptoms are not conspicuous enough to attract notice.

The practice of periodic physical examination has been established in one home. (See p. 141.) The attending physician of the institution is con-vinced that much can be done by this means to improve the health of the

[1] Non-institutional Aged Poor: Report on Aged Dependents Cared for Outside of Institutions by Private Agencies in New York City. A study directed by Neva R. Deardorff and prepared under the general direction of a committee representing The Welfare Council of New York City and others. *American Labor Legislation Review*, vol. 19, No. 2, June, 1929, p. 196.

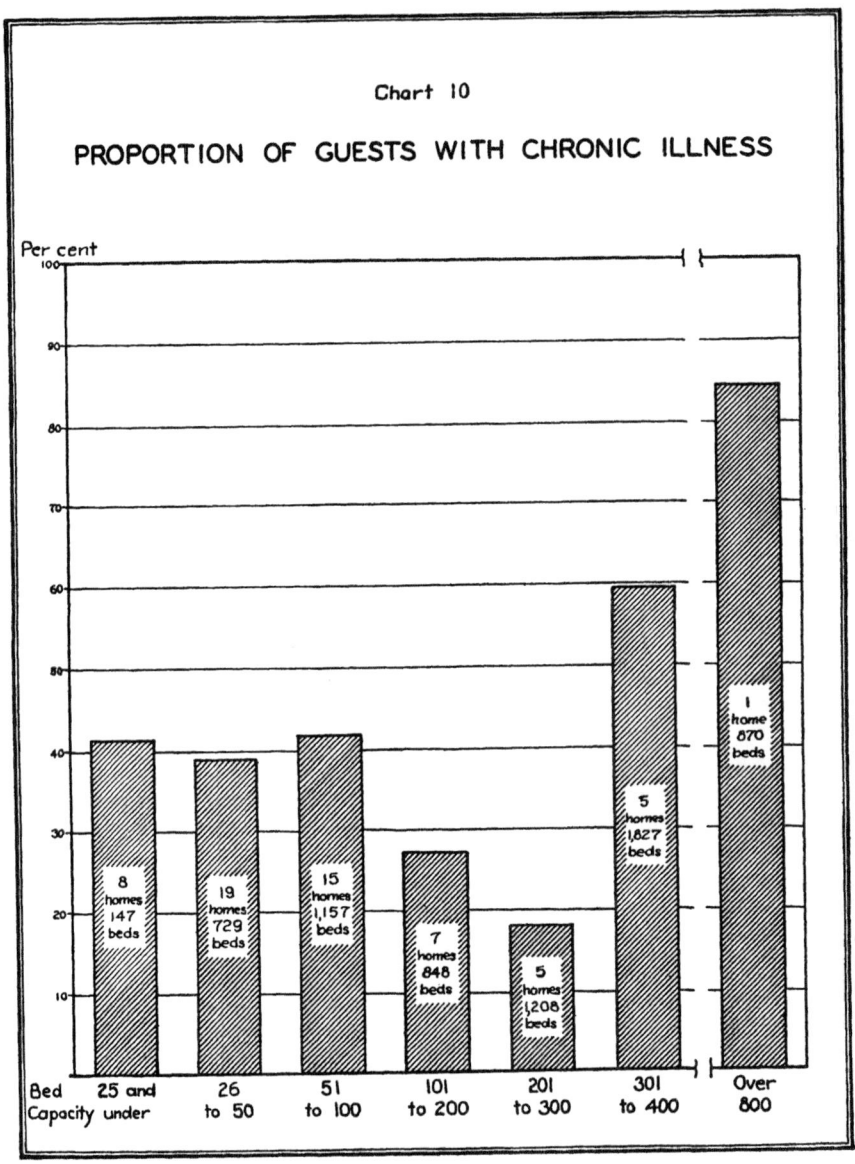

Chart 10

PROPORTION OF GUESTS WITH CHRONIC ILLNESS

guests and also that valuable contributions can be made to medical knowledge of diseases occurring in the later years of life.[2]

Although persons with mental disease are not accepted by homes for the aged, with the exception of one home, and are usually transferred to a mental hospital if the condition arises after admission, there were 405 persons, or 15.2 per cent of the chronically ill guests, who were reported to be suffering from some mental disorder. (See Appendix Table 5.) The mental abnormality had been diagnosed by a physician in the case of over half of these persons, and in the case of the rest it was sufficiently pronounced to be recognized or suspected by persons in charge. A considerably larger proportion of mental abnormality was reported among persons seventy years or over than among those under seventy years.

A majority of the older group had been actually diagnosed as mentally abnormal; but for the majority of the younger group, the condition was reported as "suspected." This seems to bear out the fact that the mental peculiarities of the guest do not receive medical attention until they become so pronounced that it is difficult to care for him.

The idea that mental conditions in old age may be improved by definite attention to the mental hygiene of old people has only recently begun to receive attention. In an interesting book on the subject, Dr. Lillien Martin, a psychiatrist, herself a woman over seventy years of age, has presented evidence of the good results of such treatment. Dr. Martin has stated her belief in the mental hygiene of old age as follows: "Modifications, change, breaking up of mental adhesions, adapting, enlarging, or developing appear as a waste of time and a futile effort since the firmly rooted conviction is that no change is possible. What we, however, have come to believe as a result of rehabilitation work with the old is that these people are just as subject to change and growth as in any other period of life, allowing always more time to effect a change in old age than in youth or childhood."[3]

Such thorough efforts to improve the mental hygiene of the aged by individual retraining, as Dr. Martin practiced it, require expert direction and skill, as well as a good deal of time and patient work; and it is not possible for many homes for the aged to consider adding such an expensive service. But much can be done even without a mental hygiene service if members of the staff are convinced that old people can be assisted to alter unfortunate habits of thinking and acting and if they make a definite attempt to learn how to help them to do so. By common sense methods this is being done in many homes, but much more could be done through more systematic efforts and some instruction of the staff in mental hygiene.

The importance of an occupational service to the mental welfare and happiness of the guests in homes for the aged has not always been recognized. No home included in the study had a systematic plan for occupational work. However, following an experiment conducted by The Welfare

[2] Zeman, Frederic D., M.D., and Lewi, Emma Weil, Periodic Physical Examinations in a Home for Aged, 1930. MS.
[3] Martin, Lillien J., and De Gruchy, Clare, Salvaging Old Age. New York, The Macmillan Company, 1930, p. 79.

Council at the request of the Section on the Care of the Aged and the Sub-section on Sheltered Workshops of the Section on Employment and Vocational Guidance in seven selected homes, a number of homes have carried on systematic occupational work; and a two-year project was undertaken under the auspices of the Welfare Council, which was financed jointly by the homes that shared in the demonstration and by funds received from other sources. Under this plan a director of occupational work and an assistant directed the work in the six homes that took part in the plan teaching guests in the homes and also marketing the products. The trade name of Dega ("aged" reversed) was adopted for the articles made; and an attempt to make marketable articles was successfully carried out. Those responsible for the demonstration believe that it has proved the value of congenial work with some remuneration in keeping the old persons happy and in giving them a sense of achievement and a feeling of still being part of the active world. The possibility of carrying on the Dega workshop as part of a joint enterprise of several sheltered workshops is under discussion.

CARE GIVEN THE CHRONICALLY ILL

Forms of Care Needed and Received

Three different forms of care are required for chronic illness:[4] (1) Medical, or "A," care. When the cause of the illness is not yet known or when the disease can be arrested and the patient's condition improved by medical skill, continuous observation and treatment by a physician is required; (2) Nursing, or "B," care. If the nature of the disease is known, the necessary treatment may sometimes be carried out by a trained nurse under the direction of a physician who sees the patient only occasionally; (3) Custodial, or "C," care. When the progress of the disease has been arrested but the patient has been left with some physical disability, he does not require medical treatment or the care of a trained nurse but does need the assistance and oversight of an attendant under the advice of a physician. A trained attendant or a person experienced in the care of the sick is usually required to give adequate "C" care to chronic patients; but for many of the aged, suffering from infirmities connected with old age rather than from the effects of a chronic disease, a simpler form of care by less experienced attendants will be sufficient. In the following table comparisons are made of the type of care considered necessary and the type of care received.

About four fifths of all guests incapacitated by chronic illness were receiving "C" care. Nearly one third of these were aged infirm persons without a specific chronic disease for whom the simplest form of custodial care was required. On the other hand nearly 5 per cent, or 111 persons, needed medical or nursing care that they were not receiving.

Very few persons, 1.6 per cent, were receiving "B," or nursing care. For nearly half of them a different form of care was indicated—several needed

[4] Boas, Ernst P., M.D., and Michelson, Nicholas, M.D., The Challenge of Chronic Diseases. New York, The Macmillan Company, 1929, p. 14.

medical care and others only attendant care. On the other hand less than a fifth of those who needed "B" care were receiving it.

Those receiving medical, or "A," care were 17 per cent of the whole number. Two thirds of them would have been equally well off with a simpler form of care. On the other hand, a third of those who actually needed medical care were not getting it. Medical service was being provided for twice as many persons as necessary, but there were 85 persons whose condition required medical attention who did not receive it. They were chiefly persons suffering from general or circulatory diseases. Those receiving medical care unnecessarily were mainly persons with diseases of the circulatory and nervous systems or infirmities of old age.

TABLE 21

CHRONICALLY ILL GUESTS IN PRIVATE HOMES FOR THE AGED CLASSIFIED
BY CARE NEEDED AND CARE RECEIVED

| Care needed | Total | CARE RECEIVED | | | | | | Not reported |
| | | Medical | | Nursing | | Attendant | | |
		Number	Per cent	Number	Per cent	Number	Per cent	
Total . . .	2,822[1]	479	16.9	44	1.6	2,297	81.5	2
Medical . . .	237	151	64.0	5	2.1	80	33.9	1
Nursing . . .	137	82	59.9	24	17.5	31	22.6	0
Attendant . .	2,384[2]	243	10.2	15	0.6	2,125	89.2	1
Not reported .	64	3	....	0	....	61	....	0

[1] Care received not reported for 2 patients.
[2] Only the simplest form of custodial care was required for 736 patients.

Of the 221 patients who needed medical care in a hospital, 110 were receiving it in homes with hospital departments and 20 in other homes able to give it satisfactorily. Forty-seven could have received it in the home, but did not; and 44 needed to be transferred to another institution. There were 16 persons who needed medical care that could be secured in a clinic.

The relation between the beginning of the illness and the time when the patient was first admitted to an institution of some kind for care on account of his illness was reported for 15 per cent of the whole number of chronically ill guests. The majority received institutional care within a year or two of the beginning of the illness. Many, however, were reported to have been ill for from one to nine years before receiving institutional care and some for as many as ten to fifteen years. (See Appendix Table 6.)

The present care in a home for the aged was the only institutional care for chronic illness ever received by the majority of about 850 guests for whom this information was reported. However, nearly a fourth had been in an institution for this reason at least once before. Nearly 5 per cent had had two previous admissions to an institution on account of their illness, and over one per cent, three or more.

Inadequacies in the Care Provided

Over a third of all chronically ill guests were receiving unsuitable care. Either their care was not of the type suited to their condition or it was inadequate as judged by the minimum requirements, given below, which were considered necessary for custodial, or "C," care for chronic patients.

(1) A working diagnosis of the patient's condition on record at the institution.

(2) General supervision of the patient by a doctor, trained nurse, practical nurse, or trained attendant.

(3) Provision for his physical well-being including assistance as needed with toilet and feeding.

(4) Facilities for resting during the day amply provided and easily accessible.

(5) Access to the out-of-doors freely available.

The table below shows the number who were receiving suitable and unsuitable care for their illness. It has been taken into consideration that the simpler form of custodial care for the infirm aged without chronic disease may be given satisfactorily in a home without the above essentials for adequate "C" care.

TABLE 22

CHRONICALLY ILL GUESTS IN PRIVATE HOMES FOR THE AGED CLASSIFIED
BY SUITABILITY OF CARE, EACH AGE GROUP

Suitability of care	AGE GROUP				
	Total	40–59	60–69	70 and over	Not reported
Total	2,822	65[1]	642	2,090	25
Suitable care . . .	1,770	54	341	1,364	11
Unsuitable care . .	989	11	243	721	14
Not reported . . .	63	0	58	5	0

[1] Includes one person thirty-four years of age.

All but two of the homes had some guests who were not receiving satisfactory care for their illness. There were 989 persons who were getting either a type of care not suited to their condition or incomplete care of the proper type. The type of care received was more intensive than necessary for 345, or more than one third of these persons. For the remainder, 644 persons, the care received was either incomplete or inadequate.

The majority of those receiving unsuitable care were in homes that did not have the facilities to give them the care they needed. Forty-four of the sixty homes had some patients who should have been in an institution with adequate facilities for caring for chronic patients. Patients who needed an adjustment of their care that could have been made within the institution were found in thirty-four homes. There were 44 homes that did not meet the minimum requirements for adequate custodial care for the chronically ill. These forty-four homes had 57 per cent of the beds and 40 per cent of the chronic patients of the sixty homes studied.

All homes for the aged are concerned with the problem of giving proper care to their guests when they become ill. They have, in addition, a further responsibility to determine what share they will take in the general movement going on in New York and other cities at the present time to provide suitable care for the dependent chronic sick of the community.

The recent Jewish Communal Survey in this city notes that "the trend today is away from the care of normal, dependent aged people in institutions, and in the direction of using such institutions for the care of the chronically sick." The conclusion is reached that the four large Jewish homes for the aged "should increasingly be devoted to the care of certain types of the chronically sick."[5]

The demands upon the homes for the aged for the care of the chronically ill will probably be increased in the near future, as the law providing allowances for the dependent aged in New York State,[6] in effect January 1, 1931, will make it possible for many who would otherwise seek admission to homes for the aged to live outside an institution. Those least seriously disabled will be most likely to take advantage of the allowance, while the infirm, for whom home care is difficult and often impossible, will continue to need institutional care. Therefore, in the future, a larger proportion of the applicants to the homes will, in all probability, be persons with chronic illnesses and incapacitating infirmities.

Referring to this situation, Dr. Boas has suggested that the homes for the aged may find it feasible to accept the chronically ill at a younger age than the age at which guests are now received. "Homes for the aged that are not occupied to capacity might well reduce the age limit of applicants for admission and admit some of the custodial group of chronic sick. This would compel them to improve their infirmary and nursing services, so that their own patients would benefit as well. In planning new community resources for the aged and the chronic sick, it will be important to bear in mind the merits of the pension system for the able-bodied aged and the advisability of restricting institutional facilities to such of the aged and of the chronic sick who actually need institutional care."[7] The possibilities of home care and foster home care for the infirm aged have been referred to in a previous section of the report.[8] (See also p. 143.)

Careful individual inquiry into the situation of each applicant for admission to a home is the only means by which the resources can be used to the best advantage and the applicants assured of care suited to their needs. One of the homes included in the study now has a full-time social worker on

---

[5] Jewish Communal Survey of Greater New York, Report of Executive Committee. The Bureau of Jewish Social Research, October, 1929, pp. 37–38.

[6] Article XIV-A of the Public Welfare Law entitled Security Against Old Age Want (Chapter 387, Laws of 1930).

[7] Boas, Ernst P., M.D., and Michelson, Nicholas, M.D., The Challenge of Chronic Diseases. New York, The Macmillan Company, 1929, pp. 78–79.

[8] See vol. 1, Chapter 1, An Orderly Advance toward the Prevention and Care of Chronic Illness, p. 32.

the staff who investigates applications. In Chicago, a number of homes for the aged adopted the plan of social investigation of applications through a joint bureau and the use of case-work methods in working out the best plan of care for each applicant. The method of investigation of applicants recommended by the Jewish Communal Survey is to obtain this service for the homes from case-working agencies. (See also pp. 147–148.)

An attempt has been made to estimate the number of persons in the census who might possibly have been eligible for care in private homes for the aged if the homes as a rule were open to the chronically ill needing custodial care. Probably the majority of those found in public institutions were properly public charges; although there are undoubtedly some striking exceptions of persons who urgently need more individual attention than they would receive in the city institutions. However, the most obvious demand for institutional care of the custodial type is for chronic patients under the care of family welfare and nursing agencies. A small number needing such care were found in private general hospitals. In addition, if the aged patients in the chronic hospitals who need only custodial care could be removed, these hospitals could then receive a larger number of those who need medical and nursing care.

There were 25 persons, sixty years or over, in private general hospitals who needed only attendant care. The community agencies reported a number of persons of sixty years of age or over not receiving suitable care at home, who needed institutional care of the custodial type. There were 80 aged infirm persons in private chronic hospitals who might equally well have been in homes for the aged. In addition, there were about 350 chronic patients, sixty years of age or over, in these hospitals who needed only custodial care, which a home for the aged could provide. Roughly speaking there were then approximately 500 persons for whom the homes might have provided, if it had been their policy to receive the chronically ill.

The private general hospitals were found to be using nearly 22 per cent of their ward bed capacity at the time of the census for chronic patients, although the care of the acutely ill is their proper function. Possibly 4 or 5 per cent of the bed capacity of a general hospital may be legitimately used for chronic patients in acute phases of illness. Allowing for this fact, there were about 200 of the chronic patients, sixty years of age or over, in general hospitals who might have been cared for in homes for the aged if it were the policy of the homes to maintain hospital departments equipped to give "A" care to the chronic sick.

If the homes were ready to receive persons under sixty years, an additional number of 200 persons between forty and sixty years, in situations similar to those just described, would have been eligible for care in homes for the aged.

That the homes for the aged could assume very little of this additional burden with their present facilities is indicated by an analysis of the reports made by the homes to the Central Information Bureau for the Care of the Aged. The central reporting system for homes for aged went into effect in

April, 1927, with a total of fifty homes reporting during some part of the following three years. During this period the average vacancies were 10.6 per cent of the capacity. Without considering two homes of fraternal organizations whose clientele is strictly limited by membership in the organization, one of which had a capacity beyond the organization's needs, the vacancies in all of the homes averaged 8.3 per cent of their total capacity. This means that over a three-year period the homes were used to about 92 per cent of their capacity.

During the period under discussion a considerable increase in facilities took place, so that a part of the 8 per cent of beds not used is probably due to the adjustments incidental to opening new wings or new homes. During this period, the average annual admissions to the homes for aged reporting were 16 per cent larger than the average annual losses.

It is to be expected that a home for the aged cannot operate to its full capacity. Different homes will vary in the extent to which they can be used to capacity, especially since some homes report their capacity without infirmary beds and others include them. Such exigencies as yearly renovations, time elapsing between the death of one guest and the admission of another, the gradual acceptance of guests for new wings of homes, or the length of time it takes to complete admissions to a new home necessarily make it impossible for the homes to be used to their full capacity.

Various estimates by superintendents of homes suggest that a home can be used to from 92 per cent to 98 per cent of its capacity. During the three-year period during which reports were made, 25 of the 44 homes were used to 95 per cent or more of their capacity. If 95 per cent is accepted as a fair standard of possible use, various adjustments by the homes might possibly increase the present capacity in use by perhaps 200 beds. Chief among possible adjustments is a greater flexibility in entrance requirements. The homes with extensive vacancies over a long period are invariably those with rigid religious, residence, nationality, or financial requirements.

It was found that the private homes with a percentage of vacancies above the average had a decidedly smaller proportion of chronic patients among their guests than the homes with fewer vacancies. It seems possible that restricted admissions in these homes have been due to the exclusion of the chronically ill. As might be expected, lower age limits for admission were found among homes with a low percentage of vacancies than among those with a high percentage.

Probably many persons not receiving suitable care at home are deterred from seeking admission to a home for the aged because they or their families know that it is difficult to find a vacancy in such an institution.

SUMMARY

1. The private homes for the aged are now caring for approximately half of all the dependent chronically ill aged of the city. It is the policy of most of the homes, nevertheless, not to admit persons incapacitated by ill-

ness. Consequently, there is no concerted plan for meeting the situation adequately.

2. Nearly half of all the guests are incapacitated by chronic illness, and 16 per cent are either bedridden or confined to wheelchairs.

The majority of the chronically ill guests have required care for their illness during nearly all of their residence in the home.

3. A still larger proportion of chronically ill guests may be expected in the future, since the recent law for allowances to dependent aged persons will permit more of the able-bodied aged to remain in their own homes.

4. Physical disabilities due to deterioration incidental to old age and to diseases of the heart were the conditions found most frequently. However, instances of almost every form of chronic disease were found.

5. No medical diagnosis was on record in the home for about one sixth of all the chronically ill guests. This occurred more frequently among the ambulatory than among the bedridden patients.

6. Although all but one of the homes attempt to exclude from admission persons with mental disease, a considerable number of the chronically ill guests (15 per cent) were found to be suffering from some mental difficulty. In most of the homes, no definite provision is made for medical attention to the mental condition of guests.

7. Among the 2,822 guests suffering from chronic illness, about 9 per cent needed medical study and treatment, 5 per cent, the care of a trained nurse; 60 per cent, the care of a trained attendant; and 26 per cent, the care of a less experienced attendant.

8. There is a great diversity among the homes in regard to their provision for the care of the sick. Four of the largest homes have hospital departments. On the other hand, 44 homes were not equipped to give adequate custodial care. Over half of the homes had patients getting an unsuitable type of care although facilities for suitable care existed in the home.

9. Persons needing medical or nursing care were not receiving it and others were receiving it for whom custodial care was sufficient.

10. More than a third of the chronically ill guests were receiving unsuitable care. A third of these were receiving more care than was necessary, and the other two thirds were receiving inadequate care.

11. It is evident that the private homes for the aged are in need of a common policy in regard to the part they should take in the care of the aged chronic sick. They are already carrying a large part of the burden. The work is being done, but it is not being done as a whole efficiently or adequately.

QUESTIONS RAISED

The private homes for the aged are facing the necessity for change in their policies in regard to the sick. They are influenced by: (1) a desire to give their chronically ill guests all the benefits of modern medicine; (2) the realization that they already have the responsibility of a large proportion of the aged chronic sick without definite policies for their care; (3) the tendency to provide means for the able-bodied aged to live in the community outside an institution; (4) pressure from the community to use their resources for the care of greater numbers of the chronically ill in need of custodial care only; and to receive persons incapacitated by chronic illness who are under the age at which guests are now admitted as a rule.

Many questions arise in considering how the homes may meet this situation, some of which follow:

(1) What system of examination will prevent the admission of persons who need a form of care that the institution is not equipped to give and at the same time indicate what care should be given to those admitted?

(2) What system of social investigation of applicants is to be preferred—a central bureau with a trained social worker in charge, service from a caseworking agency; or a trained social worker on the staff of the home?

(3) Should all homes be equipped if possible, to give adequate custodial care to aged chronics?

(4) Should all homes that are able to have one or more trained nurses on the staff, accept persons who need nursing care?

(5) Should certain homes accept no one with a chronic disease but accept the infirm aged needing the simplest kind of custodial care?

(6) Should every home have an infirmary department for the care of sick guests?

(7) Should the larger homes maintain hospital departments?

(8) Should some homes be converted entirely into hospitals for chronics?

(9) Would the homes have less hesitation in admitting persons slightly incapacitated if they had an arrangement by which, if the illness became severe enough to call for hospital care, they could readily transfer the patient to a chronic hospital?

(10) Could certain homes make arrangements with nearby clinics by which some ambulatory patients needing medical observation or treatment could be under regular supervision by the clinic?

(11) Since it is found that many guests become incapacitated soon after their admission and need the care required for chronic invalids, would it not be feasible to admit some who already are in that condition and need such care at the time of admission?

(12) If vacancies occur as anticipated in consequence of the law providing for assistance to the aged at home, would it not be desirable for the homes to lower their admission requirements to admit persons prematurely old or incapacitated by illness who are in need of institutional care?

FACILITIES OF PRIVATE HOMES FOR THE AGED IN RELATION TO THE CARE OF THE CHRONIC SICK

EXTENT AND CHARACTER OF PRIVATE FACILITIES FOR THE CARE OF THE AGED

There are 78 private benevolent homes for the aged that come within the scope of the study.[9] All except 15 were members of the Section for the Care of the Aged of the Welfare Council. This Section, formed in December, 1926, was one of the first to be organized after the Council was formed. Two official delegates are appointed by each member home to take part in the discussions and work of the Section. The homes that are not officially members of the Section often send representatives to its meetings.

At the first meeting of representatives of agencies caring for the aged called together to consider the question of organization, the discussion brought out strikingly the lack of coördination then existing in this field. It was shown that no account was kept of applicants refused admission, and therefore no one knew how many old people were not provided for. One home had had the experience of finding that old people who had applied for admission had been admitted to other homes before their applications could be acted upon favorably.

The first action of the newly organized section was the establishment, in April, 1927, of a Central Information Bureau, to serve as a clearing office for information concerning the care of the aged for both homes and applicants. Persons seeking admission to homes are advised to which homes to make applications; and the current applications and waiting lists of the homes are cleared monthly. The central reporting system of the Central Information Bureau was conducted by the Research Bureau of The Welfare Council. The homes that were members of the reporting system sent in every month their admissions, losses, and vacancies. Monthly and yearly reports analyzing these data were sent to the members of the Section. The number of homes belonging to the reporting system increased from 20 in 1927 to 52 in 1931.[10]

A special committee of the Section has prepared minimum standards for homes for the aged, which have been adopted and published.[11] Other committees are studying problems of common concern to the homes represented, such as legislation affecting the aged, occupational service, and food service. The committee on legislation coöperated in a study of non-

[9] Two other homes, Forester's Home for the Aged and Fritz Reuter Altenheim, were not listed in the Directory of Social Agencies and were not known to the Central Information Bureau when this report was written.

[10] The Welfare Council has discontinued its central reporting service for homes for the aged, as the State Department of Social Welfare instituted a system of central reporting of monthly statistics for homes for the aged throughout the state.

[11] Suggested Standards for Homes for the Aged, prepared by the Section on the Care of the Aged of The Welfare Council. Published by The Welfare Council of New York City, January, 1933.

institutional care of aged dependents in New York City,[12] and took an active part in recommending individual action by the member agencies in favor of the bill for old age assistance, which was passed by the Legislature of the state in 1930. The initial request to the Research Bureau for the study of the care of the chronically ill, of which this report is a part, came from the Section on the Care of the Aged—the result of a growing realization among the members of the Section that chronic disease is a major problem in homes for the aged.

Number and Capacity of Homes Included in the Study

In selecting the homes for the study, the official list of the Central Information Bureau for the Care of Aged was used. (See Appendix IV.) It includes all homes that were at the time incorporated in the State of New York and situated within a fifty-mile radius of New York City and beyond a fifty-mile radius when the admitting offices are in New York City and the home serves New York City clients primarily. It does not include homes for the aged blind, of which there is one in New York City, nor institutions for the aged sick only, which are discussed in the section of the report dealing with hospitals. There are a number of homes not included, in New Jersey or in New York State outside the fifty-mile radius, that also receive residents of New York City.

Information on all of the 78 homes is on file in the Central Information Bureau for the Care of the Aged. In this report, therefore, information has been tabulated for 78 homes whenever known; and the first ten tables are based upon data furnished by the Central Information Bureau, November, 1929.

A survey of facilities in further detail was made for this study in 67 homes by a field worker. Eleven homes were not studied for various reasons which follow: Three have been opened since the study was made: Braker Memorial Home, Far Rockaway Home for the Aged, and Sinnott Memorial Home for the Aged. One home, Hebrew Home for the Aged of Harlem, was temporarily closed at the time of the study; and the Victoria Home for Aged British Men and Women was in process of rebuilding. Two homes refused permission for a study of their facilities, the Home of the Little Sisters of the Poor on Bushwick and DeKalb Avenues in Brooklyn and the Webb Institute of Naval Architecture. Three homes—the New York Baptist Home, St. Catherine's Infirmary for the Aged, Amityville, L. I., and the Sons and Daughters of Liberty Home were not included because they were not listed in the Directory of Social Agencies or in current lists of the Central Information Bureau at the time of the study. The Waiting Home of the Protestant Unity League was excluded because it is a home for temporary care only. Two private organizations that give monthly allowances to aged persons in the community and care for about fifty persons were not included in

[12] Non-institutional Aged Poor: Report on Aged Dependents Cared for Outside of Institutions by Private Agencies in New York City. A study directed by Neva R. Deardorff and prepared under the general direction of a committee representing The Welfare Council of New York City and others. *American Labor Legislation Review*, vol. 19, No. 2, June, 1929, pp. 193–224.

the census. The Brooklyn Presbyterian Home for the Aged which has not yet established its home pays the board of a small number of persons in nursing homes or elsewhere. The Relief Society for the Aged assists aged persons in various ways, paying board for some of the waiting lists of the homes helping to pay admission fees, and furnishing pocket money to some in the homes.

TABLE 23

PRIVATE HOMES FOR THE AGED CLASSIFIED BY BED CAPACITY,
NOVEMBER 1, 1929, AND SEX OF PERSONS ADMITTED

Sex of persons admitted	Number		Per cent	
	Homes	Bed capacity	Homes	Bed capacity
Total	78	8,343	100.0	100.0
Men	3	924	3.9	11.1
Women	15	737	19.2	8.8
Men and women singly . . .	20	1,669	25.6	20.0
Men and couples	2	177	2.6	2.1
Men, women and couples . .	38	4,836	48.7	58.0

The census of persons suffering from chronic illness was taken in the institutions included in the study with the exception of seven homes omitted for the following reasons: Four homes refused to have the census records taken, namely, the New York Congregational Home for the Aged, the Society of St. Johnland, the United Odd Fellows Home and Orphanage Association, and the Wartburg Home for Aged and Infirm. Three homes stated that there were no chronic sick in their institutions—the French Home for the Aged, Grace Home for Aged Protestants, and the Margaret A. Howard Home. Each of the three had less than 30 guests and transferred persons with prolonged or serious illness to hospitals. The census, therefore, covers 60 homes and includes all of the larger ones having a capacity of more than 100 beds.

The 67 homes studied had a total capacity of 7,170 beds. Nine of them have since increased their capacity by a total of approximately 500 beds altogether. The capacity of the 11 homes not included for the reasons described above was 623. There were in all, therefore, about 8,300 beds for the aged provided in private benevolent institutions in or near New York City at the time of the study. There were 2,917 beds in the two municipal institutions for the care of the aged and dependent—the City Home for the Aged and Farm Colony. These two homes are discussed in the section dealing with municipal institutions and are not included in this section of the report.[13] Seven homes have under construction new wings or additional buildings that would increase the total bed capacity by about 450 beds.[14]

[13] See vol. 1, Chapter 4, The Care of the Chronic Sick in Municipal Institutions.
[14] The fourth annual report of the Central Information Bureau for the Care of the Aged of The Welfare Council of New York City, for the year ending June 30, 1931, lists all the private homes for the aged existing at that time with the bed capacity of each. Prepared by the Research Bureau, The Welfare Council of New York City. Mimeographed copy, 1931.

Twenty of the 78 homes studied are situated outside of New York City. Of the 53 within the city limits 20 are in Manhattan, 19 in Brooklyn, 11 are in the Bronx, 3 in Queens, and 5 in Richmond.

The distribution of the beds for the use of men and women is shown by Table 23.

There were more beds exclusively for aged men than for aged women. However, 93 per cent of the beds for men were in an institution exclusively for seamen.

Eleven per cent of the beds were in homes for men only and 9 per cent in homes for women only. It is not known how many of the remaining 6,682 beds can be used only for men or only for women. Nearly half of the homes, with over half of the beds, receive both men and women and also married couples. Two homes receive men and married couples, but no women alone. Twenty homes receive men and women but no married couples.

Types of Homes

Among these 78 homes studied, a great variety of types of institution is found. They represent a wide range of conditions in respect to capacity, location, admission requirements, and administration. In structure they range from the small wooden building with scant provision for comfort to the beautiful stone building whose ground floors are given over to sitting rooms, library, chapel, and dining rooms.

In size they vary from a small house for 8 guests to an institution that accommodates over 800 guests. Fourteen homes have beds for less than 25 guests. In all, 53 homes have less than 100 beds each. Twelve homes have between 100 and 200 beds for guests; 10 have between 200 and 400 beds; and 2 homes have 400 beds each. One home maintains beds for 860 guests. (See Table 24 below.)

TABLE 24

PRIVATE HOMES FOR THE AGED CLASSIFIED BY BED CAPACITY, NOVEMBER 1, 1929, AND SIZE OF INSTITUTION

Size	Homes	Beds
Total	78	8,343
Under 25 beds	14	214
25–49 beds	19	664
50–99 beds	20	1,523
100–199 beds	12	1,506
200–299 beds	6	1,449
300–399 beds	4	1,327
400–500 beds	2	800
500 or more beds	1	860

Table 25 shows roughly the types of institution found, as shown by the kind of site on which the home is situated.

The majority of the homes, 50, are situated in built-up city neighborhoods with small yards or restricted grounds around them. Four of the city homes have large grounds; 7 have no vacant land adjacent. Two thirds of all the homes are in city neighborhoods. Nearly one third are in the country, the majority of them with extensive grounds.

The question whether old people are happier in the city or in the country is often debated by those caring for the aged. The type of client the home plans to reach must be considered. It would be a serious deprivation to remove some old people many miles from their families and friends, beyond the reach of cars and subways with five-cent fares. The wrench of relin-

TABLE 25

PRIVATE HOMES FOR THE AGED CLASSIFIED BY BED CAPACITY,
NOVEMBER 1, 1929, AND TYPE OF SITE OCCUPIED

Type of site	Number		Per cent	
	Homes	Bed capacity	Homes	Bed capacity
Total	78	8,343	100.0	100.0
City site	54	6,273	69.2	75.2
No grounds	7	624	9.0	7.5
Yard	21	2,277	26.9	27.3
Grounds	22	3,083	28.2	36.9
Extensive grounds	4	289	5.1	3.7
Country site	24	2,070	30.8	24.8
Grounds	10	594	12.9	7.1
Extensive acreage	14	1,476	17.9	17.7

quishing all home ties and entering the institution is in itself a step necessitating profound readjustment. To a lonely man or woman without family ties, the home may be a haven, but to a person who has lived a normal life of usefulness among friends and family and who now sees his savings diminished and his chances of employment gone, the circumstances of entering a home often create a state of great mental distress. This condition is overcome best in an atmosphere similar to that to which he has been accustomed. The city, which affords some slight opportunity for continued employment and many opportunities for diversion, is more likely to meet the needs of such a person.

The high cost of land within the city limits must be considered. To provide adequate walks within the grounds of the institution and some outdoor exercise, it is necessary to have open land. Large grounds are essential for the homes in which guests are permitted to leave the premises only once or twice a week. An unusually wide and busy thoroughfare is a decided menace to the old people in several homes. One fine building recently built is separated from a park by a thoroughfare so congested that the superintendent has had to prohibit the guests from crossing the street. They may look upon the park from a roof garden, but they may not enjoy the pleasure of using its shaded benches.

Many homes situated in the country have beautiful grounds, maintained often by the work of the guests. Splendid walks have been made and flowers and trees have been planted. Truck gardens make possible not only a better diet for the old people but also, it is claimed, a substantial saving in the weekly budget. For diversion there are always the radio, the library, and the village "movie," as well as the activities of the community church. Many of the foreign-born guests reared in small communities, even though they have spent fifteen or twenty years in crowded tenements, revert happily to this mode of tranquil living.

The small unit, or the cottage system, has been tried with satisfactory results at Ward Manor and the Society of St. Johnland. The atmosphere of a home rather than of an institution can be created more easily in the small unit where the individual's interests can be considered rather than those of the whole group. On the other hand, there are guests who prefer the larger homes, where the freedom of a club or boarding house exists, rather than the intimate contact always present among a small group who have much leisure time.

Auspices

Of the 78 homes, 24 are under non-sectarian auspices. Fifty-four are maintained by organizations with religious affiliations, as follows: Protestant, 33; Catholic, 11; and Jewish, 10. Of the 33 Protestant homes, 23 are under the auspices of special denominations; Episcopal, 7; Lutheran, 5; Methodist, 4; Baptist, 4; Congregational, 2; and Presbyterian, 1. (See Table 26.)

TABLE 26

PRIVATE HOMES FOR THE AGED CLASSIFIED BY RELIGIOUS AUSPICES

Auspices	*Homes*	*Bed capacity*
Total	78	8,343
Non-sectarian	24	2,100
Protestant	33	2,175
Baptist	4	204
Congregational	2	95
Episcopal	7	359
Lutheran	5	259
Methodist	4	320
Presbyterian	1	50
Non-denominational Protestant	10	888
Catholic	11	1,699
Jewish	10	2,369

National groups are maintaining 18 homes, with a capacity of 969 beds, for their countrymen and descendants. Seven of these homes are for Germans, 4 for Swedish, 2 for French, 1 for Danish, 1 for Norwegian, 1 for Norwegian and Swedish, 1 for Swiss, and 1 for British. Seven of the 18 homes, with a total capacity of 541 beds, are not strictly limited to the national groups that they serve. Four German homes, with 427 beds, and 2 Scandinavian homes, with 94 beds, and 1 French home, with 20 beds, give preference to their national groups but will accept other applicants as well.

The following five homes, with 383 beds, are maintained by fraternal organizations for their members: the German Masonic Home, Long Island Independent Order of Odd Fellows Home, Sons and Daughters of Liberty Home, the United Odd Fellows Home, and the Independent Order of the B'nai B'rith Home for the Aged. The first four are non-sectarian, and the fifth is for Jewish persons only.

Admission Requirements

Age and Sex. The minimum age for admission to the private homes for the aged ranges from fifty-five to sixty-five years. The range of age requirements is shown in the following table:

TABLE 27

PRIVATE HOMES FOR THE AGED CLASSIFIED BY AGE REQUIREMENTS FOR ADMISSION

Minimum age on admission	Homes	Bed capacity
Total	87[1]	8,343[2]
No age requirements	4	122
Men	1	14
Men and women	3	108
Under 60 years	6	240
Men	1	50
Women	3	. . . . .
Men and women	2	190
60–64 years	33	4,167+
Men	5	860+[3]
Women	12	282+[4]
Men and women	16	3,025
65–69 years	42	3,167+
Men	4	. . . . .
Women	9	455+[5]
Men and women	29	2,712
70 years	1	. . . . .
Men	1	. . . . .
"Aged"	1	8
Men and women	1	8

[1] Totals more than the total of 78 homes because 9 homes have different admission ages for men and women; in 8 women are admitted 5 years younger than men; in one five years older.

[2] Totals more than the sum of the parts because 639 beds, in 9 homes having different admission ages for men and women, could not be properly distributed.

[3] Report of one home; 4 have different admission ages for men and women.

[4] Report of 8 homes; 4 have different admission ages for men and women.

[5] Report of 7 homes; 2 have different admission ages for men and women.

It is a common practice in homes that do not receive men under sixty-five years to accept women slightly younger. Under pressing circumstances, some application committees make exceptions to the rules governing age requirements for both sexes.

The analysis of the age groups within the Jewish homes for the aged made by the Jewish Communal Survey of the Bureau of Jewish Social Research points out that 25 per cent entered the homes between the ages of 65 and 69 years, 43.6 per cent entered the homes between the ages of 70 and 79 years, and about 25 per cent between 80 and 99 years. Few entered who were under 60 or over 90 years.[15]

Race and Nationality. Four homes are maintained for aged Negroes. Six homes accept both white and colored persons. Table 28 shows the number of homes and the bed capacity available for each race.

TABLE 28

BED CAPACITY OF PRIVATE HOMES FOR THE AGED RECEIVING WHITE AND NEGRO GUESTS

Group received	Number		Per cent	
	Homes	*Bed capacity*	*Homes*	*Bed capacity*
Total	78	8,343	100.0	100.0
Not restricted	6	2,044	7.7	24.5
White	68	6,223	87.2	74.6
Negro	4	76	5.1	0.9

The racial and national groups conducting homes for the aged have been mentioned above (pp. 123–124). Jewish homes have 28 per cent of the beds, and 27 per cent of the population of the city is Jewish. The beds in homes under Catholic auspices constitute 20 per cent of the whole number, and 27 per cent of the population is Catholic.[16] One per cent of the total number of beds are provided for Negroes, who constitute 5 per cent of the population.[17]

Religion. The requirements for admission to 45 of the 78 homes depend upon religious creed. The number of homes in each group and their bed capacity is shown in Table 29.

Health. Sixty-one homes for the aged, among the 67 included in the facilities study, require that the entrant must be ambulant and able to care for himself, and also that he must be free from transmissible or chronic disease. Five homes are less rigid and accept a limited number of wheelchair cases and of persons suffering from chronic disease. Only one of the homes, the Brooklyn Hebrew Home and Hospital, accepts bed cases. Nevertheless, 10 per cent of the patients found by the census were bedridden. Another 6 per cent were confined to wheelchairs.

[15] Jewish Communal Survey of Greater New York, Family Welfare Section, Care of the Aged. Bureau of Jewish Social Research, February, 1929. Mimeographed report, p. 20.

[16] Census of Religious Bodies, 1926, United States Bureau of the Census, vol. 1, pp. 646–649.

[17] Population Bulletin, second series, New York; Composition and Characteristics of the Population, United States Bureau of the Census, 1931, pp. 72–73.

Applicants to all of the homes, except the Brooklyn Hebrew Home and Hospital, must be free from mental disease. Nevertheless, 405 of the patients reported by all of the homes had some mental abnormality, either diagnosed or suspected, which is about 15 per cent of all the chronically ill guests. (See p. 109.) In the public homes for dependents, mental abnormality, diagnosed or suspected, was reported for 7 per cent of the patients.

Each applicant must receive a physical examination before he enters a home. Some institutions require two examinations, one at the time the

TABLE 29

PRIVATE HOMES FOR THE AGED CLASSIFIED BY RELIGIOUS
REQUIREMENTS FOR ADMISSION

Religious requirement	Homes	Bed capacity
Total	78	8,343
No requirement	33	3,355
Christian	35	2,619
Protestant or Catholic	2	180
Protestant	30	1,991
Any denomination	17	1,173
Baptist	3	196
Congregational	1	70
Lutheran	2	62
Methodist Episcopal	3	293
Protestant Episcopal	4	197
Catholic	3	448
Jewish	10	2,369

application is made and one just before the entrant is admitted. If the applicant is found to be ineligible for the home, there is then no need of placing his name on the waiting list, where it may remain for weeks before definite action is taken. Some homes regard this double examination as too expensive.

Fees. Thirty-one homes for the aged require admission fees ranging from $100 to $5,000. The range of fees is shown in Table 30.

Twelve of the homes charging admission are willing under special conditions to omit the fee. At times this amount is made up from funds designated for this purpose or is raised by the church. Several special funds are available for this use. The Baptist Home of Brooklyn requires a $400 deposit at the time of application in order to prohibit registration in more than one home.

In addition to the fee on admission, it is customary for the home to require transfer of property to its maintenance fund. Several homes allow the guests to withdraw a few hundred dollars for spending money before the residue of the estate is assigned to them; others refund to the entrant the interest on the amount given the home. A wise provision on the part of some homes is a probation period ranging from three to six months, at the end of which, if the entrant is dissatisfied and decides to leave the home, a weekly charge is deducted from the admission fee and the remaining fund returned to the owner. Similar arrangements apply to assigned property and insurance.

TABLE 30

PRIVATE HOMES FOR THE AGED CLASSIFIED BY ADMISSION FEES

Admission fee	Homes	Bed capacity
Total	78	8,343
No admission fee	14[1]	2,987[1]
Transfer of property to home	18[2]	1,964[2]
$150 and transfer of property at death	1	16
$200 and transfer of property	2[3]	44[3]
$300 and transfer of property	5[4]	178[4]
$350 and transfer of property	2	127
$400 and transfer of property	4[5]	252[5]
$500 and transfer of property	11	846
$600 and transfer of property	1	27
$800 and transfer of property	1	80
$1,000 and transfer of property	8[6]	342[6]
$800–$2,000 and transfer of property	1	265
$1,800–$5,000	1	307
Boarding homes at $25–$50 per month	6	318
Other	3[7]	590[7]

[1] Of these, one with 133 beds requires a donation if possible, one of 100 beds requires transfer of property if a non-member of the organization operating the home is admitted.
[2] Of these, two with 390 beds require transfer only at death, one of 8 beds requires that the guest have enough income for personal and burial expenses, three with 15, 27, and 95 beds require in addition board of $100.00 yearly, $240.00 yearly, and $10.00 weekly, respectively, if possible.
[3] One home with 14 beds requires in addition board of $5.00 a week if possible.
[4] One home of 8 beds does not require transfer of property.
[5] One home with 58 beds does not require transfer of property until death.
[6] Two homes with 54 beds do not require transfer of property.
[7] Of these, one home with 400 beds requires admission fee "according to ability to pay," two with 190 beds require that the guest have enough income for personal and burial expenses.

Members of boards and superintendents often complain that old ladies give away their jewelry and old men their real estate before application is made to enter the home. With this in mind, one home has on its admission blank the question, "What money or property have you disposed of in the last year?"

Thirty-two homes do not require an admission fee but half of these solicit the transfer of property. Only those who are entirely dependent may apply to the others. Five homes are boarding homes and therefore do not require admission fees or transfer of property.

Married Couples. Some homes will not take one member alone of a married couple. A few of the homes making no provision for couples place them in single rooms in different parts of the building; and a special concession must be made before a visit can be arranged. The hardship this entails is obvious.

In the Jewish Communal Survey, records of 724 men and 813 women in the Jewish homes were studied in relation to their marital status. It was found that 395 men and 641 women, 67.3 per cent of the whole group, were widowed; 155 men and 34 women, or 12.2 per cent of the group, were married, their spouses being cared for in other ways. Married couples numbered 53, making up 6.8 per cent of the group. About the same number were single, and a small group of 40 were either separated or divorced.[18] The Jewish homes, therefore, care chiefly for widowed men and women and for married men whose wives are being cared for in other ways.

The situation in regard to couples is similar in Massachusetts. Mr. Bardwell in the introduction to "The Adventure of Old Age"[19] gives two reasons why so few couples are found in almshouses. First, the family welfare agency considers the old couple as a unit and as long as they are well enough to live comfortably without direct supervision, support is granted; and second, in many instances in which there are children, the old mother is given a home and the father sent to the almshouse. The same reasons may be applied to many private benevolent homes.

In a study of 1,795 aged dependents cared for outside of institutions by private agencies in New York City, it was found that of 695 married persons all but seven "had managed to avoid living arrangements which would have required them to live apart."[20] The apartments provided for aged couples by the Association for Improving the Condition of the Poor are described elsewhere. (See p. 273.) Rents are moderate, and if necessary the agency pays the rent. A cafeteria is provided for those who do not wish to cook.

Social and Occupational Affiliations. Many of the homes are democratic in their policies; but if the institution attempts to foster anything like a family spirit, it is necessary that the members of the household shall be more or less homogeneous. A woman who has been a domestic servant, for example, would not be received at one institution which serves women of the professional and leisure classes.

Eight of the homes are maintained for members of a special business or professional group. One of these is for persons at some time employees of the Salvation Army. Two are maintained by the Actors' Fund for the benefit of members of that profession. The Seabury Home is conducted solely for artists, pianists, teachers, and other professional women. Sailors' Snug Harbor is maintained for sailors, and the Mariners' Family Asylum for the wives, widows, or sisters of sailors.

[18] Jewish Communal Survey of Greater New York, Family Welfare Section, Care of the Aged. Bureau of Jewish Social Research, February, 1929. Mimeographed report, p. 20.

[19] Bardwell, Francis, The Adventure of Old Age. Houghton Mifflin Company, 1926, pp. 32–35.

[20] Non-institutional Aged Poor: Report on Aged Dependents Cared for Outside of Institutions by Private Agencies in New York City. A study directed by Neva R. Deardorff and prepared under the general direction of a committee representing The Welfare Council of New York City and others. *American Labor Legislation Review*, vol. 19, No. 2, June, 1929, pp. 196, 199.

The number of homes maintained for different occupational groups is shown in Table 31.

TABLE 31

PRIVATE HOMES FOR THE AGED CLASSIFIED BY
OCCUPATIONAL REQUIREMENTS FOR ADMISSION

Type of requirement	Homes	Bed capacity
Total	78	8,343
No occupational requirements	70	7,250
Total with requirements	8	1,093
Actors . . . . ,.	2	64
Dressmakers or allied trades	1	20
Naval builders	1	50
Professional women only	1	50
Sailors	1	860
Sailors' dependents	1	32
Salvation Army workers	1	22

Residence. Residence requirements are classified in Table 32 below. Nearly half of the homes make no requirements as to residence. One fourth take persons from any part of New York City. When there is a residence requirement, it may be for an unspecified period or for a period of from three to ten years.

TABLE 32

PRIVATE HOMES FOR THE AGED CLASSIFIED BY
RESIDENCE REQUIREMENTS FOR ADMISSION

Residence	Homes	Bed capacity
Total	78	8,343
No requirements	38	3,763
New York City	19[1]	1,949[1]
Brooklyn and Long Island	5	685
Manhattan, Bronx	3[2]	523[2]
New York City and Long Island	3[3]	354[3]
Diocese of New York[4]	3	329
Manhattan, Bronx, Richmond	2	242
Brooklyn—5 years residence	2	193
Manhattan, Bronx, Westchester	2[5]	230[5]
Other[6]	1	75

[1] In two homes of 120 beds five years residence is required; in one home of 400 beds residents of Manhattan and Bronx are given preference.

[2] In two homes of 403 beds three years residence is required; in the third of 120 beds, ten years.

[3] In one home of 39 beds five years residence is required.

[4] The New York Diocese includes Manhattan, Bronx, Richmond, Westchester, and six other counties of New York State.

[5] One home of 135 beds requires ten years residence.

[6] Ninth district of the Masonic Lodge which includes New York City.

Administration

The homes present great contrasts in the amount of freedom permitted and in consideration for the individual needs and comfort of guests. The

Committee on Minimum Standards appointed by the Section on the Care of the Aged, referred to above on page 118, considered questions of both administration and construction.

The character of the administration is determined somewhat by the size and situation of the institution but most of all by the personality and ability of the matron or superintendent. In an address to superintendents of homes for the aged, Mr. Bardwell, who is Inspector of Almshouses and Institutions in the Department of Public Welfare of Massachusetts, described the qualities needed for this position: "The type of worker best suited to handle aged persons is the one who has a genuine love for old people; who inspires confidence on the part of the old; who has courage and fights for their welfare; who recognizes the importance of the proper angle of approach, who refrains from patronizing; who meets the old person on a common ground, which is his own ground; who is a good listener and who weighs what is unsaid as well as what is said. The worker should possess a sense of humor and should have a reasonable amount of the common or garden variety of sentiment, not sentimentality."[21]

In addition, the position calls for some knowledge of modern methods of conducting an institution. Some boards of directors, however, in selecting a superintendent consider only the physical needs of their guests. In some instances, the matron is looked upon by the board as a housekeeper merely. One superintendent was previously a saleswoman in a small town. Another is a former ship steward interested in providing good food at twenty-nine cents a day per person. In several institutions the superintendent does chores about the house and his wife helps with the housework.

Constant supervision and interest on the part of the board tend to raise and maintain standards. In some homes, the board has only a remote knowledge of how the home is conducted. One superintendent stated that his board had been the same for twenty years and that he never brought up anything at the board meetings that could cause discussion or dissension. The board members were busy business men, he said, and not to be bothered with details. Yet the superintendent had no authority to make improvements.

Only one attempt at any form of self-direction by the guests was found. In Boston, in a study of homes for the aged,[22] a number of matrons were asked the question, "Do you have self-government here?"; and there was a general agreement that the elderly residents were incapable of uniting in any form of self-government. In one of the most progressive of the homes in New York, it seems to have been demonstrated that the work of a committee of guests can be made effective. This home decided to give a Christmas party for twenty-five orphans in a neighboring shelter. The project was discussed from all angles by the members of the committee. A workroom was established in the basement of the home and necessary purchases

[21] The Welfare Council of New York City, Minutes of a Meeting of the Section on the Care of the Aged; Andrew Freedman Home, January 12, 1928.

[22] Eaves, Lucille, Aged Clients of Boston Social Agencies. Boston, Women's Educational and Industrial Union, 1925, p. 120.

were made by a staff member. All other activities were carried out by the aged men and women. One woman took charge of supplies, another directed the cutting out of doll dresses, etc. The old men made toys at the work bench. On Christmas Eve, one old man, as Santa Claus, distributed toys and other gifts to the children. The staff member who organized the committee said that for the first time in her experience there was a real spirit of unity and happiness in the home. That spirit is still being fostered, for the same committee under the direction of a case worker from one of the relief societies will make themselves responsible this winter for layettes, sweaters, etc., for persons who are in need of such garments. According to the staff member, her work is just beginning. A house committee is to be formed and all house problems thrashed out. "If I speak of a waste of the electric light," she said, "someone takes offence; but if the committee handles the situation, there is no such interpretation." Such a committee needs close supervision and constant stimulation; and the continued success and progress of their activities depends largely on the leadership they receive.

Clothing

All of the free homes and some of those charging fees furnish clothing for their guests. Donations of clothing are received from friends of the institution. In the larger institutions, the house tailors spend many hours renovating garments. Friends and relatives provide clothing at other times. In some of the homes charging larger fees, a guest may have enough clothing to last for years.

Most of the homes housing large numbers of guests do not provide individual clothing. After visiting several homes in which the women were sitting idle and staring into space, the field worker asked one especially intelligent looking old lady, "Would you not be happier if you sewed? Did you ever try making a nightgown by hand?" Unwittingly, a weak spot had been touched. "Sew? Sew for whom?" she said. "Once I made an apron. They put it in the wash and I never saw it again." The superintendent explained that with so many hundreds of garments it was impossible to mark and sort them. The Home for Aged and Infirm Hebrews has worked out a system to meet this situation. All clothing is marked by women assigned to the task, and each guest has a pigeon hole in the laundry. When the week's wash is completed, other women sort the clothing into allotted spaces, and it is then distributed to each person.

Spending Money

Various arrangements are made for providing guests with spending money, so that no one may know the hardship of being without carfare to go to church or money to purchase tobacco, stamps, or candy. In several homes, the inmates are paid for certain services, such as elevator, door, and kitchen service and so are provided with spending money. Other homes present a dollar to a guest before allowing him to leave the building, if it is known that he is without money. At Ward Manor, every guest has $5.00 a month for spending money. The Director sees that if the guest does not have this amount of his own money, some interested friend mails a check to him every month. In contrast with this policy, one home requires the entrant to give up all of his own money on admission, so that he must ask the superintendent for the spending money that he needs, unless some friend or relative provides a small sum for the purpose. In homes in which a fee is charged and all property assigned, it is customary to turn over a certain percentage of the interest to the guest for spending money.

Rest

Of the 67 homes, all except 4, which represent about one tenth of the entire bed capacity, reported that they had adequate facilities for patients to rest during the day. In several of them, however, the space provided for resting in relation to the number of guests is so small that it cannot be considered as adequate from the standpoint of comfort. In homes having one fourth of all the beds, facilities for rest during the day appear to be inadequate.

Personnel

No attempt was made to obtain information in regard to the total number and types of personnel engaged in conducting homes for the aged. The medical and nursing personnel only were listed. Three hundred and fifty-eight doctors give medical care either regularly or on call to the inmates of the 67 homes with 7,170 beds. Eight of them are resident physicians in four homes. Sixty-four registered nurses and 165 attendants are employed in these 67 homes. (For further discussion of medical and nursing personnel see below, pp. 139–140.)

Equipment

Sleeping Rooms. The sleeping arrangements in the 67 homes are as follows:

Single rooms only . . . . 9 homes
Single and double rooms . . . . 27 homes
Single and double rooms in addition to dormitories . . . . 17 homes
Double rooms in addition to dormitories . . . . 8 homes
Dormitories only . . . . 5 homes
Double rooms . . . . 1 home

Double rooms are used for couples and sometimes, also to good advantage, for sisters. The human equation always plays an important part in the assigning of these rooms. The Swedish Augustana Home and the Home for Aged Men and Couples in Manhattan have set aside a certain number of single rooms with doors adjoining. If these rooms are to be used by a couple, they may be kept as separate rooms or the two beds may be placed in one room and the other used as a sitting room.

Furniture for single rooms is usually provided by the home, but it is often possible for the entrant to bring a favorite chair, sewing machine, or bookcase, when there is available floor space. At other homes, the entrants are allowed to bring all of their own belongings that can be accommodated; and they seem to derive great comfort from the familiar setting.

It is impossible to create an atmosphere of home life in a dormitory. For each guest beside her white iron bed stands a white enamel wash stand with a small drawer for personal use. Although all but one home meets the legal requirements by having three feet between the dormitory beds, this space hardly allows for a comfortable chair in addition to the wash stand. In some places, small straight chairs with cushions are used between the beds and several arm chairs are placed at each end of the dormitory. Dr. E. Blum, writing on state provision for the chronically ill (including institutions for the aged) in Prussia[23] says that as the institution may demand of the inmate all the work he is capable of performing, so in turn the inmate is entitled to demand proper care on the part of the institution. He believes that rooms holding from four to eight beds should be substituted for large dormitories, and that single rooms should always be available for serious cases. He regards the provision of a dresser for storage of personal possessions an obvious necessity and the minimum to which each inmate is entitled. Of the custodial unit of a hospital for chronic diseases, which is "almost identical with a 'home for the aged and infirm,' " Dr. Boas says: "Cheerful rooms of not more than two beds each should be planned for the custodial inmates of a hospital for chronic diseases, in order to give them as much privacy as possible. Since the institution is their home for the remainder of their lives, no effort should be spared to make the whole building as livable as possible. The bedrooms must be light, the sitting rooms cheerful, the gardens well kept."[24]

An innovation found in one home is a guest room for relatives or friends of the inmates. This is particularly convenient in homes located in the outlying districts. These rooms are used constantly by visitors and at times of sickness and death they fill a real need.

Of interest also is the fact that the Home for Aged Men and Couples has placed an electric bell, known as the emergency bell, about a foot from the floor in each single room. The matron explained that aged people often collapse or fall in illness, and as their voices do not carry far, the emergency bell, which can be reached by crawling along the floor, summons the needed help. The use of this bell is seldom abused, but it so happened that while the visitor was in the home, a senile guest wishing to reprimand a chambermaid for neglecting to pick up a piece of paper pushed the button. The matron and nurse reached the room within a minute.

[23] Blum, E., M.D., Über das Siechenhauswesen in Preussen in medizinischer, juristischer, organisatorischer und finanzieller Hinsicht, Zeitschrift für das gesamte Krankenhauswesen; vol. 24, June 4, 1928, pp. 231–239.
[24] Boas, Ernst P., M.D., and Michelson, Nicholas, M.D., The Challenge of Chronic Diseases. New York, The Macmillan Company, 1929, p. 100.

Sun Parlors and Sitting Rooms. Forty-five homes provide both sun parlors and sitting rooms. Four large homes (all with more than 200 beds) that have sun parlors lack, however, adequate sitting room accommodations. Seventeen homes having no sun parlors have large sitting rooms. Only one small home has neither sun parlor nor sitting room, but it has a small enclosed porch used as a smoking room by the men. Even when both sitting rooms and sun parlors are provided, often too little space is allowed and the rooms are not comfortably arranged or furnished.

Cheerful effects have been produced in some places by the use of gay cretonnes and brightly painted furniture and by arranging the furniture to accommodate small groups. Chairs arranged along the wall sometimes give the room a forbidding look. When the sun parlor is the only sitting or lounging room in the building, there is not always ample room for all guests. The chapel or dining room are poor substitutes for the sun parlor or sitting room, yet a number of the larger homes have neglected this important feature. To see old women and men sitting or lying on large seats or hard benches is a very depressing sight.

Smoking and game rooms for the men are usually relegated to the basement or attic; but the fact that they exist makes possible many pleasant hours. One particularly understanding matron, who houses a number of old men in one wing, permits them to smoke pipes and cigars in their own rooms and she reports that she has had no fires resulting from carelessness.

Dining Rooms. The tables covered with brown linoleum and the long porcelain topped tables seating as many as twenty persons found in a few of the homes formed a sad contrast to the small round tables with their colored doilies of oilcloth or linen, surrounded by gaily painted chairs that were found in other homes. White table cloths may be a luxury, especially when old people have shaky hands and spill their food, but many homes use them at least once a day. In one home, where small white table covers are used constantly, the superintendent states that it is possible to manage with two covers a week.

One matron endeavoring to foster the spirit of a feast day was forced to use bed sheets as a substitute for table cloths. Another superintendent said, "My old ladies like to wash and change their dresses before dinner. It helps them keep up their self-respect. I always do my part by having the table extra nice."

The china used in most of the homes is of heavy porcelain, for the breakage is an important item. However, in some of the smaller homes, the same sets of dainty old china have been in use for years.

Bath and Toilet Facilities. Bathrooms and toilets seem to be well distributed throughout the buildings. In the Andrew Freedman Home each guest has either a private bath or shares a bathroom with the occupants of the adjoining suite. No uniform provision of toilets in relation to number of guests was found in the homes.

The nurse or superintendent in most of the homes checks up on the weekly bath. As large numbers of guests are unaccustomed to bathtubs, this often entails a struggle. Shower baths, sprays, and especially built tubs obviate much trouble. In one of the homes where this close supervision was not considered necessary, the matron said she felt sure that during the winter months many of the women went for weeks without bathing. Another superintendent cited the instance of an old woman who was taken suddenly ill and sent to the infirmary, where the nurse was horrified to find her skin in such a condition that oil had to be applied before she could be bathed.

Elevators. Twenty-seven homes had elevators, forty did not. A number of the institutions located in the country occupy low buildings; the able-bodied aged do not have great difficulty in using the stairs. It is, however, a decided hardship and, at times dangerous, for many aged persons to climb more than one or two flights of stairs. For this reason, the Bethany Home for the Aged, which has three stories, was installing an elevator in its building at the time of the survey. In two homes, a large dumbwaiter is used to lift the guests to the upper floors; but the inconvenience is so great that they prefer to walk, so that the conveyance is used only in emergencies.

Fire Hazards. Efforts had been made to reduce fire hazards to a minimum in all but two homes. Fire escapes, indoors and out, were abundant and fire extinguishers were placed with great frequency throughout the buildings. The two homes in question occupied old buildings and, for the sick and decrepit persons on the third floor, escape in case of fire would have been impossible. Both of these homes at the time of the study were hoping to move to new and improved quarters. One has already moved and the other has a new building under construction.

Heating. Adequate heating of the home in winter is of grave importance. The health of the guests is greatly dependent on the temperature in the building. Even the older homes, such as the Mariners' Family Asylum, built seventy-five years ago on Staten Island with a fireplace in each room and places for tapers on the wall, have installed steam heat and electric light. One physician suggests that warming the beds in cold weather will prevent much coughing at night.

Diet

Miss Lucy H. Gillett, Director of Nutrition at the Association for Improving the Condition of the Poor, in addressing a meeting of the Section on the Care of the Aged of the Welfare Council, urged that menus for the aged be carefully planned to avoid the discomfort that is caused by a poorly balanced diet. In spite of the care that should be given to menus, no home for the aged had a dietitian on the staff.

At the time of the study, diabetics in many cases were found to be getting insufficient dietetic care, with no provision for weighed diets, the usual solution being the adaptation of the regular diet in addition to injections of insulin. Since that time, a dietitian has been added to the staff in several homes; and there are at least three homes that are now giving careful attention to the dietary needs of diabetics.

In October, 1930, the Section on the Care of the Aged appointed a Food Service Committee, which worked out the problems of diet in a home for the aged with the assistance of the Department of Institutional Management of Teachers' College. A survey of five homes was made from this standpoint, and each of the homes participating was advised in regard to its particular need. In addition, general recommendations growing out of the study and balanced menus that might be generally applicable were compiled and distributed for the use of the Section.

For the sick, special light diets are often provided. Nurses and matrons endeavor to follow physicians' instructions along these lines whenever possible. The ten Jewish homes observe the Mosaic dietary laws. All of the Scandinavian homes and several others serve afternoon coffee or tea and cake. Several homes provide a glass of milk to be taken at bed time. When the simple evening meal is served as early as six o'clock, this is a great comfort. One superintendent said, "The guests in our home like meat at least once a day. They object to fish as a substitute and I can't deprive them of the pleasure of eating what they enjoy." To change the eating habits of a lifetime when they are contrary to a prescribed diet is difficult; but the old people can be appealed to on the ground of health and comfort.

Recreation

Fifty-seven homes have entertainment committees who supply regularly various forms of amusement. Ten homes have no recreation committee. In some homes little or no attempt is made to provide recreation, in contrast with other homes that give much attention to it. One home with seventeen aged people does not attempt to entertain or divert them in any way. In several of the other homes providing no entertainment for guests, amusement of any kind is prohibited.

Legal holidays are celebrated in all of the institutions, and birthdays in many of the smaller homes. A yearly tea or garden party may be a great episode in the life of the home. Pianos, radios, victrolas, and moving pictures in the home or in the neighborhood theatre, where passes are often issued, make many hours pass pleasantly. In the Hospital building at Sailors' Snug Harbor, each man has a small radio set with ear tubes attached beside his bed. In other homes, one of the guests frequently plays the piano during the evening. An old gentleman was seen in the chapel of the Home for Aged Men and Couples in Brooklyn giving instructions on the organ to his pupil, an old lady nearly seventy.

Several homes have loan book collections, others have very good libraries, where one of the guests or the matron acts as librarian. For those who do not care for books, there are magazines.

The Church Charity Foundation, one of a group of homes endeavoring to encourage every possible activity on the part of their guests, has proved that it is possible to interest old people in providing their own amusement. Ten old ladies, ranging in years from sixty-five to eighty-three had given a play called "The Sewing Circle Meets at Mrs. Martin's." Two performances of an hour and a half were given. Six weeks were spent in preparation and the guests entered into the spirit of the affair in a remarkable way. The play was given in the living room where curtains were rigged up for the stage. The old-fashioned costumes worn by the women made a charming effect. Another play, "The Strike of the Ladies' Aid," has since been given. These plays have been such a success that they are to be an annual event.

In some of the smaller homes, the guests enjoy the privilege of going out to the churches in the neighborhood. The sectarian homes conduct religious services in the chapel. The superintendent reads the service at least once a week and on Sunday a visiting minister preaches the sermon.

All homes allow guests to go out at least once a week. It is customary to leave the address of their destination in the office for obvious reasons. In many homes the guests are free to come and go at will but they are requested to be present at meal time, unless the superintendent is notified. A leave of absence is granted at times for periods of one week to six months. Places cannot be kept vacant longer than this. Certain days are set aside for visitors and in case of sickness this privilege is usually extended.

Work

In a few homes, little or no work is required of guests. Nine homes require no housework. In several of these homes the guests are too infirm to assist with the work and in others they have been unaccustomed to domestic work. "The old people complain so bitterly if they are asked to help," said a superintendent. "One old lady told me she paid $300 to get into this home (five years ago) and that the home should pay someone to clean up after her." The superintendent of one of the homes in which guests sit for hours with hands folded in their laps, gossiping or dreaming, remarked, "Our old ladies are not interested in doing anything. Our efforts have been in vain."

All but nine homes require that guests, when able, shall help care for the sleeping rooms; forty-one require, and three make optional, additional help in other household duties, such as kitchen or dining room work, mending, and care of linen. Three homes reported that guests sew or knit only for charity. The yearly bazaar given in a number of the homes is an incentive to some of the old ladies to keep busy. For example, exquisite quilts were being made for this purpose at the New York Congregational Home in Brooklyn.

The Little Sisters of the Poor realize the advantage of keeping their guests busy. Each of their institutions maintains a carpenter shop, tailor shop, a special room for upholstering, and a sewing room for the women. Nearly the same plan is carried out at the Brooklyn Hebrew Home and Hospital and at the Home for Aged and Infirm Hebrews.

In going from home to home, one gets a decided impression that where there is an attempt to fill profitably the leisure time of the guests, there is less complaining and a more wholesome attitude towards life. Mr. Folks in an article on "Home Life for the Aged," recommends that the aged should "continue occupying themselves as nearly as may be in the kind of work to which they have been accustomed, or in something resembling that as nearly as possible, having in mind increasing infirmity."[25]

Some homes permit and even encourage employment with remuneration. Nine homes make provision for giving a few inmates definite paid jobs, such as doorman, night watchman, and elevator operator. Three homes allow guests to continue their regular occupations. Fourteen give them the privilege of selling whatever handwork they make—lace, dolls, ship models, toys.

At the Andrew Freedman Home, guests are encouraged to continue their former professions. With the security of the home behind them, a limited amount of work is often possible for them and stimulates a healthy mental attitude. An interesting case was cited of a woman who, after the death of her brother with whom she had lived, had entered the Presbyterian Home for Women. Although she had never worked to support herself, she was greatly depressed by the many hours of free time in the home. Hemming napkins was first suggested. She succeeded so well at this simple task that it was found she could easily master embroidered initials. One of the large department stores was shown her work and she now earns from $6.00 to $8.00 a week. Needless to say, the woman's health, as well as her attitude toward life, improved. She is known as one of the most cheerful guests in the house.

At the time of the study not one of the homes included had a systematic plan for occupational work. However, following an experiment conducted by The Welfare Council, several homes later undertook a two-year joint project under a director of occupational work, which has been described above on pp. 109–110.

Medical Service

Examinations for Admission. All homes require at least one medical examination before admission and a few require two examinations, one upon application and the other a short time before admission.

The type of report received by the home from the doctors varies greatly. Some of the doctors omit the medical diagnosis from the report. A report on a woman later diagnosed as suffering from arteriosclerosis and myocarditis, read: "Mrs. Jones will benefit greatly by your hospitality. She needs no special care." Although no unusual form of care was required, the matron or nurse at the home could have given more intelligent care had she known these facts.

Sickness After Admission. In spite of the fact that as a rule only persons able to care for themselves are admitted to the homes for the aged, boards

[25] Folks, Homer. Home Life for the Aged. *Survey*, vol. 53, No. 2, October 13, 1924, p. 71.

of directors of homes for the aged have always had to face the problem of sickness after admission. Although operations, broken bones, and other acute illnesses may seldom occur, invariably a number of the guests have difficulty in carrying out the daily routine, simple as it may be.

The homes follow different methods of dealing with the infirm. Some homes transfer all patients needing medical and nursing care to hospitals; some transfer acute cases only and endeavor to care for the less seriously sick patient in his own room; others maintain a sick room or infirmary; and a few homes maintain a hospital floor or building.[26] (See Table 33, p. 148.)

Fifty-eight homes have what can best be termed "first aid equipment." This is made up of simple well-known remedies and a small supply of drugs. Five homes have sufficient equipment to conduct a clinic; 4 homes with hospital equipment have operating rooms, dental rooms, physiotherapy rooms, X-ray, and laboratory equipment for special tests.

In the 67 homes there were at the time of the survey 1,541 beds set apart for the care of the sick. The figure 7,170 for the total bed capacity of all the homes does not include all infirmary beds, for in a number of homes the bed capacity was apparently reported without the infirmary beds.

A few of the homes use single rooms for the care of the sick; others, double rooms; but most of the homes maintain dormitories, with the number of beds for their bedridden cases ranging from 3 to 35. In the larger homes caring for the sick in dormitories, there is at least one single room for the acutely ill.

Nearly 700 of these 1541 beds for sick guests are in the 4 homes that have hospital departments. About 500 beds are in 7 homes having an infirmary of 50 or more beds. The remaining beds, less than 400, are in 37 homes having a smaller number of infirmary beds.

Physicians. Medical service in the homes is obtained in four ways, by: (1) a resident physician; (2) a physician paying regular visits, chosen and paid by the board; (3) a volunteer physician chosen by the board, who calls once or twice a week and in emergencies; (4) a neighborhood physician chosen by either the board or the superintendent, who often, but not always, gives his services free. The choice of a local doctor is often controlled by his proximity rather than by his experience. Four homes employ resident physicians. One home only receives a daily visit from a non-resident physician in charge of its medical service. Some of the homes have no regular visiting physicians but in case of sickness call on outside doctors, who usually give their services without charge. In many of the homes, the guests are under the care of volunteer physicians, some of whom have made regular visits to the institution for as many as twenty years. (For further discussion of the care of the sick, see pp. 148–152.)

[26] The distinction between "hospital" and "infirmary" is based on equipment and care. "Hospital" in this report refers to institutions maintaining a resident physician and nursing staff; "infirmary" refers to those institutions which allocate special rooms to the sick who are cared for by a visiting physician.

Nurses. The nursing care is given by (1) registered nurses; (2) Sisters and deaconesses; (3) practical nurses and orderlies; and (4) the matron or superintendent. The latter, as a rule, has many duties that prevent her from giving much of her time to nursing. In 6 homes, not included in the above classes, registered or practical nurses are employed for short periods when needed.

Thirty-two homes employ 64 registered nurses, from 1 to 9 nurses are in each home. In 10 homes, in 9 of which there is no other nurse, the matron or superintendent has had a nurse's training. When a nurse occupies the position of matron, if she is able to give adequate assistance in caring for the sick, the situation may prove to be fortunate. In the 8 Catholic homes included in the study, Sisters nurse the sick. At Mary Louise Heins Memorial, deaconesses care for the sick and at the Church Charity Foundation a deaconess is matron. Ten homes employ practical nurses, orderlies, or trained attendants, who help in dressing, feeding, and bathing of the infirm.

Health Examination. After the applicant has passed his medical examination and has entered the institution, there is little or no medical follow-up of persons not requiring special attention. Only 6 of the 67 homes have routine examination of all inmates several times a year. A number of superintendents would consider such a check-up highly desirable and believe that much suffering could be alleviated if certain physical manifestations were noted in their beginning. Where doctors are paid for each visit, the cost of such service is prohibitive. Where doctors volunteer their services, superintendents and boards hesitate to ask for the additional time such medical examinations would require.

The opinions of two eminent physicians having a wide experience with the aged, were obtained on the question of the advisability of a periodic health examination for each guest. One physician does not think the regular routine examination given periodically would disclose many infirmities that could be corrected. Most aged persons, according to this physician, suffer from ailments due to their increasing years, and he thinks it is useless to subject the patient to the discomfort caused by repeated examinations. He says, however, that physiotherapy adds to their comfort, although it causes no lasting improvement.

The other physician expressed an opposite opinion. He believes that a periodic physical examination might easily be the means of avoiding much acute illness and consequent expense. For example, cases of enlargement of the prostate gland in old men carefully watched can be protected from a back pressure upon the kidneys, which in time may seriously involve the efficiency of the kidneys. The simple urinalysis in the cases of older diabetics may indicate the necessity for changes in diet. The care of the teeth and protection from slight wounds to the extremities are both of grave importance. In patients with varicose veins a proper support in time may avoid ulceration, hemorrhage, or the dangers of thrombosis. The prophylactic care of patients with heart disease may postpone heart failure in varying degree for many years.

Dr. Dublin, in discussing "Old Age and What It Means to the Community" at a gathering of physicians at the New York Academy of Medicine, stated that he does not feel "there is any great possibility of increasing the life span, but that the solution to the problem, if any, lies in conquering those diseases which are taking the greatest toll of old age, in preventive measures upon the part of old people, in periodic medical examination and community hygiene."[27]

At the Home for Aged and Infirm Hebrews, Dr. Frederic D. Zeman, the attending physician, has recently completed the second annual physical examination of all the guests. This is the first institution to adopt the custom of periodic physical examination. Dr. Zeman prefaces a report of his findings by pointing out the value to preventive medicine of scientific study of the diseases of later life and the exceptional opportunities for such studies to be found in homes for the aged, where old people may be observed over long periods. The benefit to the guests is shown beyond question by the reported results of the examinations. "In conclusion," the report states, "we feel that we have initiated a method of care of the aged which in each succeeding year will result in increasing benefit to our charges. Our findings clearly show that the average old person is suffering from one or more diseases, some of which are amenable to treatment; and that an institution for the aged must be well staffed with interested physicians and nurses and must be equipped with modern diagnostic and therapeutic facilities."[28]

Medical Records. No record of the physical condition of guests on admission was found in twenty-six homes. If a record of the diagnosis existed, it was kept in the home of some member of the admissions committee or in the office of the examining physician. In homes where a medical diagnosis was on record, it was rarely the result of a recent examination.

Where physicians are called in when needed, it is not customary for the doctor to leave a written record of the patient's condition with the nurse of the home. The medical charts for individual guests are kept up to date in only one home. As a rule, medicines given were recorded, not always legibly, and very few symptoms were noted. At the Home for Aged and Infirm Hebrews, where a staff physician makes examinations daily, results of every examination are entered on the records. When a specialist is consulted, his findings are added to the patient's medical record.

Expenditures and Sources of Income

There are no figures available to show current expenditures for the main-

[27] Dublin, Louis I., Old Age: An Increasing Problem. *The Survey*, vol. 56, No. 10, August 15, 1926, pp. 545–546.

[28] Zeman, Frederic D., M.D., and Lewi, Emma Weil, Periodic Physical Examinations in a Home for Aged, 1930. MS.

tenance of the 78 existing homes. Figures for 67 homes in 1926[29] give total current expenditures as amounting to approximately two and a half million dollars. The total value of property owned by 61 of these homes, on December 31, 1926, was over $28,000,000. Homes under Protestant auspices expended 41.2 per cent of the total expenditure of the 67 homes; those under Jewish auspices, 28.5 per cent; those under Catholic auspices, 17.2 per cent; and non-sectarian homes, 13.1 per cent. Of the amount expended by Protestant homes, 56.7 per cent was for homes under the auspices of churches of the following denominations: Episcopal, Methodist, Lutheran, Congregational, Presbyterian, and Baptist; 43.3 per cent was for Protestant nondenominational homes. In the same year, 1926, the city expended about $837,000 for the maintenance of the two municipal homes for the aged and infirm.

Fees and property assigned provide only a small part of the income needed to maintain one of these institutions. To this must be added membership dues, voluntary contributions, income from bazaars and entertainments, and the income from endowment funds. (For discussion of fees, see pp. 126–127.)

At the present time no inmates of private homes for the aged are being paid for by the Department of Public Welfare. In the past an occasional person was so supported as an emergency case not suitable for care in a public hospital. One woman was paid for in Peabody Home at the rate of $1.00 a day for a number of years.

The daily cost per guest in five private homes for the aged has been calculated covering all charges including insurance, interest on debt if any, and depreciation of plant and equipment. The range in daily costs per person was from 87 cents to $5.63. One of the five homes which had a hospital department fell in the middle of the scale of cost per guest.[30]

There is a small group of homes that charge board by the month or by the year. Two homes, the Society of St. Johnland and the Presbyterian Home for Aged Women charge respectively $42.00 and $25.00 a month board. The Greenpoint Home for the Aged plans to receive $100.00 a year for each year of the entrant's life. If the property assigned equals the sum judged necessary, no further step is taken. If on the other hand the property is insufficient, a friend or relative is asked to go bond to the amount of $100.00 a year as long as the guest lives. Two Catholic homes, the Home of Divine Providence and the Little Home of Divine Providence, charge a fee of $1.00 per day, whenever the guest can pay it. Braker Memorial Home, opened since the survey was made, is also a boarding home charging from $1.00 a day to $50.00 a month. In addition, two homes require board

[29] The information that follows in this paragraph was furnished by the Study of Financial Trends of Organized Social Work in New York City, conducted by the Research Bureau of The Welfare Council. The study included sixty-seven homes for the aged that drew 50 per cent or more of their total population, 1910 to 1926, from residents of New York City, exclusive of homes conducted by fraternal organizations and benefit associations. See Financial Trends in the Institutional Care of the Aged, by Kate E. Huntley. Mimeographed copy, 1930.

[30] Brown, Arthur T., Per Capita Cost in Five Homes for the Aged. The Welfare Council of New York City, Research Bureau, January, 1932. Mimeographed copy.

of $5.00 and $10.00 a week respectively, when the guest is able to pay it. Both of these homes, however, require transfer of property, and the first requires in addition an admission fee of $200.00.

It is customary for the entrant to have money or insurance covering the cost of burial. If this is not the case, most homes insist that friends or relatives meet this cost. Inhabitants of homes are never sent to the Potter's Field for lack of funds for proper burial.

The question of applying part of the funds of a home to paying board for old men and women outside of the institution has been discussed in the Welfare Council's Section on the Care of the Aged.[31] Although many of them desire the companionship and protection an institution affords, there are others who are not suited to institutional life and are much happier if subsidized in their own homes or a nursing home. Several homes are now boarding a number of persons. One of the Jewish homes in coöperation with the Jewish Social Service Association is studying the possibilities of boarding-out aged persons.

APPLICATIONS FOR ADMISSION TO HOMES FOR THE AGED

Vacancies

Until the Central Information Bureau of the Welfare Council was established, April 1, 1927, the only way to gain admission to a home for the aged was to make a direct contact with a particular home, in order to learn the possibilities for admission. Twenty-six of the 78 homes did not report their vacancies or the names of their waiting lists to the Bureau, but a sufficiently large number coöperate in these ways to make it possible to direct bureau applicants with some degree of certainty to the home most likely to meet their special needs. Another service rendered by the Bureau is the clearing of names of applicants. When duplication occurs, the homes considering the applicant are notified. When an applicant whose name has been placed on the waiting lists of several homes is admitted to one, the rest of the homes are notified.

A study of the vacancies in the 36 homes which reported them to the Bureau in September, 1929, shows that although vacancies were indicated by 15 homes, in 8 instances they were caused by death and were to be filled immediately from the waiting lists. The 39 vacancies reported by the Long Island I.O.O.F. Association Home were not available for the Bureau applicants, as the home is open only to members or wives or widows of members of the order that conducts the Home. The 108 vacancies reported by the Independent Order of the B'nai B'rith Home for Aged and Infirm did not constitute available facilities, as this fraternal order found that a larger home had been built than its clientele required, and it has since moved into a forty-bed institution. In contrast with this situation, the Mariner's Family Asylum had no vacancies during September, 1929, and never has more than two or three vacancies.

[31] Summary of minutes of a meeting of the Section on the Care of the Aged of The Welfare Council, October 22, 1931.

The 3 homes of the Little Sisters of the Poor that reported had a total of 67 vacancies. Admission to these homes is easily obtained since all indigent ambulant persons are accepted. Owing to this liberal policy, many different types of persons are admitted; some of whom find it difficult to adjust themselves to the rules of the Home and leave after a short stay.

Waiting Lists

A study of the waiting lists is a means of indicating the frequency and character of the vacancies available. The Bureau of Jewish Social Research, in its report on the homes for the aged, compares beds to be added by the building projects now on hand with the number of applications on file and states that there is no great need for further development along these lines at the present time. In contrast with these homes under Jewish auspices are the non-denominational homes with lists so long that a new applicant cannot hope to enter under two years. Ward Manor, for example, has had a waiting list nearly three times as large as its capacity; the Andrew Freedman Home, one nearly four times its capacity.

The third annual report of the Central Information Bureau of the Welfare Council analyzes the disposition of Bureau applicants over a three year period ending June, 1930. In a total of 1,452 Bureau applicants, one out of eight was admitted to a home for the aged. The average waiting period was five and a half months.

In homes where admission is dependent upon church membership for a stipulated time, usually five years prior to application, the waiting lists are small and there are frequent vacancies. This is due to the fact that the old people have moved from place to place and have not retained their church membership. For example, an old linotype worker, a very respectable man who had belonged to a Methodist Church in Brooklyn at one time in his life and had attended a Methodist Church in New York at another time, was eligible for neither of the homes supported by his church. Being ineligible and having quarreled with his only daughter's husband, he was spending his entire income for shelter in a cheap boarding house in Brooklyn.

In the homes supported by the churches, there are usually strict limitations upon the use of the endowment funds, so that these homes are very much restricted in the type of applicants they can accept. The applicants whom they are obliged to refuse then turn to the non-denominational Protestant homes. For this reason, these institutions have long waiting lists. There are several of the Protestant homes, such as the Congregational, Presbyterian and Episcopal homes, with as many as fifty names on their waiting lists.

The homes basing their admission requirements on former occupations or professions, as well as those serving fraternal orders, are able to accommodate all applicants within a short time. Of the homes limiting admission to a national group, the Swiss homes, at the time of the survey, had a waiting list of 10; the three Swedish homes, 22; the three German homes, 20; the Danish homes, 20; the Swedish and Norwegian homes, 15 to 20. Figures for the French home are not known and for the British home were not obtained.[32] Two homes have endeavored to obviate the difficulty arising from a prolonged period pending the applicant's entrance by paying a regular monthly stipend in cases where the applicant has not enough money to maintain himself in his accustomed way until a vacancy occurs. Several of the homes do not consider the applications in the order filed, but are governed by the needs of the person applying. Other homes rigidly consider each application in the order in which it is received.

The majority of the homes require a person to wait until he is sixty-five years of age before he files his application. As the waiting period is sometimes as long as two years, the funds intended for the entrance fee are often spent for maintenance by the time there is an opening in the home. It is a question whether it would not be advisable to receive applications at an earlier age.

Of the homes making a racial distinction, the matron of the Brooklyn Home for Aged Colored People stated that fifty additional beds could be filled at any time; and the A. Clayton Powell Home, which serves members of the Abyssinian Church primarily, had several vacancies.

The records kept by most of the application committees are so meager that it was impossible to gather the data on the length of time that expires between the date of application and the date of entrance. The Jewish Communal Survey secured this information for the occupants of the Jewish homes for the aged, with the exception of 20 per cent of those admitted in previous years, when adequate records were not kept. Deducting this group, one third of the guests were admitted after waiting less than a month, 86 per cent were admitted in less than three months, and only 5 per cent waited for six months or longer. The median length of time of waiting for those known was thirty-five days. At the same time it is interesting to note that of those who died, who left, who were transferred, or who were dismissed from the homes during the period July 1, 1926, to June 30, 1927, 4.6 per cent had been in the home less than one year. Fifty-two and eight-tenths per cent of those leaving the institutions had been there for less than two years. One might, therefore, expect to find the population of the home greatly changed every three years.[33]

Death is the main cause for this large turnover. A few old persons are discharged for antisocial behavior. At times relatives or friends come forward and arrange for a guest to withdraw from the home and return to his intimate circle. The question of transfer to a hospital or more suitable institution is discussed on pp. 148–149.

Rejections

All homes for the aged reject applicants unable to meet the special requirements set forth by the board. (See pp. 124–129 above.) A study was

[32] The Victoria Home representing this group was excluded from the study as the institution was changing its location.
[33] Jewish Communal Survey of Greater New York, Family Welfare Section, Care of the Aged. Bureau of Jewish Social Research, February, 1929. Mimeographed report, pp. 16–17.

made of the disposition of 177 persons who made formal application for admission to the Home for Aged and Infirm Hebrews during the year 1927, with the following results:

Total	177
Accepted by Committee	136
Entered home	127
Failed to enter	9
Application not considered	12
Withdrawn	11
Patient died	1
Rejected	29
Ineligible	20
For medical reasons	7
For other reasons	13
Unwilling to comply with regulations	9

The seven ineligible for medical reasons were rejected by the doctor for the following causes: (1) incurable, referred and admitted to Beth Abraham Home for Incurables; (2) needed too much care, diagnosis: arteriosclerosis, hypertension, myocardial insufficiency, bilateral varicose veins, elephantiasis, conjunctivitis, and spondylitis deformans,—disposition unknown; (3) advanced pulmonary tuberculosis, possible lung tumor, hypertensive cardiovascular disease, referred to Jewish Social Service Association for better placement; (4) severe paralysis agitans, disposition unknown; (5) acromegaly, general arteriosclerosis and senility, referred to Jewish Social Service Association for better placement; (6) senile, unable to answer questions, disposition unknown; and (7) hypertensive cardiovascular disease and mental deterioration, disposition unknown.

The thirteen who were ineligible for other reasons were rejected for such reasons as the following: in the case of five applicants the family was able to give care; one man was untruthful and had left another home because he refused to bathe; one man was not "deserving," he had deserted his family and owned over $3,000 in mortgages; three persons did not meet residence requirements; one was under age; one was "undesirable," he was untruthful, had deserted his wife ten times, had been convicted for forgery and served a term in prison; one was blind and was referred to the proper agency.

Nine applicants refused to meet the requirements in the following ways: one failed to assign property; in the case of four applicants, the son or daughter refused to call in order to make the necessary adjustments; one refused to trim his beard; two refused to answer questions or be examined; one refused to go into a ward.

Nine applicants failed to enter after their applications were accepted: one couple heard the home was not "kosher"; one application was dropped for lack of address; five persons refused to enter for no obvious reason, and one withdrew the application because friends helped her to maintain her apartment a little longer.

Eleven withdrew their applications for the following reasons: one had

$600 and a son able to care for her; one who left after waiting fifteen minutes for the doctor to arrive, had a son able to care for her; one wished to enter after an eye operation; one did not return to be examined by the doctor; seven withdrew the application for no obvious reason. One died before the application was considered.

The fact that eleven applications were withdrawn is an indication of how difficult it is for the aged to cut loose from their accustomed environment to enter a home. The withdrawal of the application and failure to comply with the committee's requests often indicate a last effort for continued independence on the part of the applicant.

When each of the homes was visited, the superintendent was urged to refer all rejections to the Central Information Bureau, where, in turn, an endeavor is made to guide the applicant to an appropriate institution or to a family welfare organization. Many homes now coöperate with the Central Information Bureau to this extent; others go further, referring applicants if their waiting lists are unduly long or if the applicant does not meet the obvious requirements. As a result of this interchange of information, many of the homes have come to see the necessity of keeping better records. Upon request, the Central Information Bureau has drawn up forms upon which a minimum amount of detail can be recorded. Only by keeping adequate records will it ever be possible to know to what extent the needs of the aged of the community are being met.

At times the Central Information Bureau is hard pressed to find places for diabetics requiring a weighed diet or for senile persons. Such applicants must of necessity resort to private nursing homes and sanitariums or to state institutions.

Investigation

Applications for admission are investigated in various ways. In the majority of the homes, whatever investigation is required is made by a member of the Board, usually the Chairman of the admissions committee. Several homes have applications investigated by a social worker. The guests of Ward Manor are selected from among the clients of the Association for Improving the Condition of the Poor which maintains this home, and therefore their applications have been investigated by social workers of this agency. A social worker of the Swiss Benevolent Society inquires into applications for the Swiss Home. For Braker Memorial Home, social investigations are made by the welfare director of the Protestant Welfare League. The Home for Aged and Infirm Hebrews has added to its staff within the last few years a social worker who is in charge of investigations for admission of guests. The Miriam Osborne Home arranges for an investigation by a social worker in special cases.

One of the recommendations of the Jewish Communal Survey was that the initial social investigation of applications to homes for the aged should be made by a case work agency[34] and that the admissions committee base its decision upon the information thus obtained.

---

[34] *Ibid.*, p. 6c.

Another method is in use in Chicago. A joint admission and investigation bureau for several homes was opened in April, 1930, under the auspices of the Section on the Care of the Aged of the Chicago Council of Social Agencies. Here the problems of applicants are given attention by the method of case work, with the result that a satisfactory solution is found whenever it is possible.

CARE OF THE SICK IN HOMES FOR THE AGED

In 18 of the 60 homes in which the census was taken, 50 per cent or more of the guests of the home were reported chronically ill. In 5 homes, 80 per cent or more were so reported. A high proportion of chronic sick was found in both small and large homes. In the homes of intermediate size, having between 100 and 300 beds, the proportion of chronic sick in every case was under 40 per cent.

Types of Care

In some homes, guests who become sick are always sent elsewhere for care. Other homes provide for the care of the sick in some way within the institution. The homes that make provision for the care of the sick fall into three groups: (1) homes caring for minor illness in guests' own rooms; (2) homes maintaining an infirmary; (3) homes maintaining a hospital.

The following table shows the types of provision made for sickness.

TABLE 33

PROVISION FOR CARE OF THE SICK IN PRIVATE HOMES FOR THE AGED, EACH BOROUGH AND METROPOLITAN AREA OUTSIDE OF NEW YORK CITY, JULY, 1928

Borough	Total homes	Homes that transfer sick patients		Homes that provide care for sick patients			Homes that have hospitals or infirmaries				
		All patients	Operative and mental patients	Hospital	Infirmary	Patients' rooms	Hospital or infirmary beds	Doctors Resident	Other[1]	Nurses	Attendants
Total . .	67	5	62	4	45	13	1,541	8	350	64	165
Manhattan .	19	2	17	1	14	2	525	1	141	24	39
Bronx . . .	7	0	7	1	2	3	263	1	27	11	32
Brooklyn . .	18	1	18	1	14	3	424	1	129	6	52
Queens . .	3	0	3	0	2	1	27	0	6	1	3
Richmond .	5	0	5	1	1	3	203	5	6	9	29
Outside New York City	15	2	13	0	12	1	99	0	141	13	10

[1] These are made up of both general practitioners and specialists; also those who visit regularly and those who are on call at irregular intervals.

Several of the homes that transfer patients to private hospitals have special beds maintained by the hospital for the use of their guests. The forms of medical service employed in the various homes and the number of beds allotted to the care of sick guests have been discussed also on pp. 138–139.

Cases of broken bones, severe mental conditions, or those requiring major operations, are usually sent to an appropriate hospital. Minor surgery is at times performed in the hospital of the home, and occasionally it is feasible to set a broken bone without hospitalization, but such instances are rare.

Cases of mild mental deterioration are always permitted to remain in the home; but pronounced cases of mental illness are not kept. The Brooklyn Hebrew Home and Hospital is the only private benevolent home for the aged maintaining a locked ward; but violent patients are transferred to Kings County Hospital. Bellevue Hospital admits mental patients from the Manhattan homes and Kings County Hospital cares for those from Brooklyn. After a period of observation, both of these hospitals usually transfer the patient to one of the state institutions for mental diseases.[35]

Five homes transfer all chronically or acutely ill patients who require prolonged nursing care or supervision. Sixty-two homes transfer only patients requiring a serious operation and those whose mental condition makes them a menace to the institution.

It is of interest to note the attitude of the guests toward transfer to a hospital when ill. The more intelligent among them realize the advantages of treatment in a hospital, but others believe they are being sent away to die. Several superintendents reported that it was at times very difficult to persuade a guest to move into the hospital or infirmary of the home, much less to an outside institution. A situation in contrast to this was found at the Actors' Fund Home, when it was on Staten Island. It was said that the old people were so fond of staying in bed for breakfast and of being petted and nursed that there was a constant demand for infirmary beds. As the applications for the home increased, and as there was a very coöperative hospital adjacent to the home, the infirmary was converted into ordinary sleeping quarters. The health of the home improved immediately.

Homes Caring for Minor Illness in Guests' Own Rooms

Eighteen homes for the aged permit the guest when ill to remain in his own room. Five of these have a trained nurse as a member of the staff; 3 employ a practical nurse; 9 have no nurse, but 4 homes in this group employ a nurse if necessary, either at their own or the patient's expense.

The French Home for the Aged is a part of the French Hospital and the old people are under the medical supervision of the Hospital's staff and are nursed by the Sisters; but cases of chronic illness are transferred to Bellevue Hospital and other public institutions, as the Hospital treats only acute diseases.

[35] When a patient who has assigned property to the home is transferred to a state hospital for mental diseases, a stated monthly sum for board is deducted from the amount of his property and if there is a balance, which rarely happens, it is returned to the proper guardian or administrator.

The Bethany Home, one of five homes that neither employ a nurse nor have one on the staff, is incorporated under the same charter as the Bethany Deaconess Hospital, but the medical staff of the Hospital does not supervise the guests in the Home. They are cared for by the volunteer services of a physician in the neighborhood; and if they need hospital care they are transferred to the Bethany Deaconess Hospital or other institutions.

The St. Philip's Home, which has no resident nurse, calls on the Henry Street Visiting Nurse Service when the need arises.

Homes Maintaining an Infirmary

Forty-five of the homes for the aged maintain infirmaries. The beds in each home utilized for the care of the sick vary from one to 122. A number of homes care for the sick in small wards, others in single rooms. One small room is usually used as a dispensary where patients are examined and from which medicines are distributed. The infirmary is usually a small room in a quiet part of the building. The white iron beds, clean counterpanes, and simple furnishings, in addition to the first-aid equipment, are the distinguishing features of the room. At times, a wing of the building is converted into the infirmary. At other times, an entire building is used as an infirmary.

Thirty of these homes are under the supervision of a resident trained nurse and a visiting physician. Included in this group are a number of homes whose matrons are trained nurses. The matron is usually assisted by practical nurses in caring for the sick.

Ten of the homes maintaining infirmaries are under the supervision of a visiting physician and a practical nurse. The German Evangelical Home cares for the largest number in this group. Its infirmary of fifty beds, occupying a separate building, is under the supervision of a practical nurse assisted by two untrained attendants. In addition to the fifty persons receiving medical care in the infirmary at the time the home was visited, fifteen guests were confined to beds in their own rooms in the adjoining building, and each needed some supervision and care. The size of the task precludes the possibility of much individual care.

Five homes maintaining an infirmary have neither nurses nor attendants on the staff, but employ them when needed. The A. Clayton Powell Home, supported by the Abyssinian Church, employs a nurse's aid trained in the Red Cross nursing class, whenever nursing care is needed.

Homes Maintaining a Hospital

Four homes maintained hospitals supervised by resident physicians and registered nurses.[36] The hospitals range in size from 70 to 218 beds.

The Brooklyn Hebrew Home and Hospital admits applicants over sixty, who may have almost any type of disease. Most of the patients under care, however, are not acutely ill. Medical charts had not been kept for patients up to this time, but they were to be installed. In fact, supplementary medi-

---

[36] A number of other homes have since added or set aside for the purpose from 25 to 100 hospital beds each.

cal examination in some cases was necessary before the diagnosis could be recorded in the census of the chronic sick. There are a good X-ray apparatus and a fluoroscope, as well as a clinical laboratory where minor tests can be carried out. The physiotherapy department is inadequate to serve 375 guests. Diabetics do not get weighed diets. A large staff of visiting specialists call daily at the institution, and a dentist and oculist call regularly every week. The nursing staff is composed of 2 nurses, and of 16 female and 2 male attendants. Similar conditions exist in the Home of the Daughters of Israel and in the Home of the Daughters of Jacob. All three of these homes care for their sick in large wards. Small rooms adjoining the wards are maintained for the acutely ill or dying.

Sailors' Snug Harbor maintains a 200-bed hospital. The resident physician is aided by 3 resident internes, and an oculist who calls weekly. Patients are sent out for dental work. As no women are employed at the Harbor, 9 male graduate nurses, 17 orderlies, and 10 porters compose the attendant staff. A medical chart is kept of every patient, as well as one for each of the other 600 guests.

Insufficiencies in Medical Care

A wide range of practice is found in the care of the sick. The group of homes providing neither sick rooms nor nurses are giving inadequate care. There are, however, only a small number of homes in this class. The large majority of the homes are endeavoring to minister to all the needs of their guests. Many institutions are not ignorant of their shortcomings in giving the sick adequate care but are hampered by lacks of funds.

The fact that twelve homes for the aged were extending their provision for the chronic sick at the time of the survey, by increasing the number of beds for the sick, indicates that the boards of these institutions are directing their attention toward this problem and are aware of the need of additional physical care for the old people in their charge. The Miriam Osborne Home had a new infirmary building under construction which has since been completed. The top floor is used to house cases of illness, the second floor will eventually be given over to chronics and the first will be utilized for other guests requiring slight supervision. On each floor there is a sun parlor. The Menorah Home has recently completed an addition of a million-dollar building, which increases the capacity of this home to 150 beds and provides additional space for the sick. The new wings added to the Andrew Freedman Home make more room available for infirmary use. The new building of the Church Charity Foundation will enable the management to convert the old hospital for acute diseases into one for chronic diseases sometime in the future. The United Home for Aged Hebrews also has plans for a hospital for the use of the chronically ill aged.

The medical service in homes for the aged is frequently given by physicians no longer under pressure to earn an income, who are seeking to give service without regard to the fees attached. This type of gratuitous service cannot always be relied upon to be systematic and thorough. A small group of paid physicians are giving painstaking and adequate service. In order to secure the services of alert and competent doctors, the home must provide facilities for adequate nursing, for making laboratory tests, and for keeping suitable medical records.

SUMMARY

For the care of the aged there were about 8,300 beds in 78 institutions provided by private organizations of New York City.

The homes have been coördinated since 1927 through the Section on the Care of the Aged of the Welfare Council. The Section conducts a Central Information Bureau. A central reporting system, to which 56 homes sent monthly reports of their admissions, rejections, and losses was carried on in The Research Bureau of the Welfare Council until January, 1933, when it was discontinued because the State Board of Social Welfare had begun a system of monthly reporting of statistics for all homes for the aged in the state. Other projects of the Section were the development of minimum standards for administration, a study of food service, and an experiment in occupational work.

Approximately 70 per cent of the homes and 75 per cent of the beds were maintained by organizations with religious affiliations; and the remainder, 30 per cent of the homes and 25 per cent of the beds, were under non-sectarian auspices.

There were 33 homes under Protestant auspices, 11 under Catholic auspices, and 10 under Jewish auspices.

Less than 100 beds were specially provided for Negroes; but about a fourth of all the beds were in homes that have no race restrictions.

Eleven per cent of the beds were for men only, 9 per cent for women only; the remainder were in homes that receive both men and women. Married couples were received in over half of the homes.

National groups maintained 22 per cent of the homes and 11 per cent of the beds. Fraternal organizations maintained 6 per cent of the homes and over 4 per cent of the beds.

The homes vary in size from a small cottage to a great institution and in location from a city street to a large country estate.

Some single rooms were found in two thirds of the homes; double rooms also in about two thirds; and dormitories in more than a third. Nine homes had only single rooms, and one home only double rooms. Five homes had only dormitories.

Many of the homes were well equipped with adequate and attractive sitting rooms and dining rooms, with elevators, bathrooms, and fire escapes. Many, however, are lacking in one or more of these important requirements for the health and comfort of their guests.

The entire personnel engaged in maintaining the homes for the aged is not known. Sixty-four nurses and 165 attendants were found to be employed in the 67 homes studied.

Medical care was given by 358 doctors most of whom served only on call. Eight are resident physicians.

No two of the 67 homes studied are conducted in the same way. It is extremely unlikely that similar standards of maintenance should ever be found among them in view of the fact that their governing boards represent at least seven national groups, three religious faiths with many sects, and a great variety of occupations from day laborer to bank president.

A wide range of conditions also result from the great diversity of requirements for admission, the use of dormitories or single rooms, the difference in medical and nursing care, and the differing population of the homes.

Striking contrasts were found in the administration of the homes in regard to the type of person selected as superintendent, attention to physical order and charm in the institution, and care for the comfort and personal well-being of the guests.

Most of the homes admit persons sixty years or over; a few admit persons between fifty-five and sixty; and several have no age requirements. Women are admitted at an earlier age than men.

With few exceptions, only those who are able to take care of themselves and free from active disease are accepted. Cases of mental disease are excluded, if recognized, in all but one home; but a considerable number of cases of mental abnormality were found in the census. Sickness that occurs after admission is dealt with in various ways summed up below (page 154).

The admission fees ranged from $100 to $5,000 in 39 homes. In 32 homes, no fee was charged; but in 17 of these homes, transfer of property was required and in 2 of the homes the guest was expected to have an income sufficient for personal expenses and burial. The majority of the homes required that property owned shall be transferred to the home. Five homes charged a small amount for board.

Most of the homes have no stated admission requirements limiting them to persons of a particular social group. Only 11 were maintained for a particular group—members of a fraternal organization or persons with a certain occupation.

Residence requirements for admission applied in a little over half of the homes, and in the majority of these the only requirement was residence in New York City. Other homes serve one or more boroughs.

The homes for the aged under private auspices are spending, at the lowest estimate, over a million and a half dollars annually for maintenance. Admission fees and property assignments from guests constitute a relatively small part of the amount spent. The greater part consists of contributions and income from invested funds. Further information on this subject will be found in the report of the Study of Financial Trends of Organized Social Work in New York City, conducted by the Welfare Council's Research Bureau, to be published shortly.

Provision of work for guests is inadequate in most of the homes. In some, the guests spend many vacant hours. In the majority, no opportunity is offered for earning money.

A number of the sheltered workshops are providing employment for persons suffering from greater handicaps than many of the idle ones in the homes for the aged. The same type of occupation will not do for all—for the American-born woman who lived the sheltered girlhood of fifty years ago and for the peasant who knew the hardships of European farm life. To find the best work for each group is a task for an expert teacher.

Many questions are yet to be considered, such as whether guests should be encouraged to obtain work to be done in the home or outside and whether part of their earnings should go to the home.

Recreation is amply provided for in all except a few homes in which it is almost entirely neglected.

No home employed a trained dietitian regularly at the time of the study. Several homes have since added a dietitian to the staff. A committee of the Section for the Care of the Aged of the Welfare Council has made a study of problems of diet in homes for the aged.

There is no recognized standard of medical service in homes for the aged. Any arrangement may be found from expert service and hospital facilities to no medical oversight and a doctor called only in case of sickness. The medical examination on admission may be thorough and carefully followed up with the care and treatment likely to give the guest the greatest possible comfort or it may be cursory and unrelated to the guest's régime of life in the home. Only one home had instituted the practice of periodic health examination of all guests.

A preliminary examination when the application is made prevents much hardship, for if found ineligible the applicant is saved the long wait for a vacancy to occur and can make other arrangements. Some homes find this double examination too great an expense. It should be possible for several homes to combine to secure this service either from a private physician or from some centrally situated clinic.

Applications for admission are usually investigated by a member of the Board. Five homes, however, employ the services of a trained social worker to make the social investigation.

Among the 67 homes studied, all but 5 made provision of some kind to care for their guests if they became ill. In these 5 homes, all cases of illness were transferred to a hospital. In all homes, some patients are transferred to hospitals when special types of care are required, particularly mental cases and cases for operation.

The homes gave medical care to their guests in a variety of ways—4 homes maintained hospitals of 50 to 200 beds; 45 assigned to this purpose special rooms or wards equipped as an infirmary; and 13 cared for sick guests in their own rooms.

About one fifth of the homes were increasing the number of beds they devoted to the care of the sick. In addition to the need for an increased number of beds for the sick, in the majority of the homes there is also need for improvement in the type of medical and nursing service provided.

CHAPTER 4

Convalescent Homes in Relation to the Care of the Chronic Sick

SECTION A

THE CHRONIC SICK IN CONVALESCENT HOMES

RELATION OF CHRONIC AND CONVALESCENT CARE

THE emphasis of convalescent care is upon rehabilitation, both physical and social, rather than upon amelioration of a permanent condition or adjustment to a permanent handicap. A convalescent home, as defined by the Sub-committee on Surgical Convalescence of the Public Health Committee of the New York Academy of Medicine, is "a place where patients who are recovering from an acute illness may spend the time necessary for them to return to economic efficiency. . . . The time element should be elastic. The only criterion for admission to a convalescent home should be the probability that the patient will in time completely regain his or her strength and not become a permanent burden or inmate of such a home."[1] Convalescent care, therefore, strictly speaking, is not a part of care for chronic illness.

Convalescent facilities may be in demand, however, for the care of persons with chronic illness as defined in this study for the following types of illness:

(1) Acute forms of disease or injuries occurring in persons who suffer also from a chronic disease. The problem of convalescence is similar for these patients and for others suffering from the effects of acute illness.

(2) Acute and recurrent manifestations of a chronic condition that require hospital care. Cardiac patients are the outstanding example. Convalescence for them means not only rehabilitation after an acute illness but also, in most cases, an adjustment to the limitations of the functional capacity of the heart.

(3) Chronic conditions that do not prevent the patient from making a complete or partial recovery and returning to his normal activities. Orthopedic cases are the outstanding example of such conditions.

Aside from the convalescent care required for chronic patients who may be expected to return to an active mode of life, there is the further question of the use of convalescent facilities for the care of chronically ill persons permanently incapacitated, who will require prolonged or life-long care. The general convalescent homes, moreover, are often forced because of the lack of suitable provision for the chronic sick to receive patients suffering from

---

[1] Institutional Convalescence: Standards for the Care and Management of Convalescent Homes. A report of the Public Health Committee of the New York Academy of Medicine. Reprinted by the Sturgis Reserve Fund of the Burke Foundation, 1925, p. 10.

chronic illnesses that call for active medical study and diagnosis or for treatment of a kind that convalescent homes are not equipped to provide.

The general policy of convalescent institutions, other than the special homes for cardiac and orthopedic patients, is not to accept the chronic sick; and a few homes adhere rigidly to this rule. Nevertheless, 28 per cent of the beds in the twelve general convalescent homes studied were in use for chronic patients. There seems to be no consistent use of the facilities of convalescent homes in behalf of the chronic sick.

Although there is some demand for convalescent care for persons with chronic diseases to recuperate from acute conditions, it is on the whole comparatively small. In general, if the chronic hospital were able to do its full duty, the patient would be ready to go home on discharge from the hospital and would not need the convalescent institution. A good chronic hospital has all the facilities that a convalescent institution has and more. It has occupational and recreational therapy, opportunities for exercise out-of-doors; and it aids the patient in learning to adjust himself to his condition.

Convalescent homes should formulate a policy in regard to the chronic sick which would define the types of chronic condition, if any, that should be received. At present, there is a disposition to use the general convalescent homes as a temporary shelter for persons for whom other agencies have not been able to make plans. Children are often sent to convalescent homes suffering from malnutrition because of lack of food or bad feeding habits in the family and when improved return to the same conditions. All chronic patients require long-time planning, which should be started as soon as possible. It is doubtful, for example, whether convalescent facilities would be required for diabetic patients if medical social service facilities were adequate for their care. Even after spending some time in a convalescent home, the diabetic patient without medical social service on returning home is very likely to fail in keeping up his dietary régime.

The convalescent institutions for children and young persons suffering from cardiac and orthopedic diseases have functions and problems distinctly different from those of convalescent homes, which are for recuperation after acute illness. Both cardiac and orthopedic patients often need long intensive care requiring special equipment and educational facilities. In the orthopedic homes especially, children receive care that is essentially a part of the medical treatment, so that these institutions strictly speaking offer an extension of hospital care rather than convalescent care.

The present practice of classifying these institutions as "convalescent homes" is misleading. The institutions caring for children with orthopedic disorders keep many of them for long periods, in some instances during their entire childhood, and therefore, are essentially child-caring institutions. They should be conducted according to the standards of child care and training developed for such agencies[2] and with the facilities required for the education of normal children and vocational guidance of handicapped chil-

[2] Detailed Standards of Children's Aid Organizations and Outlines of Standards of Children's Protective Societies and Institutions. New York, Child Welfare League of America, Inc., December, 1929.

dren, as well as special equipment for orthopedic treatment. In some instances, however, the teachers employed do not meet the requirements of the Board of Education. And, as a rule, these institutions do not have the staff necessary for maintaining contact with the homes of the children while they are in the institution and for fostering natural healthy relationships with their families. Visiting rules usually permit the parents to visit only once a month. There is no preparation of the home for the child's return; and when a child has reached the age limit of the institution, usually sixteen years of age, he is sent home without provision for his future or training for

TABLE 34

CHRONIC PATIENTS IN CONVALESCENT INSTITUTIONS CLASSIFIED BY AGE, EACH TYPE OF INSTITUTION

| Age | Total | | TYPE OF INSTITUTION | | | | | |
| | | | General | | Orthopedic | | Cardiac | |
	Number	Per cent	Number	Per cent	Number	Per cent	Number	Per cent
Total	886	100.0	267	100.0	508	100.0	111	100.0
Under 16 years .	632	71.9	94	35.2	440	87.6	98	89.1
16–39 years . . .	142	16.2	72	26.9	58	11.6	12	10.9
40–59 years . . .	84	9.6	80	30.0	4	0.8	0	0
60–69 years . . .	16	1.8	16	6.0	0	0	0	0
70 years and over	5	0.6	5	1.9	0	0	0	0
Not reported . .	7	.....	0	.....	6	.....	1	.....

earning his living. The result is that these badly handicapped children, after years of protection and kind care, are suddenly left without guidance in situations in which they and their families are helpless.

CHRONIC PATIENTS IN CONVALESCENT HOMES

The census of chronic illness was made in all of the orthopedic homes serving New York City patients with the exception of two situated in New Jersey, in all of the cardiac homes, and in over a fourth of the general convalescent homes. Nearly 900 chronic patients, about 4 per cent of the entire census, were reported by the 24 institutions studied. About 500 were in orthopedic homes; over 100, in cardiac homes; and over 250, in general convalescent homes.

Social and Economic Status

The large majority of the chronic patients in convalescent institutions were children and young persons. Table 34 shows the age distribution for the three types of homes. Nearly three fourths of the whole number were under sixteen years of age; nearly four fifths were under twenty-one years of age; and all but 12 per cent were under forty years of age. In the special orthopedic homes, there were few adults. The cardiac homes had a few young persons sixteen years of age or over. In the general convalescent homes, 59 per cent were twenty-one years of age or over and 38 per cent were forty years of age or over.

The percentage of males (52 per cent) and females (48 per cent) in convalescent institutions was nearly the same as in the total census. Males

TABLE 35

CHRONIC PATIENTS IN CONVALESCENT INSTITUTIONS CLASSIFIED BY DIAGNOSES, EACH TYPE OF INSTITUTION

Diagnosis	Total	TYPE OF INSTITUTION		
		General	Cardiac	Orthopedic
Total	886	267	111	508
Orthopedic diseases	449	22	2	425
Poliomyelitis	138	2	0	136
Tuberculosis of spine and joints	196	8	0	188
Rickets	11	1	0	10
Diseases of bones and organs of locomotion . .	83	11	0	72
Malformations	21	. . .	2	19
Circulatory diseases	193	63	101	29
Cardiac	182	52	101	29
Other	11	11	0	0
Neurological diseases	103	68	2	33
Chorea	67	52	2	13
Other	36	16	0	20
Rheumatism	36	18	5	13
Respiratory diseases	25	24	0	1
Digestive diseases	15	15	0	0
Non-venereal diseases of the genitourinary system	14	14	0	0
Cancer	12	12	0	0
Other	39	31	1	7

predominated in the general convalescent homes and females in the orthopedic and cardiac homes, particularly in the latter, where 56 per cent of the children were girls. This is due to the fact that a larger percentage of the cardiac convalescent facilities have been provided for girls than for boys.

Negroes were over 3 per cent of the patients in convalescent institutions—4 per cent in orthopedic homes, less than 1 per cent in cardiac homes, and about 2 per cent in general homes. The fact that this is a smaller percentage of Negroes than was reported in the total census bears out the fact that there is a shortage of convalescent facilities for Negroes.

The proportion of Protestant patients in convalescent institutions was considerably less, of Catholics, slightly less, of Jewish patients, much larger than in the total census of the chronic sick.

All but 3 per cent of the patients in convalescent institutions were wholly dependent for their care and maintenance upon resources other than their own personal income and three fourths were wholly dependent upon public or private aid.

Medical Condition

In the special orthopedic homes, 82 per cent were suffering from orthopedic disorders. In the special cardiac homes, 91 per cent were cardiac patients. In general convalescent homes, over a fourth were neurological patients, most of whom had chorea; nearly a fourth were suffering from circulatory diseases, largely heart disease; 9 per cent were suffering from respiratory diseases, 8 per cent from orthopedic disorders, and 5 per cent from cancer. Table 35 shows the diagnosis of patients in the various types of institution.

Nearly half of these chronic patients in general convalescent homes suffered from conditions for which the special cardiac and orthopedic homes are intended. Although the cardiac home is best adapted to the care of patients with chorea, the majority of the chorea patients were in general convalescent homes. Apart from those with cardiac and orthopedic diseases, the chronic patients in general convalescent homes were 0.6 per cent of the whole census.

Duration of Care

All but 6 per cent of the patients in the general convalescent homes had been under care for less than three months; and two thirds had been under care less than a month. Of those under care three months or longer, only one patient had been under care as long as a year. In the cardiac homes, more than half of the patients had been under care less than three months and only four persons longer than a year. In orthopedic homes, more than half had been continuously under care over three months and more than a fourth over a year; and thirty persons had had five years or more of continuous care. Many of the children in the orthopedic homes had been there for a much longer period than the census records show, as the time under care was reported from the date of the last admission and many of these children are returned from time to time to hospitals for further treatment.

In one orthopedic home, half of the forty children reported had been there for four years or longer and sixteen had been there as long as five years. One child had been in the institution over ten years. Most of the children who had received four years or more of care were between thirteen and eighteen years of age. In the general convalescent homes, nearly half of the patients had been ill for less than a year and a fifth for five years or longer. In both cardiac and orthopedic homes, less than 10 per cent of the patients had been ill under a year and about half had been sick five years or longer.

Patients in general convalescent homes and orthopedic homes are usually admitted after a period of hospital care. Only seven of these chronic patients had received no previous institutional care for their illness. Cardiac children, however, not requiring hospital care, are sometimes sent directly to convalescent institutions from clinics. In general convalescent homes, only one person, in orthopedic homes, 8 per cent; and in cardiac homes, one fifth had not been in an institution previously. Ten per cent of the whole number had been in institutions five or more times—4 per cent of those in general homes; 10 per cent, in cardiac homes; and 13 per cent, in orthopedic homes. Twelve per cent of all the persons who had been institutionalized more than once had never been in any type of institution except a convalescent home. This was particularly true in cardiac homes, where nearly a third had not previously been in any other type of institution.

In general, the previous institutional care had been comparatively recent and of comparatively short duration. Except in orthopedic homes, where 5 per cent had been in an institution at least ten years previously, no patient had had institutional care so long before. Twelve per cent in all homes and

TABLE 36

CHRONIC PATIENTS IN CONVALESCENT INSTITUTIONS CLASSIFIED BY
CARE NEEDED AND CARE RECEIVED, EACH TYPE OF INSTITUTION

	CARE RECEIVED							
	General			Cardiac	Orthopedic			
Care needed	Total	Medical, clinic	Attendant	Medical, clinic	Total	Medical, clinic	Nursing	Attendant
Total . . .	267	252	15	111	508	311	191	6
Medical . . .	250	248	2	111	311	306	5	0
Hospital . .	6	6	0	7	11	11	0	0
Clinic . . .	244	242	2	104	300	295	5	0
Nursing . . .	0	0	0	0	172	0	172	0
Attendant . .	17	4	13	0	25	5	14	6

17 per cent in orthopedic homes had had institutional care five or more years earlier. Half of the patients in all homes and three fourths in general homes had first been institutionalized within the year.

A third of all the patients had had less than three months of institutional care—51 per cent in general homes and 22 per cent in orthopedic homes. Nearly three fourths had had less than a year of institutional care; and in general convalescent homes this was true of all but two patients.

Care Needed and Received

Since patients in convalescent institutions generally remain under the medical supervision of the sending agency, they were regarded as receiving clinic care during their stay, with the exception of those in orthopedic homes that are country branches of orthopedic hospitals, where the care given is expert nursing care under the supervision of physicians. Only 24 persons in convalescent institutions, less than 3 per cent, were thought to be in need of hospital care. Only 42 persons, either in general convalescent homes or in orthopedic homes, needed attendant care and of these over half were receiving a more skilled type of care. All of nearly 200 patients who required nursing care were receiving it; and of the 650 who needed clinic care only two did not receive it.

All but 4 per cent of the patients in convalescent institutions were regarded as receiving a suitable type of care. This 4 per cent was made up of the small number who needed hospital care and those who received clinic care although they needed only attendant care.

SUMMARY

1. Chronic patients may require convalescent care for (1) acute forms of disease occurring in addition to the chronic condition, (2) for acute manifestations of a chronic condition requiring a period of hospital care, or (3) for chronic conditions that do not prevent the patient from recovering sufficiently to return to his normal activities.

2. Convalescent institutions are of two different types: (1) special institutions equipped for the care of chronic conditions, such as cardiac or orthopedic disorders; and (2) general convalescent homes serving primarily persons recovering from acute illness. It is a question whether institutions of the former group should be classified among convalescent homes, as the service for which they exist is distinctly different from that of the general convalescent home.

3. The 900 chronic patients reported by convalescent institutions of both types are about 4 per cent of the total number of chronically ill persons in the census. Over half were in orthopedic homes, about an eighth in cardiac homes, and nearly a third in general homes.

4. Chronic patients in convalescent institutions were largely young persons. In cardiac homes, they were all children or young persons under eighteen. In orthopedic homes, all but 12 per cent were children under sixteen years of age. In the general convalescent homes, 35 per cent were children; and the large majority were in the middle years, only 8 per cent being sixty years of age or over.

5. In the general convalescent homes, nearly a fifth of the chronic patients were suffering from chorea; a fourth, from circulatory diseases; and 8 per cent, from orthopedic disorders. Nearly half, therefore, were suffering from conditions usually cared for in special cardiac and orthopedic homes.

6. The cardiac and orthopedic homes should be equipped to carry out the standards of care and training approved for other child-caring agencies.

7. Although the general policy of general convalescent homes is to refuse the chronic sick, over a fourth of the bed capacity of these institutions was occupied by chronic patients.

8. A relatively small number of chronic patients need convalescent care, since as a rule a plan for permanent readjustment should be begun as early

as possible. If chronic hospital facilities were adequate, convalescent institutions would probably receive few demands for the care of persons with chronic diseases.

9. The policy of general convalescent homes in regard to the chronic sick should be more carefully formulated, in order to define the chronic conditions that would be benefited by convalescent care and should be received.

SECTION B

FACILITIES OF CONVALESCENT HOMES IN RELATION TO THE CARE OF THE CHRONIC SICK

The discussion of facilities for convalescence that follows includes a brief account of the organization of this field and the extent of convalescent services in New York City and a more detailed description of the facilities of the twenty-four convalescent institutions studied, which reported patients included in the study of the chronic sick. (See Appendix V-a.) Half of this group of twenty-four institutions are general convalescent homes intended for recuperation following acute illness, and the other half are either cardiac or orthopedic homes caring for these types of chronic disease.

CENTRAL ORGANIZATION OF CONVALESCENCE SERVICES

The coördinating body in the field of convalescence in New York City is the Section on Convalescent Care of the Health Division of The Welfare Council, in which fifty-five institutions are represented. At the time the Section was organized, in July, 1927, the Convalescence Service of the Hospital Information and Service Bureau of the United Hospital Fund had been in existence for about two years. The Advisory Committee of the Convalescence Service became the Executive Committee of the Section.

The Committee on Public Health Relations of the New York Academy of Medicine formulated Standards for the Care and Management of Convalescent Homes and suggested the formation of an Advisory Committee on Convalescence in 1925. Under its auspices a meeting of representatives of convalescent homes and social service departments was held. At this meeting a resolution was passed endorsing the standards and it was proposed that an Advisory Committee on Convalescence be established under the auspices of the Hospital Information and Service Bureau of the United Hospital Fund. This committee was appointed by the Advisory Committee of the Hospital Information and Service Bureau and met for the first time in October, 1925.

A standard application card was prepared and published by the Advisory Committee of the Convalescence Service in June, 1927. A small advisory information service for the general public has been conducted since 1925. In October, 1927, an information and placement service was begun.

In April, 1929, the Section on Convalescent Care of the Welfare Council and the Convalescence Service of the Hospital Information and Service Bureau jointly adopted minimum standards for convalescent homes which were later published for distribution.[3] They represent a higher standard than the practice of a number of homes. They are not yet used as a basis

[3] Minimum Standards for Convalescent Homes. Adopted by the Section on Convalescent Care of The Welfare Council and the Convalescence Service of the Hospital Information and Service Bureau, United Hospital Fund of New York. New York City, The Welfare Council, December, 1928.

for admission to the Section but rather as a measuring rod for the use of the homes themselves in judging and grading their own work.

The Convalescence Service of the Hospital Information and Service Bureau serves as a central information bureau on convalescent facilities. Its secretary is the sole admission officer for one group of homes; for another group of homes, she may admit although the homes also maintain their own admitting offices; and a third group of homes notify her daily of their vacancies. The social agencies of the city, therefore, have a central source of information in regard to current vacancies, type of patient accepted, and admission requirements of the different homes.

The New York Tuberculosis and Health Association, through the Committee on Convalescent Care of its Heart Committee, serves as the admitting agent for convalescent homes for cardiac children. The cardiac convalescent work is thereby coördinated with the other activities of the Heart Committee—research, vocational guidance, and clinic supervision.

TYPES OF CONVALESCENT HOME

The fifty-eight convalescent institutions of the city[4] are divided into three groups: (1) for cardiac conditions; (2) for orthopedic disorders; and (3) for persons recovering from acute illnesses. The special homes for cardiac and orthopedic convalescence serve largely children. The general convalescent homes serve both adults and children. They vary extensively as to the type of patient they accept. Some take only medical patients and therefore accept no patients requiring surgical dressings. Many are equipped to give simple dressings; a few to give more difficult ones. Some of the general convalescent homes accept cardiac patients and others do not. Only a few can give bed care. Two of the homes that have been included among those providing general convalescence accept only adolescent, undernourished children, to whom they are equipped to give long-time care.

These fifty-eight convalescent institutions have a year-round capacity of nearly 3,100 beds and in the summer an additional capacity of about 1,000 beds. There is also a group of summer homes with a capacity of about 700 beds, making a total of nearly 5,000 beds for convalescent and fresh air work for the sick in New York City. In this discussion of convalescent homes in relation to the care of the chronically ill, only homes that are open all the year are considered.

Table 37 below shows the bed capacity of the homes and indicates whether they care for adults or children. Forty-five per cent of the homes are for children only, about 31 per cent for adults, and about 24 per cent for both adults and children. The beds are almost equally divided among the three groups, about one third in each.

In a discussion of convalescent homes, mention should be made of the practice of providing convalescent care in foster homes. The growing tendency to place children with chronic disorders in private family homes

---

[4] See Appendix V-a, made for this study, for a list of convalescent homes included in the census of the chronically ill and Appendix V-b for a list of those not included.

selected for this purpose has been referred to in other sections of the report. The Children's Hospital in Boston has made use of this method in coöperation with child-caring agencies. In New York, the Speedwell Society, established in 1902 as an organization for the convalescent care of children under twelve years of age, more particularly babies and younger children, has always used foster homes entirely. The New York Foundling Hospital has a boarding-out department for children under school age requiring medical supervision. The New York Nursery and Child's Hospital conducts a Foster Home Service for Dependent Children, who receive medical care when needed.

TABLE 37

CONVALESCENT HOMES IN NEW YORK CITY CLASSIFIED BY
BED CAPACITY AND TYPES OF PATIENT SERVED, 1928

Type of patient	Homes	Bed capacity
Total homes	58	3,080
General convalescence	44	2,353
Adults	18	990
Children	14	659
Adults and children	12	704
Orthopedic	10	597
Children	8	382
Adults and children	2	215
Cardiac: children	4	130

The system of the Speedwell Society, which is unique, is well known. A number of approved homes in a certain district, fully equipped by the Society for the care of a sick child, constitute a unit. In nine such units, there are 244 available beds. The medical and nursing supervision is carefully systematized and thorough. Dr. Henry Dwight Chapin, who is responsible for this plan, recently stated his conclusions in regard to its value as follows: "During the twenty-nine years of its operation, the Speedwell plan has proved that carefully systematized boarding out is superior to any mass handling of these cases; also that the ordinary, plain American home, by the carefully controlled environment the Speedwell plan has inaugurated, can be safely and satisfactorily utilized in much remedial work for children."[5]

STANDARDS

Standards of convalescent service in New York City are far from uniform. The minimum standards, as adopted jointly by the Convalescent Section of the Welfare Council and the Convalescence Service of the Hospital Information and Service Bureau in April, 1929, represent a minimum goal rather than minimum performance.

Of the fifteen requirements in the minimum standards, five deal with the plant—its lay-out, location, sanitation, equipment, and fire protection—

[5] Chapin, Henry Dwight, M.D., Convalescent Care for Hospital Babies. Reprinted from the *Journal of the American Medical Association*, vol. 98, January 2, 1932, p. 2.

and suggest a country location with enough land for outdoor recreation and exercise, a cottage type of building permitting the care of patients in small groups, and privacy for adults in single rooms or cubicles. The minimum personnel requirements are at least one graduate nurse in attendance at all times and at least weekly examination of all patients by the attending physician. Further requirements refer to food, recreation, the patient's daily routine, provision for emergency medical treatment, and equipment for special types of cases. The remaining five points have to do with admission and discharge regulations, records, and the relation of the convalescent home to the sending agency in regard to responsibility for social investigation and for follow-up and to the use of a Central Information Bureau.

COSTS

It is generally conceded that the cost of convalescent care is much less than that of hospital care. Dr. Corwin, in 1924, estimated that the annual expenditure in New York City for convalescent homes was approximately two million dollars.[6] During the same year, the expenditures for the member hospitals of the United Hospital Fund alone totaled nearly twenty million dollars.[7] He estimated that the daily cost per patient was in the neighborhood of $2.00.[6] During the same year, the daily cost per patient in the general hospitals of the United Hospital Fund was $5.60, and that of all its member hospitals was $4.81.[7] In 1928, the Convalescence Service of the United Hospital Fund estimated, from reports made by various convalescent homes, a daily expenditure per patient of $2.25, which represents about the same increase in cost per patient that the general hospitals of the United Hospital Fund showed in the same period.

HOMES INCLUDED IN THE STUDY

At a joint meeting of the Advisory Committee of the Convalescent Service of the Hospital Information and Service Bureau of the United Hospital Fund and the Section on Convalescent Care of the Welfare Council in April, 1928, the value of a census of persons chronically ill in convalescent homes was discussed; and it was agreed that it would be of interest to know to what extent convalescent homes are used for the care of patients suffering from chronic illness.

Twenty-four homes in the metropolitan area of New York were selected for study. (See Appendix V-a.) They were selected because they were thought to have the largest number of cases of chronic illness. All the existing homes for orthopedic patients, eight in number, and for cardiac patients, four in number, were included. The twelve general convalescent homes in which it seemed likely that the largest proportion of cases of chronic illness would be found, were indicated by the secretary of the Hospital Information

---

[6] Corwin, E. H. L., The Hospital Situation in Greater New York. New York, G. P. Putnam's Sons, 1924, pp. 283–284; 295–296.
[7] United Hospital Fund of New York, Forty-Sixth Annual Report, New York, 1926; Statistical Report for the year ended June 30, 1925.

Bureau's Convalescence Service, on the basis of her experience and of the information contained in the Directory of Social Agencies.[8]

This group of institutions does not represent the total number of convalescent homes in which chronically ill persons receive care. Taking into consideration, however, the scattered locations of the remaining thirty-four convalescent homes and the small percentage of chronic patients cared for, neither the time nor expenditure necessary to make an inclusive study of the entire group seemed warranted. But the fact that these thirty-four homes also were caring for a small number of patients with chronic diseases should not be forgotten.

Four of the twenty-four institutions included in the census, maintained for cardiac children, were doing intensive follow-up work and it was decided to include their active cases in the study. Census records were also taken for a group of cardiac children, each of whom was receiving vocational guidance from the Cardiac Vocational Guidance Service of the New York Tuberculosis and Health Association and medical supervision from a cardiac clinic. (See also Chapter 5, dealing with Cardiac After-Care Services.)

Contact with the convalescent homes was made by a letter outlining the purpose of the study and requesting an interview with the executive in charge of the home. At the interview, further details of the census taking were discussed and arrangements made for a recorder to collect the data relating to those suffering from a chronic disease. No effort was made to gather information in regard to the facilities of the various institutions, as these data are currently on file in the office of the Convalescence Service of the Hospital Information and Service Bureau of the United Hospital Fund.

In the census of the chronically ill in the twenty-four homes selected, all persons were included who had been incapacitated by disease for three months or longer and were likely to be ill for an indefinite period, with the exception of mental patients and those with tuberculosis of the lungs. In the organizations working with cardiac patients, records were taken only of persons falling within the cardiac classifications IIa, IIb, and III,[9] that is,

---

[8] Directory of Social Agencies of the City of New York, 37th Edition, 1929. Published by The Charity Organization Society, in Coöperation with The Welfare Council and other agencies, New York, 1929.

[9] The following five groupings are approved by the American Heart Association, Inc., and are used in cardiac clinics to indicate the degree of incapacity of each patient:

CLASS I
    Patients with organic heart disease, able to carry on ordinary physical activity without discomfort. (Excluded from census.)

CLASS II
    Patients with organic heart disease, unable to carry on ordinary physical activity without discomfort; (a) activity slightly limited; (b) activity greatly limited. (Included in census.)

CLASS III
    Patients with organic heart disease and with symptoms or signs of heart failure when at rest, unable to carry on any physical activity without discomfort. (Included in census.)

CLASS E
    Patients with abnormal signs or symptoms not believed to be due to organic disease. (Excluded from census.)

CLASS F
    Patients without circulatory disease, but considered "potential" because of the presence or history of an etiologic factor which might cause cardiac disease. (Excluded from census.)

(The above classification is taken from "A Nomenclature for Cardiac Diagnosis, Approved by the American Heart Association," adopted, 1923. Distributed by the Heart Committee of the New York Tuberculosis and Health Association.)

those whose cardiac disability was sufficient to restrict their physical activity.

The twenty-four institutions serving convalescents that are included in the census have a total capacity of 1,602 beds or 53 per cent of the total year-round capacity of all homes. The general convalescent homes studied have 943 beds or 40 per cent of the capacity of the total homes of this type.

Special Convalescent Homes

For Cardiac Patients. There are four convalescent homes serving cardiac convalescents: Irvington House, Martine Farm, Nichols Cottage, and Pelham Home for Children, organized and maintained for boys and girls hav-

TABLE 38

ORTHOPEDIC CONVALESCENT HOMES FOR CHILDREN AND ADULTS
CLASSIFIED BY BED CAPACITY, 1928

Patients served	Total homes		Homes in study			
					Chronic patients	
	Number	Capacity	Number	Capacity	Number	Per cent
Total	10	597[1]	8	529[1]	508	96.0
Children	8	382[1]	6	314[1]	299	95.3
Children and adults . . .	2	215	2	215	209	97.2

[1] One home of 100 beds assigns 50 beds to other than orthopedic services.

ing, or suspected of having, organic heart disease. The capacity of these four homes is 130 beds, 85 per cent of which were occupied by the chronically ill at the time of the census.[10] The fact that functional and potential heart disorders, other than chorea and rheumatic fever, are excluded from the census accounts for the difference between the whole number in the homes and the number of records taken.

Of these four homes, one with 6 beds is exclusively for boys from 10 to 16 years of age, one of 30 beds is exclusively for girls from 6 to 14 years of age. The other two accept both boys and girls, one of 70 beds taking 40 boys and 30 girls between 6 and 16 years of age and the other having 7 beds for boys from 6 to 10 years and 17 beds for girls from 6 to 16 years.[11] There are in all 53 beds for boys and 77 beds for girls.

For Orthopedic Patients. Eight convalescent homes are organized and conducted for the care of orthopedic patients, largely children. They are: Blythedale Home for Crippled Children, Wavecrest Home maintained by the Brooklyn Children's Aid Society, Convalescent Home for Hebrew Children,[12] Evelyn Goldsmith Home for Crippled Children, Breezy Point (coun-

[10] In addition, Campbell Cottages of New York Hospital have twenty beds for cardiac children.
[11] Beginning in January, 1930, this home used its facilities for boys and girls in whatever ratio the demand indicated.
[12] Fifty beds are used for orthopedic patients and fifty for general convalescent care.

try branch of the Hospital for Joint Diseases),[13] House of St. Giles the Cripple (Garden City Home), New York Orthopedic Dispensary and Hospital (country branch),[13] and Robin's Nest, maintained by the Association for the Aid of Crippled Children. The capacity of these eight homes is 529 beds—314 devoted exclusively to children and 215 to both adults and children. The census found 508 chronically ill persons occupying 96 per cent of their total bed capacity. Two homes for orthopedic patients, with a total of sixty-eight beds, were not included in the census because they are situated in New Jersey, although they accept New York City patients.

All of these homes accept children; two accept children of any age; one accepts them at three years; three accept them at four years; two accept them at six years. Five of the homes make the upper age limit for accepting children variously from ten to fourteen years.

General Convalescent Homes

The remaining twelve convalescent homes are organized for the care of persons recovering from acute illness, for whom the period of convalescent care ranges usually from two weeks to eight weeks. Of these twelve convalescent homes, the three conducted by the Children's Aid Society— Elizabeth Milbank Anderson Home, Martha Home, and Milbank Memorial—caring for 240 children stated that they receive convalescents from practically all acute conditions—medical, surgical, post-contagious, tubercular bones and glands without abscesses, and chorea. They do not accept severe cases of mental disease, cardiac patients as such, or patients with chronic and communicable diseases. However, records of sixty-nine patients, representing 29 per cent of their total capacity of 240 beds, were secured in the census of chronic sick children in these homes. Children with a chronic ailment needing prolonged care limit the turnover; and if these children are given preference, the bed space for those recovering from acute illness is considerably diminished.

Campbell Cottages, conducted under the auspices of the New York Hospital, for boys and girls up to the age of sixteen, admits general medical and surgical convalescents in addition to children with chorea, asthma, and heart disease. Seventeen, or 20 per cent of the eighty-six beds in the institution, were used for chronic patients at the time of the census.

St. Luke's Convalescent Hospital, which accepts patients referred from the hospital, was caring for 25 patients with chronic disease, representing 29 per cent of its capacity, at the time of the census.

Fifteen of the 25 beds in the Bikur Cholim Convalescent Home were occupied by chronically ill persons. Since there is only one doctor on call and no graduate nurse in the Home, it is not prepared to give care for chronic illness. Hebrew Convalescent Home reported 30 of its 45 beds occupied by patients having a chronic disease. There is one graduate nurse in residence and a physician calls daily. Patients are permitted to return to the clinics from which they were referred for treatment as often as necessary. The

[13] Takes only patients with bone tuberculosis.

Jewish Home for Convalescents is maintained for general convalescent and post-operative cases, and yet 33 of its 65 beds were occupied by patients having a chronic disease.

Isabella Home has 28 beds for convalescent patients in addition to provision for the aged who receive permanent care. Thirteen beds were occupied at the time of the census by patients considered chronically ill. The physician visits daily but no graduate nurse is employed. As all patients are ambulant, many of them are permitted to seek employment prior to leaving the institution.

TABLE 39

GENERAL CONVALESCENT HOMES FOR CHILDREN AND ADULTS
CLASSIFIED BY BED CAPACITY, 1928

Patients served	Total homes		Homes in study			
					Chronic patients	
	Number	Capacity	Number	Capacity	Number	Per cent
Total	44	2,353	12	943	267	28.3
Children	14	659	5	376	78	20.7
Adults	18	990	5	463	150	32.4
Children and adults . . .	12	704	2	104	29	27.9

Burke Foundation is one of the largest and most adequately equipped convalescent homes in the country. Its director states that "more than 25 per cent of the 6,000-plus patients yearly admitted to the Burke Foundation's country repair institution are in the chronic class."[14] At the time of the census, 59 of its patients, representing 19 per cent of its total capacity, were reported as suffering from chronic illness.

The capacity of the 12 general convalescent homes studied is 943 beds, or about 40 per cent of the beds for general convalescence in the 44 homes of this type in the city. Twenty-eight per cent of the beds in the homes studied were occupied by chronic patients, as Table 39 shows.

Of the 12 general convalescent homes in the study, 5 are for children, 5 for adults, and 2 for both. The Children's Aid Society arranges for children of all ages from three up to be cared for in three homes, but it reserves two homes for older boys and uses the third for girls and small boys. Another home accepts only boys from certain grades in school. In the two homes accepting both adults and children, there are no limitations as to the age of the children.

ADMISSION REQUIREMENTS

Medical Examination

Admission to all convalescent homes is dependent upon a physician's recommendation. Three of the 24 convalescent homes studied are country

[14] Brush, Frederic, M.D., The Interrelations of Chronic and Convalescent Care. The Sturgis Reserve Fund of the Burke Foundation, January 4, 1927, p. 3.

branches of hospitals and the transfer of patients needing convalescent care is direct. In 9 homes, the entrant must be examined by the admitting physician of the home. Five of these require in addition the report of the sending agency's medical examination.

Nine homes accept the medical examination and diagnosis of the sending agency. Two homes accept the medical examination of the hospital referring the patient in some instances and make their own examination in others. One home is operated by a hospital largely for its own patients. When it accepts other patients, it does not reëxamine any but cardiac patients.

Physical Condition

Convalescent homes maintained for medical cases do not admit persons requiring special care or dressings. Of the convalescent homes that accept surgical cases, not all are equipped to supply dressings.

Of the 24 convalescent homes included in the study, 6 admit cardiac patients; 12 admit patients recovering from medical or surgical conditions, 4 of which do not take cases requiring surgical dressings; 8 admit orthopedic cases.

Of the 6 institutions taking cardiac patients, 4 are cardiac homes for children, 1 is a general convalescent home for children, and the remaining institution, Burke Foundation, assigns 75 beds to adult cardiac patients of either sex as the need arises.

Relation to Hospital Discharge

In general, the convalescent homes studied accept hospital patients immediately upon discharge. There are some exceptions—the four cardiac convalescent homes do not accept children who have had acute rheumatic fever or chorea until six weeks after hospital discharge; Burke Foundation does not accept cardiac patients until two weeks after hospital discharge, but for all others preference is given to those seeking admission immediately upon discharge.

Age and Sex

Of the 24 homes included in the census, 15 accept children only; 5 accept adults only; and 4 accept both children and adults. Of the 19 providing for children, 1 accepts no boys; and 4 accept no girls. In the homes for boys, the admitting age varies from infancy to ten years. The upper age limit varies from eight years to fourteen or sixteen years. Nine of the homes take boys only up to twelve years; and the other 9 accept older boys.

The homes accepting girls, accept them over a wider age range than in the case of boys. In 5 of the 15 homes for girls, the youngest admitting age is six years; and in the others, it ranges from infancy to four years. The upper age limit is from ten to twelve years in 4 homes, and from fourteen to sixteen years in the others.

Of these 19 convalescent homes, 11 accommodate 341 boys of varying ages from three to sixteen years; and 8 accommodate 301 girls, varying in age from three to sixteen years. Four homes with 189 beds for children and 3 homes with 299 beds for adults and children make flexible arrangements for separate provision for boys and girls. Of the 130 beds in the 4 cardiac homes, 77 beds are for girls and 53 beds for boys.

Five convalescent homes accept adults only. There is no division of the number of males and females accommodated in two of these homes with 90 beds. The 3 remaining homes provide care for 199 men and 174 women. Four additional homes accept adults and children; and 1 has 8 beds for mothers with children. The other 3, all conducted under the auspices of hospitals, accept men and women in whatever proportion the demand for beds requires.

Race

Campbell Cottages, Wavecrest, and the three convalescent homes conducted by the Children's Aid Society of New York, admit colored children Reed Farm accepts colored mothers and babies.[15] A number of the other homes do not exclude colored children, but they stipulate that they shall not be admitted singly. This requirement necessarily limits the facilities for this particular group.

The greatest unmet need for convalescent care is the lack of provision for caring for the adolescent Negro boy. The Children's Aid Society's Milbank Memorial Home, with 65 beds, for boys from ten to sixteen years of age, is the only home taking older boys that admits Negroes as freely as other boys.

Residence

The Children's Aid Society of New York does not admit children into its convalescent homes from outlying sections of the city, because it requires a home investigation in all cases. In all other instances, the 24 homes included in the study make no residence restrictions.

VACANCIES, WAITING LISTS, AND REJECTIONS

The existing vacancies in convalescent homes at any one time are fairly accurately known at the office of the Hospital Information and Service Bureau and at the New York Tuberculosis and Health Association, which is the admitting office for the four cardiac children's homes.

Waiting lists are kept in a number of convalescent homes. However, as the convalescent period lasts only a short time, the placing organization usually accepts for its client the first available opening rather than place him on a waiting list.

The Convalescence Service of the Hospital Information and Service Bureau, United Hospital Fund, furnished the following data on admission to convalescent homes, from figures on patients referred to the Service during the three months, April, May, and June, 1928, which cover the census period. Of 850 patients referred for placement from various organ-

---

[15] In November, 1931, this institution became a home for cardiac boys and accepts Negro boys.

izations during the period, 771 patients, or 90.7 per cent, were placed in 33 convalescent homes. Of this number, 68 were placed in 20 of the homes included in the study.

For the same period, the New York Tuberculosis and Health Association furnished the following information for the four cardiac homes, of which the total bed capacity was 143 beds. During the three months, the homes were used to 89 per cent of capacity. During the period, 258 applications were received for convalescent care and a waiting list of 167 applicants was carried over from previous months. Of this total, one fourth of the applicants were placed in homes during the period; two thirds, or 281, were still on the waiting list at the end of the period; and a small percentage were rejected or their applications were cancelled after being put on the waiting list.

Of the 30 children whose applications were cancelled, 21 dropped out because they had waited so long that the parents or social workers had made other arrangements for their care. Three were cancelled by the social worker because they were "un-coöperative" or because, when the vacancy occurred, the parents did not wish them to be sent away. Two of the applicants were too ill for convalescent care and 4 had died when vacancies occurred.

Since the homes had during this period a bed capacity of 143 and a waiting list of 281, it is obvious that many cardiac children have a long wait before they can be admitted to the convalescent home. However, the largest number of applicants are received during the spring months, 34 per cent of the total for the year 1928. During the entire year 1928, 57 per cent of the applicants were admitted to the homes; the applications of 20 per cent were cancelled before they were reached on the waiting list; and only 20 per cent were still on the waiting list at the end of the year, as opposed to two thirds at the end of the period studied.

MEDICAL CARE

Two homes, Burke Foundation and The Country Branch of the New York Orthopedic Hospital have resident physicians. All of the 24 homes have a visiting consultant staff. In some instances, the physicians pay weekly or bi-weekly calls and in other institutions, they visit only when sent for.

Nearly all of the homes studied, except those for cardiacs, accept patients requiring surgical dressings. All of the 8 orthopedic homes are prepared to give dressings. Of the 12 general convalescent homes, 7 accept dressing cases, 5 do not.

NURSING CARE

Three institutions, Bikur Cholim Convalescent Home, Surprise Lake Camp, and Isabella Home do not have graduate nurses resident in their respective institutions. The other 21 homes employ a total of 66 graduate nurses. In some of the homes, 1 nurse acts as both superintendent and nurse. Burke Foundation and the Country Branch of New York Orthopedic Hospital have each 7 nurses.

Physiotherapy

All of the homes for the convalescence of orthopedic patients have physiotherapy equipment. They are all equipped to give massage treatment for the retraining of muscles. Of the homes for general convalescence studied, one, St. Luke's Convalescent Hospital, has physiotherapy equipment.

Occupational Therapy

Occupational therapy broadly defined is any activity prescribed for the purpose of promoting recovery from the effects of illness. The results at Burke Foundation, over a period of fourteen years, indicate the benefits that may be derived from occupational therapy. Many of the convalescent homes organized later than Burke Foundation have included occupational therapy as part of the daily routine.

In the seventh annual report of the Burke Foundation, the daily régime at the institution is sketched. The first days are almost completely given over to rest. Then follows a period of one or two hours of prescribed therapeutic occupation, which often grades first into longer hours of paid work at a modest wage and later into regular employment in the institution or vicinity while still under treatment. Recreational therapy is applied in a variety of forms, indoors and outdoors, throughout the day; and means of making it increasingly effective through skilled application and new developments are continually studied. Mechanical physical therapy is used to some extent but the main dependence is upon normal constructive activities in play, light work, and exercise and upon new interests and ambitions. There is a careful avoidance of fostering the habit of invalidism in dealing with convalescent patients.[16]

Of the homes studied, St. Luke's Convalescent Hospital and Campbell Cottages, among the general homes have occupational therapy service. In Campbell Cottages it is, of course, limited by the age of the children accepted. The cardiac and orthopedic homes have occupational therapy. In the latter group of homes it is directly designed for the retraining of muscles.

Recreation

Recreation in many forms is provided in the various convalescent homes. Through the schoolroom, workshop, library, moving pictures, and radio, the diversion so essential for the patient recuperating from a long illness is provided. In some of the homes, the recreation program is closely related to occupational and physical therapy. In the Convalescent Home for Hebrew Children, for example, some of the members of a patient's band played in it in order to exercise leg and foot muscles that needed retraining. At this home and at the Wavecrest Home, of the Brooklyn Children's Aid Society, situated on the seashore, swimming is an important part of recreational therapy.

[16] The Winifred Masterson Burke Relief Foundation, Seventh Annual Report, 1925–1927, p. 13.

At the Burke Foundation, the extensive grounds make it possible to provide a variety of outdoor sports, such as baseball, tennis, and golf. Here also concerts, theatricals, and dances are organized by patient talent. Emphasis is upon normal social group life. At the three homes of the Children's Aid Society of New York, in Westchester County, the emphasis is upon outdoor recreation and nature study. Country walks, with a counsellor, are organized in small groups of children with equal endurance. At Irvington House, there is a Garden Club and a Nature Museum started by an East Side boy to whom Irvington House gave his first experience of country life.

Special Diets

Few convalescent homes provide more than an ordinary simple diet. In no home is the food weighed or the menu planned to suit special diet cases. The social service departments of hospitals have particular difficulty in placing patients needing a "special diet" such as those suffering from nephritis, diabetes, and post-operative gastric ulcer.[17] The group of homes studied makes no provision for the care of patients requiring special diet.

Education

In institutions dealing with children over a prolonged period, standardized schools are provided. In some instances, the school within the convalescent home is treated as an annex to one of the city schools and teachers are supplied by the New York City Department of Education. In other instances, the children are sent to a school in the neighborhood of the convalescent home. However, since only the regular grade school work is provided in this way, there is little opportunity for special vocational training of the handicapped, such as is found in orthopedic homes.

SOCIAL SERVICE

The principle on which convalescent homes accept patients for care is that the patient shall remain under the medical and social care of the sending agency while in the convalescent institution. Therefore, convalescent homes have not developed social service departments, although there is sometimes a trained social worker in the admitting office. The sending agency supplies social information to the homes, prepares the home for the patient's return, and is responsible for post-convalescent medical and social follow-up.

Since the convalescent period is an incident in the complete medical care of the patient, it will probably continue to be the practice for the clinic or hospital to keep the patient under care during his convalescence. The need for social service in convalescent homes, therefore, is limited, provided the medical agencies using convalescent homes maintain an adequate social

[17] Corwin, E. H. L., The Hospital Situation in Greater New York. New York, G. P. Putnam's Sons, 1924, p. 288.

service personnel. Only in homes that care for patients over a period of months or years, would it be necessary to have a social service staff in order to keep in active contact with the patient's family and to build up the resources for his readjustment after convalescence.

ADEQUACY OF FACILITIES

Among the outstanding lacks in convalescent care at the time of the census were facilities for men and for Negroes, particularly for the adolescent Negro boy. Burke Foundation, on February 1, 1930, made an attempt to correct the shortage of beds for men by increasing its total facilities by 15 beds and by so rearranging its facilities as to care for 210 men instead of 140 formerly cared for, and to care for 105 women instead of 160 formerly cared for. It has also made 15 beds recently added available for use by either men or women as the demand arises. In addition, it has for a number of years been appropriating $10,000 annually for the work of the New York Urban League in securing convalescent care in boarding homes for Negroes. At the present time, the New York Urban League has acquired a farm house overlooking the Hudson about thirty-five miles from New York City, which it plans to convert into a convalescent home as soon as money for the project can be raised.[18]

The necessity for homes for children with chronic asthma is being urged by Mt. Sinai Hospital, where special studies have been made of this condition in children. "In the light of this experience, it would appear that the most logical and humane solution would be the creation of homes especially adapted to the needs of this type of asthmatic child. The social service department of Mount Sinai Hospital has recognized this need and has recommended the establishment of such a home to take care of those children attending the allergy clinic who are in need of environmental treatment. . . . Until newer methods of treatment are advanced which will successfully control or free this group of children from asthma, the establishment of a 'home' where a child with chronic refractory asthma can be kept for at least six months is regarded as a humane, urgent, and economic necessity as well as a therapeutic measure of definite value."[19] A Sub-committee of the Advisory Committee on Convalescent Care of the United Hospital Fund submitted a report, in 1930, advocating the establishment of such homes, one for children and one for adults.[20]

The Convalescence Service of the Hospital Information and Service Bureau estimates that additional beds are needed for cardiacs of all ages; for adults needing special diets, such as those with nephritis or diabetes; for women and boys and girls with an asthmatic condition; for boys and girls

[18] Convalescent Need for Negroes in New York, The New York Urban League, September, 1931.

[19] Peshkin, Murray M., M.D., Asthma in Children. IX. Role of Environment in the Treatment of a Selected Group of Cases: A Plea for a "Home" as a Restorative Measure. Reprinted from the *American Journal of Diseases of Children*, vol. 39, April, 1930, pp. 6; 8.

[20] News Notes: Report of the Sub-committee on Convalescent Care for Asthmatic Patients. *Hospital Social Service*, vol. 21, No. 3, March, 1930, p. 261.

with chorea; and for Negro adults. This conclusion was reached after an analysis of patients referred to the Convalescence Service for convalescent placement and the extent to which vacancies existed for their care. There were no vacancies, either for the types of diseases mentioned above or for acute medical and surgical cases, for nearly a fourth of the boys referred, for a fifth of the men and girls referred and for 11 per cent of the women referred.[21]

In regard to cardiac convalescent facilities, the Committee on Convalescent Care of the Heart Committee has not yet arrived at a conclusion as to the value of the type of care now being given. It is studying the whole question and will not make recommendations for extension of facilities until it also has recommendations as to the type of post-hospital care required for cardiac children. Its decision to coöperate in the medical direction of the new Irvington House, which will function to some extent as a preventorium for rheumatic fever sufferers, is a step in the movement to give children susceptible to rheumatic fever a similar type of care to that which is given to children susceptible to tuberculosis.

The cardiac facilities for boys have recently been increased by Reed Farm of 20 beds, which in November, 1931 was given over to the care of cardiac boys from ten to sixteen years of age, both white and colored.

The facilities now existing for various types of convalescence are inadequate partly because of the inflexibility of admission requirements and partly also because of the inadequate standards of care in some homes. Each home decides for itself what age groups and which sex it will accept. It is possible that there are enough beds to meet the demand if the homes were able to operate flexibly. However, there is likely to be a surplus of beds for younger girls together with an acute shortage for adolescent boys, and an excess of beds for women together with a shortage of beds for men. An extension in other homes of Burke Foundation's policy to use some of its beds for either men or women as the demand arises would extend facilities without further capital expenditure.

Furthermore, some homes are more freely used by social agencies than others because the agencies have learned from experience that their patients convalesce more successfully in some homes than in others. The general acceptance of the minimum standards already laid down for convalescent homes would increase the present effective bed capacity.

A further need that has been stressed is for municipal convalescent facilities. Dr. Adrian V. S. Lambert, chairman of the Convalescent Section of the Welfare Council and of the Convalescence Service of the Hospital Information and Service Bureau has repeatedly pointed out this need.[22] At present there are no municipal facilities except a semi-official convalescent home of 60 beds for vaginitis. The city government has heretofore maintained that the need for facilities for the acutely ill has been too pressing to permit

[21] Clarke, Grace M., The Convalescent Field in Greater New York. *Hospital Social Service*, vol. 25, No. 1, January, 1932, pp. 65–70.
[22] Minutes of Quarterly Meeting of the New York City Visiting Committee, April 15, 1931, and of the Annual Meeting, December 3, 1931.

a development of convalescent facilities, particularly in view of the fact that there had never been an acute shortage of private facilities, which are open to patients in municipal hospitals. This contention is to some extent borne out by this study, which has found a great need for additional municipal facilities for the care of chronic patients. If the city should develop convalescent facilities before more adequate provision is made for the chronic sick, it would be difficult to keep the new institution from being used to a great extent for chronic service. The New York City Visiting Committee has a committee that is studying the various aspects of the problem of municipal convalescent facilities, with a view to making a recommendation to the municipal Department of Hospitals on the advisability of establishing a convalescent home.

Another lack in the convalescent field, which affects both chronic and acute patients who need care, is a central admissions bureau for the convalescent homes. Dr. Adrian V. S. Lambert, in the address just referred to, outlined a plan for a central admissions bureau that should both facilitate the use of homes by a quicker filling up of vacancies and a decrease of improper placements and also reduce the cost of examinations for admission. Without such a system, it is difficult either to use convalescent homes as fully as possible or to measure exactly what the needs are.

SUMMARY

1. The Convalescence Service of the United Hospital Fund serves as a central information bureau on convalescent facilities. Its executive committee is also the executive committee of the Section on Convalescent Care of the Health Division of the Welfare Council, which is the coördinating agency for convalescent work.

2. The minimum standards for convalescent homes adopted by the above agencies have not yet been put into effect in all homes.

3. The cost of convalescent care is less than half the cost of hospital ward care.

4. All special cardiac and orthopedic homes were included in the study and a sample of general convalescent homes, consisting of 12 homes having 40 per cent of the total bed capacity of general convalescent homes.

5. The outstanding lacks in convalescent care in New York City judged by the demands for this service are: facilities for Negroes, particularly adolescent boys; for men; for persons of all ages with cardiac disorders; for adults needing special diets; and for persons convalescing from asthma or chorea.

6. A central admission bureau would facilitate a more complete use of the convalescent homes and would also decrease the cost of admission examinations.

7. The question of a need for municipal convalescent facilities has been raised by the Advisory Committee on Convalescence of the United Hospital Fund, and is being studied by a special committee of the New York City Visiting Committee. One of the problems involved is whether in the development of municipal facilities, the needs of chronic patients should take precedence over the needs of convalescents.

8. The inadequacy of chronic facilities causes a demand for convalescent facilities and, to some extent at least, a misuse of the general convalescent homes.

CHAPTER 5

Cardiac After-Care Services

DEVELOPMENT OF AFTER-CARE SERVICES

RECOGNITION of the importance of controlling heart disease among children led to the organization of after-care services to fill the gaps in social service and follow-up work in this field. At the time of the study, these agencies in New York City included the Cardiac Vocational Guidance Service of the New York Tuberculosis and Health Association and the after-care services of the cardiac convalescent homes,[1] the most extensive of which is the After-Care Committee of Irvington House.

The first organized work of this kind was begun in 1920, when the Public Education Association formed its Cardiac Vocational Guidance Committee, in order to guide and supervise the vocational training and placement of children with heart defects and as an integral part of its purpose "to compile and study data collected from this work, with the hope of securing new scientific material for future work with children." Children were referred for vocational guidance by cardiac clinics and convalescent homes, by the Board of Education when children in school were found to have heart defects, and by the Board of Health whenever children were refused working papers because of heart disease. Children under the care of the Vocational Guidance Service were required to be also under the care of a recognized cardiac clinic; and much of the agency's effort was employed in keeping children under clinic supervision.

The Cardiac Vocational Guidance Service, between 1924 and 1927, also supervised special trade classes established by the Board of Education. These classes were given up in 1927 on recommendation of the Guidance Service, which found that cardiac children could safely attend the regular trade schools provided by the Board of Education. In the same year, the Public Education Association transferred its vocational guidance work to the New York Tuberculosis and Health Association; and at the end of 1930 the work of the Vocational Guidance Service was discontinued, because the conclusion had been reached that cardiac children do not require a type of vocational service different from that required for other children. The recommendation was made to the Board of Education that a sufficient number of vocational counsellors should be provided in the public schools to meet the needs of all children; in which case the special needs of cardiac children would be covered.

Irvington House since its opening in 1920 has had an After-Care Committee primarily for follow-up of the cardiac child after convalescence. Every effort is made to keep the child under clinic care and to make the records useful as a contribution to research in the cardiac field. The medical

[1] For discussion of homes for children with cardiac disease, see Chapter 4 and also vol. 1, Chapter 3, The Special Problems of Some Main Groups of Chronic Diseases, p. 152.

reports secured semi-annually from the clinic record of each child are used by the Research Service of the Heart Committee of the New York Tuberculosis and Health Association in its studies of heart disease. In 1928, a special arrangement was made for examination by a private physician of all children whom it was impossible to keep in attendance at a clinic. Since that time this non-clinic group has been kept under supervision and attempts have been made to get a physical examination every six months. In 1931, when the work of the Cardiac Vocational Guidance Service had been given up and the Board of Education had increased its vocational counsellors by only five, instead of the additional fifteen recommended by the Vocational Guidance Service and other social agencies, the After-Care Committee of Irvington House set up such a service for children under its care. This is definitely regarded as a temporary measure to be discontinued as soon as the service in the public schools is adequate.

In addition to these two after-care services, Martine Farm and Nichols Cottage, both under the same management, and Pelham Home, to some extent, follow up the children who have received convalescent care and make an effort to bring them back to the clinic if they fail in their attendance.

In 1928, when the census of chronic illness was made, children were being referred to the Cardiac Vocational Guidance Service from various sources. All cardiac convalescent homes discharging children thirteen years of age or over and the social service departments of the 54 cardiac clinics referred boys and girls in order that the courses selected in school or the work at which they were employed might be approved or suggestions for change might be made. The Department of Health also referred children to whom working papers were denied because of organic heart disease. Often these children had not previously known of their cardiac condition and had to be referred to a cardiac clinic. The boy or girl who has once planned to leave school, whether on account of a dislike of school or of financial pressure at home, is apt to be particularly difficult to guide when his handicapped physical condition necessitates a change in his plans. Every effort was made to readjust the school life of such children.

The Board of Child Welfare has called attention to the problem of further schooling for cardiac children when they become of working age but are unable to work: "The prevalence of heart disease among the children has been noted and calls attention to the importance of education beyond the elementary grade for this group. As such children cannot become wage-earners when at the age of sixteen, the allowance has been discontinued, the loss of income in the home is the cause of great distress. Frequently scholarships are secured but, unfortunately, are not always available. This problem is a serious one and is recommended to the consideration of the Board."[2] It should be possible to plan for these children in advance, before they reach the working age. If they get to the point of applying for working papers, they and their families are faced with disappointment and the necessity for a complete readjustment of their ideas for the future.

[2] The Board of Child Welfare of the City of New York, Thirteenth Annual Report, 1928, p. 10.

THE CENSUS IN AFTER-CARE SERVICES

The after-care services of the cardiac convalescent homes and the Cardiac Vocational Guidance Service reported 878 children and young persons under twenty-five years of age in the census of the chronic sick, or 4 per cent of the total number of chronically ill persons in the study.[3] Ninety-five per cent of the 878 children were suffering from cardiac diseases and 5 per cent were suffering from chorea, rheumatism, or orthopedic disorders. Fifty-three per cent were under sixteen years of age and the remainder were between sixteen and twenty-five years of age. Two thirds were of working age, that is, fourteen years or older.

A large proportion of the patients under the care of cardiac after-care services had suffered from their disease for a long time. In 59 per cent, the onset of the disease had occurred at least five years earlier. Of all the patients under forty years of age in the whole census, 50 per cent had been sick so long.

Nearly all of these patients had had institutional care, nearly half of them at least once. Over a fifth had been three or more times in an institution because of their cardiac condition. The average number of admissions was nearly two, only a little lower than the average for all the chronic sick in the census, which was over two per patient.

The length of time since the patient had first had care in an institution for his condition was much shorter for this group than for other patients in the census. Of the children, 8 per cent had been in an institution at least five years earlier; and in the total census, 29 per cent of the children had had institutional care at least five years earlier. Among the younger adults, 26 per cent in after-care agencies and 33 per cent in the total census had been in an institution at least five years earlier; but only 12 per cent of those in after-care agencies had first been institutionalized within the year compared with a third in the total census.

[3] The organizations working with cardiac patients were asked to report only persons whose cardiac disability was sufficient to restrict their physical activity, or those falling within the cardiac classifications, IIa, IIb, and III, among the following five groupings approved by the American Heart Association and used in cardiac clinics to indicate the degree of incapacity of each patient:

CLASS I
    Patients with organic heart disease, able to carry on ordinary physical activity without discomfort.

CLASS II
    Patients with organic heart disease, unable to carry on ordinary physical activity without discomfort; (a) activity slightly limited; (b) activity greatly limited.

CLASS III
    Patients with organic heart disease and with symptoms or signs of heart failure when at rest, unable to carry on any physical activity without discomfort.

CLASS E
    Patients with abnormal signs or symptoms not believed to be due to organic disease.

CLASS F
    Patients without circulatory disease, but considered "potential" because of the presence or history of an etiologic factor which might cause cardiac disease.

(The above classification is taken from A Nomenclature for Cardiac Diagnosis, Approved by the American Heart Association, adopted, 1923. Distributed by the Heart Committee of the New York Tuberculosis and Health Association.)

The patients of after-care agencies naturally were almost all clinic patients. Only 15 required hospital care and of these 11 were getting clinic care. Of those who needed clinic care, about 1 per cent were getting a less skilled type of care. Less than 3 per cent, therefore, were getting unsuitable care. Another 6 per cent had unsuitable homes; and for a large number whose home care was reported to be satisfactory, a full report of home conditions was not secured. All but 2 per cent of these patients were at home.

PRESENT STATUS OF AFTER-CARE SERVICES

Since the special cardiac after-care services have grown up largely because of the inability of already existing agencies to provide complete service for cardiac children, they do not expect to develop their services further. Vocational guidance for cardiac children is not now considered a specialized service, but rather a specialized function within a general service for all public school children. What is being done in this field for cardiac children is merely by way of protecting one special group from the consequences of inadequate public provision in the schools.

The same is true to some extent of the after-care services of convalescent homes. Cardiac and other convalescent homes coöperate with agencies who refer patients to them for convalescence on the principle that the patient during his convalescence shall remain under the medical and social care of the sending agency. If this were carried out, there would be no reason why the convalescent home should set up a service either for returning delinquents to clinics or for getting medical care for those who are unable or unwilling to attend clinics. But medical agencies at the present time do not have sufficient social service personnel to do thorough follow-up work nor sufficient evening clinics to take care of the working child or adult. If the medical agencies extended their service over the post-convalescent period, the need for after-care service by convalescent homes would no longer exist.

CHAPTER 6

The Care of the Chronic Sick by Nursing Services

SECTION A

THE CHRONIC SICK UNDER THE CARE OF NURSING SERVICES

THE RELATION OF CHRONIC ILLNESS TO THE WORK OF THESE AGENCIES

THE sick cared for at home greatly outnumber those treated in hospitals. It is estimated, on the basis of facts disclosed by sickness surveys, that about 16 per cent of all cases of incapacitating illness in New York City are hospitalized.[1] In this city, therefore, where approximately 150,000 persons are disabled by illness at any one time,[2] probably over 125,000 persons are sick at home at any one time. A large proportion of them are treated by private physicians and nursed by relatives or private nurses; but many are dependent upon visiting nurse service.

The proportion of all the sick who need the care of a visiting nurse cannot be estimated at the present time with any degree of accuracy. An estimate of nursing service needed in cities with a population of 50,000 persons showed that one visiting nurse was needed for every 5,000 persons of the population to give bedside care to the sick.[3] If the same standard were applicable in New York, 1,200 nurses would be required for the care of the sick. However, this standard is not a reliable basis for estimating the needs of New York, as many conditions that affect the situation are different in so large a city.

The nurses giving some form of nursing care in the home of the patient in this city numbered nearly 700 at the time of the study, in 1928.[4] (See also p. 223.) This number includes the visiting nurse, who is a trained public health nurse giving complete nursing service—both educational and bedside nursing; the public health nurse doing only educational work; and the practical nurse giving only bedside care. In addition to the nurses who care for the sick in the community, some whose duties are largely educational health work, those who supervise orthopedic patients, and those engaged in maternity service are included in the above figure.

The census of the chronic sick in the care of medical and social agencies

[1] Davis, Michael M., Clinics, Hospitals and Health Centers. New York, Harper and Brothers, 1927, p. 6.
[2] Davis, Michael M., and Jarrett, Mary C., A Health Inventory of New York City: A Study of the Volume and Distribution of Health Services in the Five Boroughs. The Welfare Council of New York City, 1929, p. 1.
[3] Community Health Organization: Revised Plans for Communities of 100,000 and 50,000 and a New Plan for 30,000 Population, edited by Ira V. Hiscock. American Health Congress Series, vol. 6, Part 4, American Public Health Association, 1927, pp. 85–86.
[4] New York City, early in 1931, has between 1,500 and 1,600 nurses engaged in all forms of home visiting service including health service and care of the sick, approximately two fifths from the Department of Health and the remainder from voluntary agencies.

shows that the community nursing agencies are bearing a large part of the responsibility for the care of chronic illness. The 6,400 patients found under the care of nursing services,[5] represent over 30 per cent of all patients in the entire census.

Many chronic patients requiring skilled nursing can be suitably cared for at home provided that regular visits from a nurse can be assured; otherwise, expensive hospital care must be provided, possibly over a long period. However, the chief duty of the nurse is to respond to calls for assistance in acute and dangerous illness. In periods of seasonal epidemics, the professional ethics of the nurse demand that she shall attend the acute cases of illness at the shortest possible notice. She is then obliged to lengthen the interval between visits to patients in a less acute condition. Members of the family or neighbors are called in to relieve her of whatever tasks she can be spared. The nurse continues supervision of such patients and instructs the family or neighbors in the care of the patient. This emergency situation may grow to be a permanent arrangement. The question whether the services of the nurse can be dispensed with in a particular case may in this way be decided by expediency rather than by the needs of the patient. The fact that there is no hope of complete recovery or even marked improvement for many of these chronic patients inevitably causes their needs to be subordinated to the demands of the acutely ill.

There is no clear policy in regard to the types of advanced illness that are suitable for home nursing care and those that require institutional care. There is a difference of opinion, for example, among cancer specialists on the question of advisability of home care for advanced cancer cases. Some physicians think that the patient not only cannot be given suitable care at home unless a nurse is in constant attendance, but also that the presence of such a patient in an incommodious home is too great a hardship for the family. Other physicians believe that through modern methods of treatment, it is possible even in very poor homes to arrange for suitable care, with the help of a visiting nurse and that both patient and family are apt to be happier than they would be if the patient were sent to a hospital for chronic diseases. Particularly with reference to patients who no longer require medical treatment but need daily or frequent attention, either from a nurse or from a trained attendant, there is no settled policy as to whether a community should make provision for care at home or in an institution.

The majority of orthopedic patients after discharge from an institution need further treatment and nursing supervision over a long period. It is neither humane nor efficient to give a patient the benefit of the skill of an orthopedic surgeon and then allow him to relapse into his former condition for lack of proper supervision. The reëducation of muscles is often the most important part of the cure. Exercises must be regular if permanent benefit is to be expected, and they must also be planned especially for the individual. The orthopedic nursing services are also called upon to meet a

[5] This figure includes sixty-eight patients reported by two visiting doctor services of North Eastern Dispensary and Northern Dispensary of New York City. Both of these services refer outdoor medical cases needing nursing care to the Henry Street Visiting Nurse Service.

variety of needs not directly connected with medical or nursing care, such as special educational services, vocational guidance, and transportation. The effectiveness of any nursing organization dealing with orthopedic patients depends, therefore, partly upon other related activities over which it may have no control.

The amount of service that nursing agencies devote to the chronic sick is affected by the expansion of nursing service in the field of maternity work and the extensive educational programs conducted by health agencies, in which the public health nurse is an indispensable agent. The educational work of nursing agencies has a direct relation to the prevention and mitigation of chronic illness; but it also reduces the amount of service that can be given to nursing the chronic sick.

One of the difficulties that the public health nurse meets in giving care to the chronic sick in their homes is that often the service required is mainly in the nature of housework rather than nursing. The nurse's visits may be essential for some special service or for general supervision of the patient's care, but in addition to the service that is properly hers, there is often much to be done in the way of cleaning or cooking. This the nurse cannot attend to without neglecting her own duties and depriving other patients of skilled nursing care. This situation arises particularly among patients who live alone; but it occurs also among those living with families in which all of the adult members must work in order to contribute to the family income. The time of a visiting nurse after years of expensive training is too valuable to be absorbed by household services.

This kind of help can be given by a visiting houseworker or a practical nurse, who has been selected and trained for this purpose. There is no clear distinction between the duties of these two types of worker. On the whole, patients who require mainly personal attention because of their infirmities will need the practical nurse, and those who require mainly help with household tasks that they are not able to perform will need the visiting houseworker.

The term "visiting houseworker" is to be distinguished from the term "visiting housekeeper." The latter "is most commonly used to designate workers who have had training in home economics and give demonstration instruction, chiefly in the home, in cooking and other household operations and in budgeting and household management."[6] Her services are usually required for the education of an incompetent or ignorant housewife, regardless of whether there is a chronic invalid in the family. Although, in some instances, this service may be of value in a household in which it is necessary to make readjustments because a member of the family has become chronically ill, visiting housekeeper service is intended primarily for educational rather than for custodial purposes; and it is not directly related to the care of the chronically ill. However, some organizations prefer to use the term "visiting housekeeper" for the capable but untrained woman engaged

[6] Nesbitt, Florence, Visiting Housekeepers and Home Economists. In The Social Work Year Book, 1929. New York, Russell Sage Foundation, 1930, p. 465.

to go to a family daily and keep house in the mother's place during the latter's absence or illness.

Many families are able to pay moderate charges for both the nursing and the housework necessary to insure treatment and comfort for the chronic invalid. They do not wish to receive these services as charitable assistance, and yet they cannot afford the usual private rates. The Henry Street Visiting Nurse Service began in 1926 to offer hourly nursing service at a moderate cost. (See p. 228.) A similar service was established in Brooklyn in 1928, as a branch of the regular service of the Nurses' Official Registry of Brooklyn. A visiting housekeeper service has been conducted by the Jewish Social Service Association for several years to provide competent women to care for homes in which there are children if the mother is bedridden or absent through illness or for any other reason. (See also pp. 273–274.)

By a recent ruling of the Commissioner of Licenses, adopted upon the recommendation of the special committee on Nursing of the Medical Society of the County of New York, five classes of nurses are created for home nursing service: "registered nurses (as under present law); non-registered nurses (from non-registered schools, with two years' hospital training and a diploma); trained state hospital nurses (as under present law); undergraduates (nine months' hospital training), or trained attendants (care from the State); and practical nurses (all miscellaneous nurses)."[7]

In several other communities, household help and attendant nursing services have been organized in various ways. The first organization in the country to train attendant nurses to relieve graduate visiting nurses when possible was the Mutual Aid Association of Brattleboro, Vermont, over thirty years ago, prompted by the need for such assistance among families of moderate means in cases of illness not requiring the services of a trained nurse. "For such patients it was not only economical but also often an essential part of the healing process that the household machinery should run continuously and smoothly."[8] The service is for mildly ill, convalescent and chronic patients; and the maternity service is limited to postpartum care. The Household Nursing Association in Boston conducts a training school for attendant nurses. The service is intended for families able to pay moderate rates for private service for chronic or mildly ill patients. The care of the home is considered to be as important a part of the duty of the attendant nurse as the care of the patient. In the first six weeks of the course, the aim is to teach the pupil household management including the buying and cooking of food for the patient and family. She then goes to a hospital for a year of training in bedside nursing. Six months of supervised field duty follow the hospital training during which time

[7] *Better Times Weekly Welfare Bulletin,* The Welfare Council of New York City, vol. 13, No. 27, April 4, 1932, p. 3.

[8] Peebles, Allon and McDermott, Valeria D., Nursing Services and Insurance for Medical Care in Brattleboro, Vermont: A Study of the Activities of the Thomas Thompson Trust, with an Evaluation of the Nursing Program by Violet H. Hodgson, and Katherine Tucker. Publications of The Committee on the Costs of Medical Care: No. 17, Chicago, 1932, p. 14.

the attendant nurse is placed on private cases and collects her own wages of $21 a week.

The administrative control of such services presents difficulties. Individual attendant nurses working independently may be called upon by the family physician to nurse in forms of illness for the care of which their training has not fitted them. Some evidence was found in Brattleboro that "the attendant is giving service to cases which call for more preparation and a higher degree of skill than her qualifications warrant."[9]

The community nursing organizations of the city are fully aware of their difficulties in providing regular and adequate nursing service for chronically ill persons. The Committee on Public Health Nursing of the Welfare Council's Section on Health Administration and Education, in April, 1928, drew up the following statement of some of the problems involved in caring for the chronic sick:

"1. Because of the increased demand for the services of trained visiting nurses for acutely ill patients during certain seasons of the year, the chronic sick do not receive adequate care. Could a supplementary group of workers be developed to care for chronically ill patients who do not require skilled care?

"2. Many chronically ill patients do not receive adequate care in their homes because the only persons who might care for them are the breadwinners. Would it not be as economical to subsidize the breadwinner's earnings or to pay for a part-time attendant, and so keep the patient at home, as to pay the cost of a hospital bed?

"3. Many chronically ill patients refuse institutional care for various good reasons. Could a plan be devised to board out chronic patients in private homes?

"4. Physicians sometimes order special treatment for this type of patient, such as massage, electric treatments, and baking. What provision could be made so that these patients might secure such treatments through temporary hospitalization or through workers sent out from the hospital to their homes?"

In regard to the first question, the possible need for a service of trained attendants or houseworkers to relieve visiting nurses, the study has shown that, in all probability, about 10 per cent of the adults with chronic illness under the care of nursing agencies, or about 200 persons, could have been adequately cared for at home by workers much less skilled than the trained visiting nurse. In the census in other groups of agencies, approximately 100 additional persons were found, needing custodial care, for whom the best solution for adequate care was probably the services of a practical nurse or visiting houseworker in the home. About two thirds of these 300 persons were receiving skilled nursing care although they needed only attendant care. The remainder were receiving inadequate care or were in unsuitable homes. In addition, among about 700 patients in the whole census who were not being properly cared for at home but did not need hospital care, there were no doubt many for whom the alternative for

[9] *Ibid.*, p. 14.

institutional care would have been the services of a visiting houseworker. There are no doubt others not known to welfare agencies who are also in need of this type of service.

In considering the second question, whether it would be more economical to provide assistance in the home than to care for the patient in a hospital, the cost of custodial care in a chronic hospital must be compared with the cost of attendant care by a trained attendant under supervision of a nursing agency. The daily cost per person in the custodial section of Montefiore Hospital is estimated to be about $2.50. If $5.00 a day is regarded as reasonable compensation for a trained attendant or visiting houseworker, patients needing less than four hours of service daily can be cared for at home less expensively from the standpoint of the welfare agencies than in an institution, if the family is otherwise able to provide for the patient's needs.

The advisability of boarding-out chronic patients in private homes, the third question, depends largely upon the character of the nursing or boarding homes available for this purpose. The Department of Hospitals licenses nursing homes in one or two family houses but not in multiple dwellings. At least one family service agency has made a practice of boarding from six to eight of its infirm aged clients in the home of a nurse and others in the home of another capable woman. The nursing agencies had under care about 150 persons in homes not suitable for their care who needed only custodial care, which could have been given in a private nursing home. Of about 100 persons who needed to be in institutions for non-medical reasons, two thirds reported their opposition to institutional care as the reason for not being in an institution. Provision for many in these two groups could no doubt have been made in this way, if facilities existed for boarding-out. The cost of board in a nursing home runs as low as $15.00, although it varies with the standard of living as well as the amount of care that the patient requires. It may not be more than the minimum rate in a well-equipped custodial institution.

To answer the fourth question, concerning the possibility of giving special treatments in patients' homes or through temporary hospitalization, it would be necessary to study the requirements of individual patients with reference to the periods for which treatment is required and the location of the hospitals from which it can be obtained, as well as the number and geographical distribution of patients needing such treatments. Opportunities for temporary hospitalization for this purpose would be increased if the chronic patients found by the census in general hospitals could be cared for in chronic hospitals. Beds that might be used for chronic patients needing treatment for a short time are occupied for long periods by patients who belong in a hospital for chronic diseases. About 200 of the patients found in general hospitals needed only custodial care, and probably many of them could have been cared for at home if sufficient home nursing facilities for chronic patients had been available, thereby releasing additional beds for temporary hospitalization.

CHRONICALLY ILL PERSONS UNDER CARE

The census found 6,401 chronic patients under the care of nursing serv-ices, which is 31 per cent of those reported by all agencies. Of this number, 404 persons were reported as being under the care of a family service agency as well as of a nursing agency. These were nearly all clients of the Association for Improving the Condition of the Poor receiving service from both the nursing and the family service departments of this agency; and in tabulations of the total number of persons in the census, these patients

TABLE 40

CHRONIC PATIENTS OF NURSING SERVICES CLASSIFIED BY
RACE AND SEX, EACH AGE GROUP

Race and sex	Total	AGE GROUP					
		Under 16	16-39	40-59	60-69	70 and over	Not reported
Total	6,401¹	4,318	945	544	284	264	46
Male	2,994	2,222	406	193	86	69	18
Female	3,404	2,095	539	350	198	195	27
White	5,943	4,040	848	501	275	238	41
Male	2,785	2,078	365	180	82	62	18
Female	3,158	1,962	483	321	193	176	23
Negro	334	220	60	30	4	17	3
Male	146	114	20	8	0	4	0
Female	188	106	40	22	4	13	3
Not reported	124¹	58	37	13	5	9	2
Male	63	30	21	5	4	3	0
Female	58	27	16	7	1	6	1

¹ Includes three for whom sex was not reported.

were attributed to the nursing department. The remaining 149 patients, for whom nursing services shared the responsibility with other agencies were distributed as follows: more than half, with convalescent homes; over a third, with hospitals; and the remainder, with after-care agencies, private homes for aged, or agencies for sheltered work.

Age, Sex, and Race

Over three fourths of the chronically ill reported by nursing agencies were in the period of childhood or youth. Over two thirds (68 per cent) were children under sixteen years of age, over four fifths of whom had some form of orthopedic difficulty. Fifteen per cent were between the ages of sixteen and forty years, over half of whom were under twenty-one years of age. Twice as many persons were found between forty and sixty years of age as between sixty and seventy years of age. The number of persons seventy years of age and over was somewhat smaller than the number of those between sixty and seventy years of age. The percentage of persons in each age period is shown in Chart 11.

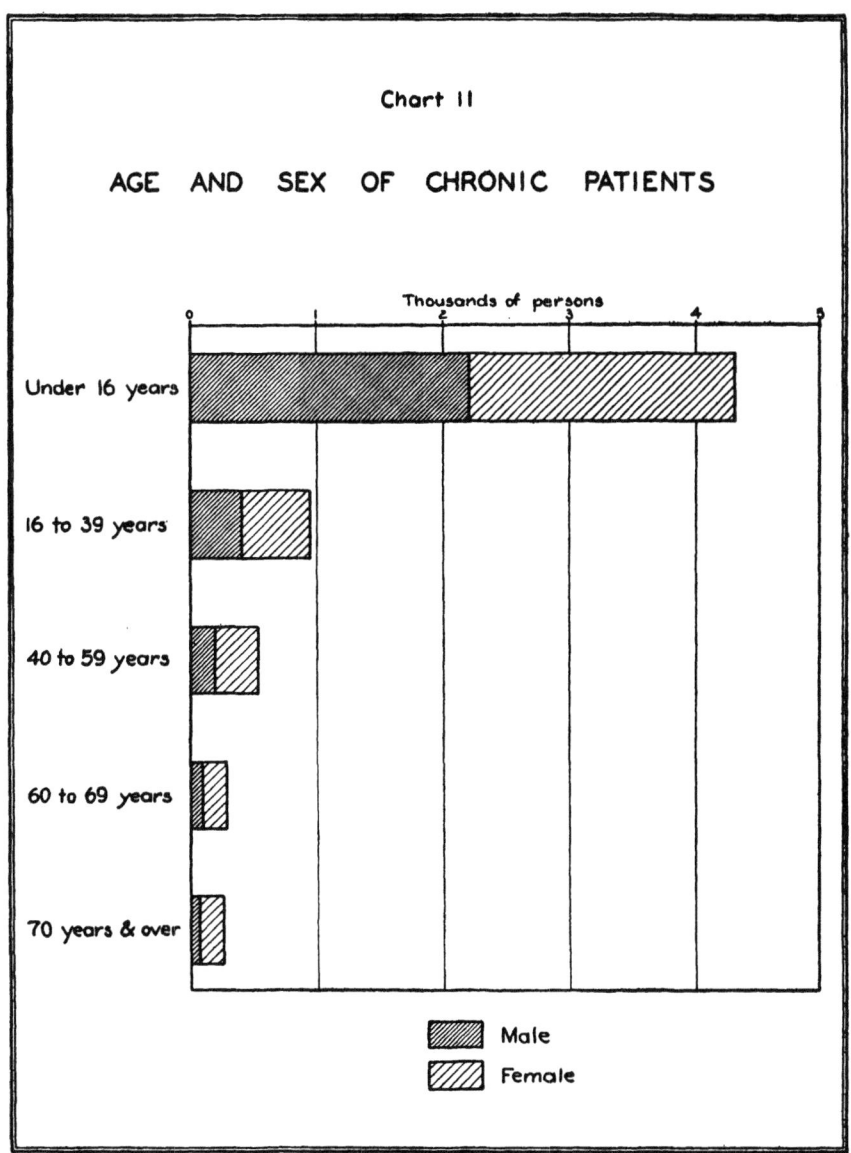

Chart 11

AGE AND SEX OF CHRONIC PATIENTS

Among the 4,300 children, there were about 100 more boys than girls. In the older ages, there were about 500 more women than men. Among both white persons and Negroes, who were 5 per cent of the whole number, there were more males among the children and more females among the adults, as seen in Table 40 above.

Residence

Somewhat less than half of the chronic patients reported by the nursing agencies were Manhattan residents. Less than a fourth came from the Bronx and less than a fifth from Brooklyn. Seven per cent came from Queens and less than 1 per cent from Richmond. Over 4 per cent lived outside of New York City, most of whom were persons from neighboring states attending the clinic of Memorial Hospital for the Treatment of Cancer or the New York Orthopedic Hospital's out-patient department for observation, corrective exercises, or dressings. The percentage of patients residing in each borough in relation to the percentage of the population in the borough is shown in Table 41.

TABLE 41

NUMBER AND PERCENTAGE DISTRIBUTION OF CHRONIC PATIENTS OF NURSING
SERVICES AMONG THE DIFFERENT BOROUGHS, IN RELATION TO POPULATION

Residence	Patients		Per cent of population[1]
	Number	Per cent	
Total	6,401	100.0	100.0
Manhattan	2,940	45.9	28.9
Bronx	1,479	23.1	17.5
Brooklyn	1,202	18.7	36.8
Queens	443	6.9	14.5
Richmond	36	0.6	2.3
New York City—borough unknown	17	0.3	. . . . .
Other parts of New York State	157	2.5	. . . . .
Outside of New York State	116	1.8	. . . . .
Not reported	11	0.2	. . . . .

[1] Estimates of the United States Bureau of the Census for July 1, 1928, based upon the Census of 1930.

Both Manhattan and the Bronx have a much higher percentage of the patients than of the population, especially the former borough. In Brooklyn, on the contrary, the percentage of patients receiving this type of care is only half as large as the borough's percentage of the population; and in the other two boroughs it is less than half.

Agencies extending their service to all boroughs reported 29 per cent of the patients. (See Table 42.) Those covering Manhattan, the Bronx, and in one instance Richmond reported 42 per cent. Those limiting their service to Manhattan reported 12.8 per cent; to Brooklyn, 12 per cent; to Queens, 4 per cent.

Diseases

The children, constituting 68 per cent of all the chronic patients of nursing agencies, were reported mainly by the special orthopedic nursing services. Four fifths of all the children under sixteen years of age reported by nursing services were suffering from orthopedic diseases; so that over half of the patients of these agencies were children with orthopedic difficulties. Chart 12 shows the main forms of disease found among children and adults.

TABLE 42

CHRONIC PATIENTS REPORTED BY NURSING SERVICES IN THE DIFFERENT BOROUGHS

Borough served	Number	Per cent
Total	6,401	100.0
Manhattan	776	12.1
Brooklyn	817	12.8
Queens	256	4.0
Manhattan and Bronx	2,543	39.7
Manhattan, Bronx and Richmond	155	2.4
All boroughs	1,854	29.0

Poliomyelitis was the cause of one half of the orthopedic conditions among the children. Nearly 10 per cent of the children had non-pulmonary tuberculosis; 8.5 per cent, spinal cord diseases; 5 per cent, heart disease. Eight per cent with rickets were reported mainly by the Bureau of Educational Nursing of the Association for Improving the Condition of the Poor, which was carrying on special preventive work for children with this condition at the time of the census. Other diseases were found among the children in smaller numbers. The diagnoses reported for persons of different ages are given in Appendix Table 7.

The diagnosis of over one third of the younger adults was poliomyelitis. Other forms of disease found most frequently among the adults were cancer, rheumatism and arthritis, circulatory diseases, paralysis, and fractures. A small number of ill-defined diagnoses were reported in each age group except the aged. Five persons were reported whose condition was undiagnosed.

Nearly a third of all patients with cancer in the census were reported by nursing agencies. Nearly a third of all the fractures were reported by the nursing agencies. Since a third of all persons in the census were reported by nursing agencies, these two conditions occurred among their patients with the same frequency as in the whole group. Patients with rheumatism and arthritis were a fifth and patients with diseases of the nervous system were over a fifth of all those suffering from these conditions.

Mental Abnormality

The nursing agencies reported the mental condition of 90 per cent of their patients. No other group of agencies reported this information for

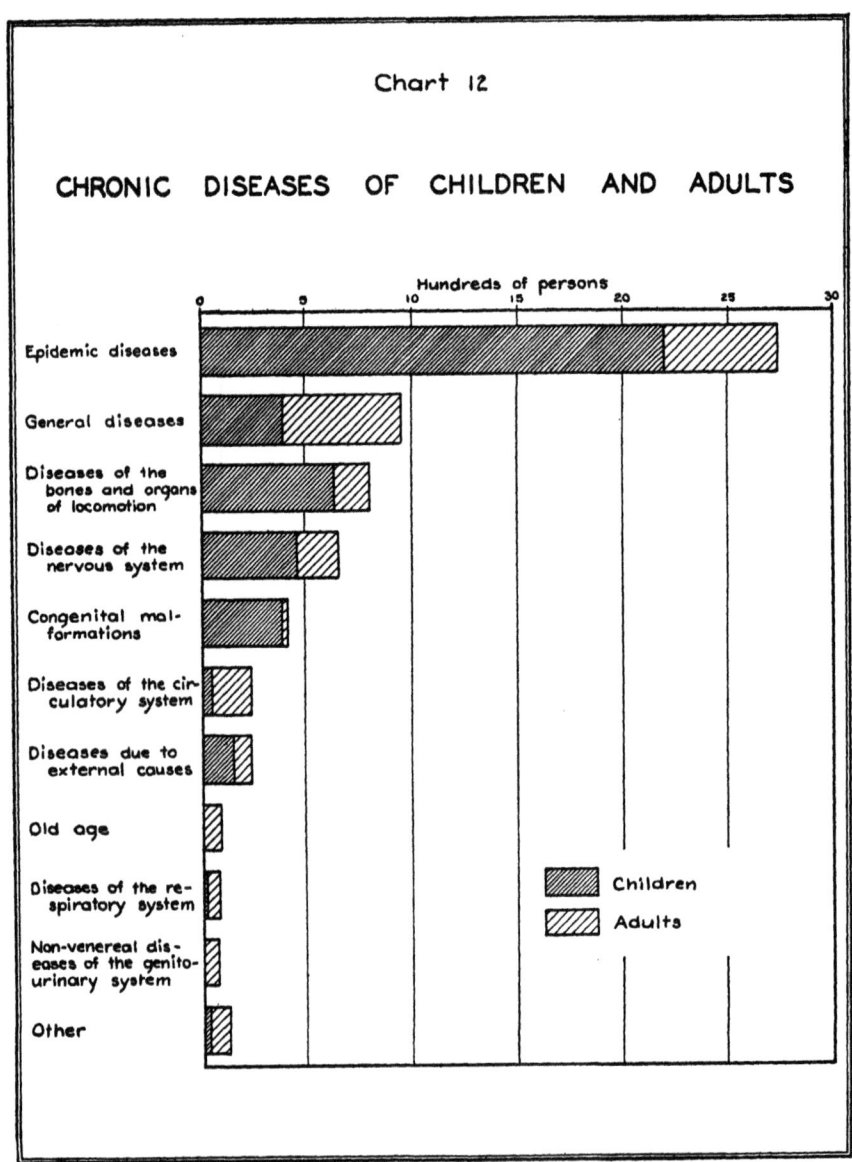

so large a percentage of patients. The proportion of persons reported to be mentally abnormal was lower than in any other group of agencies. Some mental abnormality was found in 6.4 per cent of the patients, in over two thirds of whom it was not diagnosed but suspected only. (See Table 43.) This is in contrast to 24.4 per cent of the chronically ill clients of family service agencies reported as having a mental disorder, in two thirds of whom it was not diagnosed but suspected.

TABLE 43

CHRONIC PATIENTS OF NURSING SERVICES CLASSIFIED BY
MENTAL ABNORMALITY, EACH AGE GROUP

Age	Per cent reporting	MENTAL ABNORMALITY			
		Total	None	Diagnosed	Suspected
Total	90.6	5,798[1]	93.6	2.1	4.3
Under 16 years	93.9	4,055	93.7	2.3	4.0
16–39 years	90.5	855	95.6	1.6	2.8
40–59 years	78.1	425	90.1	0.9	9.0
60–69 years	77.1	219	93.6	1.8	4.6
70 years and over . . .	79.2	209	89.5	2.4	8.1
Not reported	35	35	34	0	1

[1] Mental abnormality not reported for 603 persons.

It may be expected that mental difficulties will be noted more frequently by the family social worker, whose understanding of the client's personality is fundamental to her attempt to assist him, than by the nurse, who is responsible primarily for his bodily welfare. Recently some of the more progressive nursing organizations have recognized the importance of mental health in promoting efficiency and happiness by establishing a mental hygiene advisory service within the organization. By this means the nurses learn to recognize some of the signs of unhealthy mental states and to teach some of the principles of mental hygiene.

There was more recognized mental disorder among the chronic patients in middle life than among any other age group except the aged. The lowest percentage of diagnosed cases, however, was in the middle-aged group. The percentage of diagnosed cases was the same among the children and the aged.

Length of Care

The periods of continuous care given by the nursing agency to their chronic patients, as shown in Table 44 for persons of each age group, varied from less than three months, for nearly 12 per cent, to fifteen years or more, for less than 1 per cent. A patient might also have been under the care of the nursing agency for an earlier period not reported.

The probable duration of the future care required is indicated to some extent by the prognosis for recovery from the illness, which was reported for about half of the patients—41 per cent of the children and 66 per cent of the adults. For 26 per cent of the children under sixteen years of age, and also for all young persons under twenty-one years of age, and for 9 per cent of the adults over twenty-one years of age, the prognosis was said to be favorable. A higher percentage of persons with a favorable prognosis was reported by the nursing services than by any other group of agencies.

Some persons in each age group had been under care for a period as long

TABLE 44

CHRONIC PATIENTS OF NURSING SERVICES CLASSIFIED BY
PERIODS OF CARE RECEIVED, EACH AGE GROUP

Period of care received[1]	Total	AGE GROUP					Not reported
		Under 16	16–39	40–59	60–69	70 and over	
Total	6,265	4,280	920	544	284	244	43
Under 3 months	11.6	6.9	12.4	29.9	32.2	25.0	19
3 months and under 1 year	24.4	22.9	22.6	34.6	34.4	25.4	8
1 year and under 2 years	14.6	15.8	10.5	11.8	14.6	15.2	5
2 years and under 3 years	10.2	11.6	7.0	7.3	6.4	9.1	4
3 years and under 4 years	8.6	10.0	6.6	5.5	1.9	7.4	1
4 years and under 5 years	6.7	7.9	4.0	3.7	3.4	5.7	3
5 years and under 10 years	16.6	18.1	20.7	6.5	6.4	10.2	3
10 years and under 15 years	6.8	6.8	13.0	0.6	0.4	0.0	0
15 years and under 20 years	0.4	0.0	2.7	0.2	0.4	2.0	0
20 years and over	0.1	.....	0.5	0.0	0.0	0.0	0

[1] Time under care was not reported for 136 persons.

as ten years. The largest percentage receiving long periods of care was among persons between sixteen and forty years and the next largest was among children, due to the fact that a majority of the patients of these ages were suffering from orthopedic disorders. It is probable that most of the cases of poliomyelitis among the younger adults occurred in the 1916 epidemic. Less than half of the children suffering from poliomyelitis were old enough to have had the disease during this epidemic.

A large proportion of persons between forty and seventy years of age had been under care less than a year. Otherwise no great differences appear in the length of care given to persons of different ages, up to a period of five years. Beyond five years, a decidedly larger proportion of patients under forty years of age is found, owing to the long-time care required by orthopedic patients, who were over two thirds of all patients reported by nursing agencies and over three fourths of those under forty years of age.

Visits Received from Nurses

The number of visits made to the chronic patients during the time they had been under care is shown in Table 45. The home nursing services of hospitals are not included in this tabulation because the nurse sees the patient when he comes to the hospital clinic and, therefore, does not make as many visits to the home as would otherwise be necessary.

A little over a fourth of the patients had received less than 10 visits from the nurse; two thirds had received fewer than 50 visits. Only 14 per cent received 100 or more visits, of whom 50 patients received 300 or more visits, and 6 patients 500 or more visits. A larger proportion of the patients in Manhattan had received 50 or more visits than in other boroughs.

TABLE 45

NURSE'S VISITS TO CHRONIC PATIENTS CLASSIFIED BY BOROUGH

Nurse's visits	Total[1]		Manhattan	Bronx	Brooklyn	Queens	Other[2]
	Number	Per cent					
Total	3,669	100.0	1,580	1,089	789	175	36
1–9	967	26.4	21.3	25.2	34.2	44.0	9
10–19	627	17.1	16.5	19.0	15.2	18.9	6
20–29	409	11.1	11.8	14.1	6.2	10.3	2
30–39	280	7.6	7.7	8.8	5.5	8.6	5
40–49	209	5.7	6.4	6.0	3.4	7.4	3
50–99	657	17.9	20.9	18.0	13.8	9.1	6
100–199	381	10.4	12.0	8.2	12.2	1.7	3
200–299	89	2.4	2.2	0.4	6.1	0.0	2
300–499	44	1.2	1.1	0.2	3.0	0.0	0
500 and over . . .	6	0.2	0.1	0.1	0.4	0.0	0

[1] The number of nurse's visits was not reported for 224 patients of agencies for which this item was tabulated, and for 2,508 patients of agencies that did not record the information in this way, the item was omitted.

[2] Includes Richmond, 11; New York City, borough unknown, 11; New York State, 8; residence not reported, 6.

Information on the average frequency of the nurse's visits was obtained for 3,658 patients, about 60 per cent of the total number. (See Table 46.) Data on this point from two services were not used, because visits by nurses and patients' visits to clinics were not differentiated. In the records of the Association for Improving the Condition of the Poor, visits for health service were not distinguished from visits for social case work, so that these figures also were not used in this connection. Of patients for whom this information was known, 14 per cent were visited on an average of at least once a week, nearly 50 per cent were visited once a month or oftener, 42 per cent were visited at least once in three months but not as often as once a month, and 9 per cent were visited less frequently than once in three months.

Of the patients of the Henry Street Visiting Nurse Service for whom the information was reported, 53 per cent were visited as frequently as two or three times a week; 30 per cent were visited once a week; and only eight patients were visited less frequently than once a month. The patients of the Brooklyn Visiting Nurse Association for whom the information was reported, were distributed as follows: 12 per cent were visited on an average oftener than once a week; 16 per cent, once a week; another 31 per cent, at least once a month but not as often as once a week; an additional 22 per cent, at least once in three months but not as often as once a month; and 9 per cent, at intervals of six months or longer. This Association has a special service for orthopedic patients, many of whom do not require frequent visiting, and this may account for the fact that its patients show a lower percentage visited at short intervals. The Association for the Aid

TABLE 46

NURSE'S VISITS TO CHRONIC PATIENTS BY FREQUENCY

Frequency	Number	Per cent
Total	3,658[1]	100.0
Three times a week	150	4.1
Twice a week	110	3.0
Once a week	265	7.3
Once in two weeks	367	10.0
Once in three weeks	447	12.2
Once in four weeks	471	12.9
Once in six weeks	690	18.9
Once in three months	838	22.9
Once in six months	242	6.6
At intervals of more than six months . . .	78	2.1
Every week at least	525	14.4
Every month at least	1,810	49.5
Every three months at least	3,338	91.3

[1] Frequency was not reported for 2,743 patients.

of Crippled Children visited 41 per cent of its patients once a month or oftener; another 53 per cent at least once in three months but not as often as once a month; an additional 5 per cent at least once in six months but not as often as once in three months; and a few at longer intervals.

Home Conditions

A little over two fifths (41.6 per cent) of the adults were married. Nearly three fifths (58.4 per cent) were either single, widowed, or divorced. A larger percentage of men than of women were married. The number of unmarried women was nearly twice as large as the number of unmarried men. There were 257 women of sixty years of age and over and only 49 men of this age who were unattached. In the age group forty to fifty-nine years, there were 114 women and 22 men unattached. Among the younger adults, the number of unmarried men and women is more nearly equal.

There were 180 persons, of whom 48 were children, who had no home of their own and were living in some temporary way at the time of the census. Some of them were receiving temporary care in institutions.

Three aspects of the home conditions of the patients were considered—

physical conditions such as space and sanitation, the make-up of the family with reference to their ability to care for a chronic invalid, and the reciprocal attitudes of the members of the family and the patient. The home conditions of a fourth were not reported. The percentage of unknown home conditions is largest among the children and younger adults. This is believed to be due to a lack of the information on the records from which the schedules were made and the recorders' failure to obtain it in other ways and not to lack of knowledge of the home conditions on the part of the nurses.

TABLE 47

CHRONIC PATIENTS OF NURSING SERVICES WITH HOMES CLASSIFIED BY HOME CONDITIONS

Situation reported	HOME CONDITIONS							
	All conditions		Physical condition		Family make-up		Family attitude	
	Number	Per cent	Number	Per cent	Number	Per cent	Number	Per cent
Total . .	6,221[1]	100.0	6,221	100.0	6,221	100.0	6,221	100.0
Suitable . .	3,846	61.8	4,210	67.7	4,232	68.0	4,176	67.1
Unsuitable .	171	2.7	471	7.6	355	5.7	470	7.6
Unknown . .	1,453	23.4	1,540	24.7	1,634	26.3	1,575	25.3

[1] This includes 751 or 12.1 per cent of homes in which there were various combinations of suitable, unsuitable, and unknown factors.

The extent to which the home conditions were suitable for the care of the chronic patient is shown in Chart 13 for different age groups. No striking differences occur in the proportion of unsuitable homes among persons of different ages. The smallest proportion of unsuitable homes, however, was found among persons sixty years of age and over.

Each of the three factors considered in judging the suitability of the home for the care of the chronic patient was found to be satisfactory in about the same proportion of homes as shown in Table 47.

Financial Status

Income. The economic condition of the patients under the care of nursing agencies probably does not differ from that of the whole number of chronically ill persons in the census. Therefore, the information on incomes has not been tabulated separately for these patients.

In the total census, among adults outside of homes for the aged, 40 per cent had a personal income derived from their share in the family income, a subsidy from a social agency, earnings, or, in a few instances, from savings, pensions, insurance, or compensation. Of 400 persons for whom the amount of the personal income was reported, four fifths had less than $25.00 a week at the time of the census of the chronic sick in the spring of 1928.

The amount of the family income was reported for about 5,000 persons

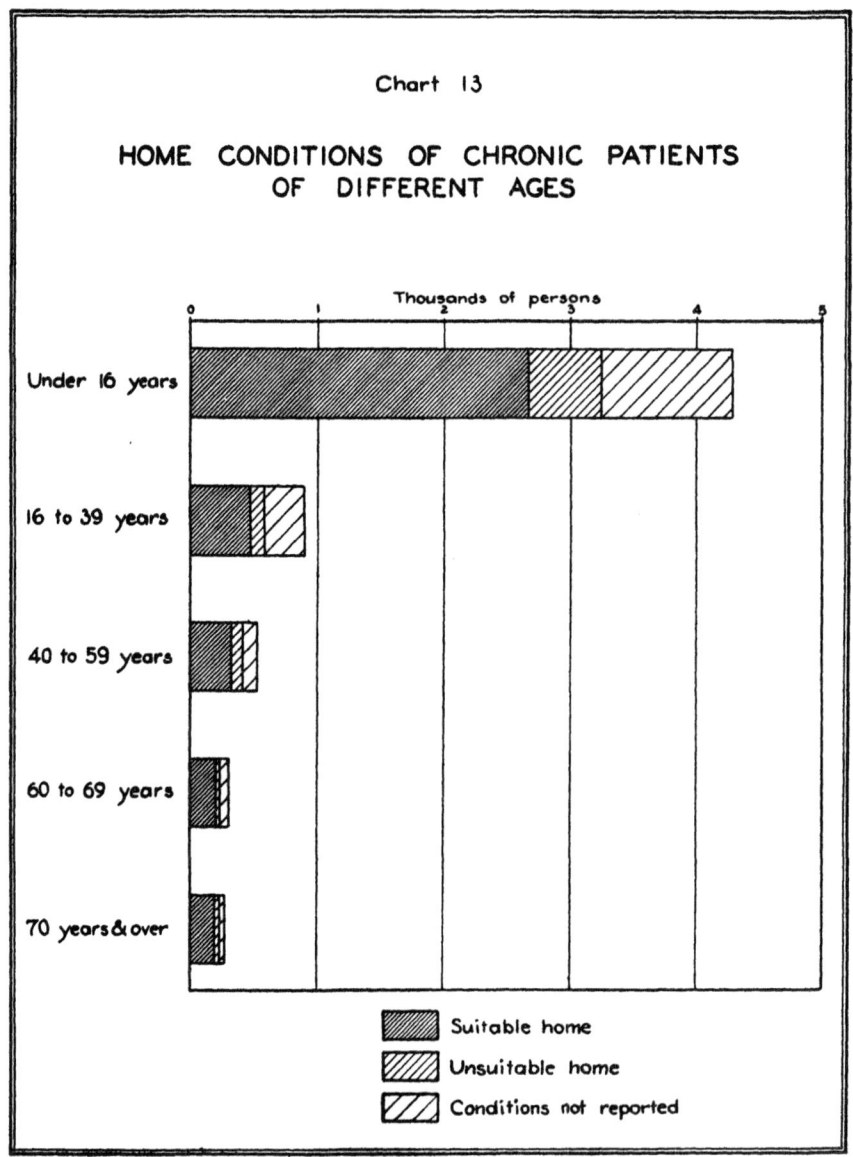

Chart 13

HOME CONDITIONS OF CHRONIC PATIENTS
OF DIFFERENT AGES

in the whole census, 85 per cent of whom had a weekly income of less than $50.00. Assuming a regular weekly income, 71 per cent of the families with five or more members had an annual income below $2,150, the amount required in 1928 to maintain a family of five persons.[10] The average per capita weekly income per person was $6.67, and the average family consisted of five persons.

TABLE 48

CHRONIC PATIENTS OF NURSING SERVICES CLASSIFIED BY TYPE OF
DEPENDENCY, EACH AGE GROUP

Type of dependency	Total	AGE GROUP						
		Children under 16	Adults					Not reported
			Total	16–39	40–59	60–69	70 and over	
Total	6,035[1]	4,181	1,818	861	474	253	230	36
Patient wholly dependent .	4,714	4,164	544	419	40	35	50	6
Public aid only	22	12	10	3	4	2	1	0
Private aid only	166	82	84	19	16	20	29	0
Private, family or friends	4,101	3,703	394	358	10	10	16	4
Public and private aid .	25	9	16	5	9	1	1	0
Public and private, family or friends	400	358	40	34	1	2	3	2
Patient partly dependent .	1,321	17	1,274	442	434	218	180	30
Private aid only	1,209	9	1,171	416	393	197	165	29
Private, family or friends	50	7	42	7	15	12	8	1
Public and private aid .	57	0	57	17	26	9	5	0
Public and private, family or friends	5	1	4	2	0	0	2	0
Not reported	213	11	192	73	63	29	27	10

[1] In this total 153 duplicate records of patients receiving care from another type of agency as well as from a nursing agency are excluded.

Dependency. The need for care and supervision by the nursing agency was regarded in itself as a form of dependency, so that all of the patients were to this extent "dependent." Of 1,800 adults, for whom this information was obtained, 30 per cent were wholly dependent; but only a fifth of these were wholly dependent upon public or private agencies, as the remainder were assisted in part by relatives or friends. Of those partly dependent, only 4 per cent were receiving assistance from their families. Of the children, 97 per cent were dependent upon their families—89 per cent assisted by private agencies and 8 per cent by both public and private agencies.

The number of persons dependent upon assistance from different sources appears in Table 48.

[10] See also vol. 1, Chapter 2, The Chronically Ill Persons Found by a Census in Medical and Social Agencies, pp. 77–79.

The smallest percentage (13.8 per cent) of those wholly dependent, with the exception of the children, was in the age groups sixty to sixty-nine years. The largest percentage (48.7 per cent) was among persons sixteen to thirty-nine years of age, about half of whom were under twenty-one years of age.

INADEQUACIES IN THE COMMUNITY'S FACILITIES FOR CARE

Types of Care Needed and Received

Active medical attention, or "A" care, was required for 92 per cent of the chronically ill patients of the nursing agencies—99 per cent of the children and 79 per cent of the adults. Two per cent required only skilled nursing, or "B" care—6 per cent of the adults and less than 1 per cent of the children. Attendant, or "C" care, was required for 6 per cent. A fifth of those needing attendant care required only the simpler form of attention suitable for aged persons suffering from infirmities of old age rather than from a chronic disease. The forms of care needed by persons of different ages is shown below in Table 49.

TABLE 49

CHRONIC PATIENTS OF NURSING SERVICES CLASSIFIED BY
CARE NEEDED, EACH AGE GROUP

Age group	Total[1]	Medical			Nursing	Attendant	Aged
		Total	Hospital	Clinic			
Total	6,237[2]	92.0	11.9	80.1	2.1	4.8	1.2
Under 16 years . . .	4,192	98.6	9.5	89.1	0.4	1.0	0.0
Adults	1,999	78.6	16.6	62.0	5.6	12.1	3.7
16–39 years	934	94.6	15.5	79.1	2.3	3.1	0.0
40–59 years	537	78.6	20.9	57.7	6.1	15.3	0.0
60–69 years	271	65.7	17.7	48.0	11.4	22.9	0.0
70 years and over .	257	34.2	10.9	23.3	10.1	26.9	28.8
Age not reported . . .	46	31	10	21	4	11	0

[1] In this total 153 records of patients receiving care from another type of agency as well as from a nursing agency are excluded. Their age distribution is as follows: under 16 years, 126; 16 to 39, 11; 40 to 59, 7; 60 to 69, 2; 70 and over, 7.
[2] Care needed was not reported for 11 persons.

The large majority of persons of all ages under seventy years of age required "A" care. Of those seventy years of age or more, over half required only "C" care; and more than half of these needed only the simpler form of attendant care.

The percentage of those in each age group who were receiving the different forms of care is shown in Table 50. Eighty-two per cent received medical care—91 per cent of the children and 64 per cent of the adults. Ten per cent received nursing care—less than 2 per cent of the children and more than a fourth of the adults. About 6 per cent of both children and adults received attendant care. Over 1 per cent of the children and 3 per cent of the adults were receiving no particular care for their illness, although they were reported as under the supervision of a nursing agency.

Comparison of the type of care the patient needed and the type he was receiving (see Table 51) shows that 88 per cent of those needing "A" care were receiving it—92 per cent among children and 77 per cent among adults. But 6 per cent of those who required "A" care were receiving only

TABLE 50

CHRONIC PATIENTS OF NURSING SERVICES CLASSIFIED BY
CARE RECEIVED, EACH AGE GROUP

| Age group | Total[1] | CARE RECEIVED | | | | | |
| | | Medical | | | Nursing | Attendant | None |
		Total	Hospital	Clinic			
Total	6,085[2]	82.1	1.6	80.5	10.0	6.0	1.9
Under 16 years . . .	4,089	91.3	1.6	89.7	1.6	5.7	1.4
Adults	1,951	63.7	1.5	62.2	26.7	6.5	3.1
16–39 years	899	83.5	2.0	81.5	8.2	5.8	2.5
40–59 years	524	53.1	1.5	51.6	38.7	4.2	4.0
60–69 years	276	45.3	0.7	44.6	46.7	5.1	2.9
70 years and over .	252	35.3	0.4	34.9	45.2	15.5	4.0
Age not reported . . .	45	16	1	15	24	5	0

[1] In this total 153 duplicate records of patients receiving care from another type of agency as well as from a nursing agency are excluded. These 153 cases are distributed as to age in the following groups: under 16, 126; 16 to 39, 11; 40 to 59, 7; 60 to 69, 2; 70 and over, 7.

[2] Care received was not reported for 163 persons.

"C" care, and 2 per cent were getting no care for their illness. Of the patients in need of "B" care, 87 per cent were receiving it; 3 per cent were receiving only "C" care; and 10 per cent were receiving clinic care. Of those needing "C" care, 22 per cent were receiving it; 18 per cent were getting "A" care; 55 per cent, "B" care; and 5 per cent, no care for their illness. A much larger proportion of patients received the type of care that their condition called for among those needing medical and nursing care than among those needing attendant care. This was to be expected, since nursing agencies as a rule have not undertaken to provide the custodial type of care for chronic patients.

A small percentage of the whole number of patients, 1.6 per cent, or 98 persons, were in hospitals at the time of the census; and another 10 per cent were considered to be in need of hospital care. Of all who needed hospital care, 12 per cent were not receiving any medical care, three fourths were getting either clinic care or nursing care with clinic supervision, and the remainder were in hospitals. The number needing hospital care who were not receiving it is particularly large in the age group forty to fifty-nine years.

Of nearly 4,900 patients who were receiving medical care in clinics or from private physicians, 7 per cent needed hospital care, 91 per cent needed clinic care, and 2 per cent needed less than medical care. Of those who needed clinic care, 94 per cent were receiving it, a few persons were in hospitals, and 6 per cent were receiving either attendant or no care.

Of the 80 persons who were receiving no care, 24 needed care in orthopedic clinics, most of whom were children suffering from the end results

TABLE 51

CHRONIC PATIENTS OF NURSING SERVICES, CHILDREN AND ADULTS,
CLASSIFIED BY CARE NEEDED AND CARE RECEIVED

Care needed	CARE RECEIVED				
	Total[1]	Medical	Nursing	Attendant	No care
Total					
Total	6,085	82.1	10.0	6.0	1.9
Medical	5,586	87.9	5.3	5.0	1.7
Nursing	127	9.5	87.4	3.1	0.0
Attendant	363	18.2	54.8	22.3	4.7
Not reported	9	5	0	0	4
Under 16 years					
Total	4,089	91.3	1.6	5.7	1.4
Medical	4,034	92.1	1.3	5.2	1.4
Nursing	12	5	7	0	0
Attendant	43	13	5	23	2
Adults					
Total	1,951	63.7	26.7	6.5	3.1
Medical	1,522	77.4	15.4	4.5	2.7
Nursing	111	6.3	90.1	3.6	0.0
Attendant	309	17.1	60.2	17.8	4.9
Not reported	9	5	0	0	4

[1] Care received not reported for 163 persons.
[2] This total includes 45 persons whose age was not reported.

of poliomyelitis whose parents had not taken advantage of the treatment offered. The Association for the Aid of Crippled Children reported 35 persons whom it had not been able to keep under care, either in a clinic or a hospital. This organization often continues its efforts for months in order to persuade families to keep their children under medical supervision.

The patients receiving nursing care at home who were in need of medical attention in a hospital were suffering chiefly from general diseases and diseases of the circulatory system. The patients receiving "C" care but needing "A" care were mainly those suffering from conditions resulting from epidemic diseases. Aged persons and those suffering from general diseases and diseases of the nervous system made up the group of 280 patients receiving "A" or "B" care although less skilled care would have been adequate for their needs.

Persons Receiving Unsuitable Care

Half of the patients of the nursing services were reported to be suitably cared for both from the medical and social standpoint. For another 22 per cent the medical and nursing care was reported to be satisfactory but the home conditions were not recorded. Twenty-eight per cent of the patients were reported to be cared for unsuitably from either the medical or social standpoint or both. For 13 per cent of these, however, the un-

TABLE 52

CHRONIC PATIENTS OF NURSING SERVICES AT HOME AND IN INSTITUTIONS
CLASSIFIED BY SUITABILITY OF CARE RECEIVED, EACH AGE GROUP

Suitability of care received	Total[1]		AGE GROUP						Not reported
			Children under 16	Adults					
	Number	Per cent		Total	16–39	40–59	60–69	70 and over	
Total	6,112	100.0	4,112	1,954	906	528	268	252	46
Suitable care . . .	3,069	50.2	56.0	38.2	38.8	36.6	40.0	38.5	17
At home	2,902	47.5	52.8	36.5	36.2	35.0	39.6	37.7	15
In institutions .	167	2.7	3.2	1.7	2.5	1.5	0.4	0.8	2
Unsuitable care . .	1,713	28.0	22.3	39.5	28.4	47.1	46.2	55.6	24
At home	1,701	27.8	22.2	39.1	28.2	46.8	45.5	55.2	24
In institutions .	12	0.2	0.1	0.4	0.2	0.4	0.7	0.4	0
Medical and nursing care suitable, home not reported	1,330	21.8	21.6	22.3	32.8	16.3	13.8	5.9	5
Not reported . . .	136	.....	80	56	28	9	14	5	0

[1] In this total, 153 duplicate records of patients receiving care from another type of agency as well as from a nursing agency are excluded. These 153 patients are distributed as to age in the following groups: under 16 years of age, 126; 16 to 39, 11; 40 to 59, 7; 60 to 69, 2; 70 and over, 7.

suitability of the care lay only in the fact that the patient was receiving a more skilled type of care than he required. The suitability of the care received by children and adults is represented in Chart 14.

Among the different age groups, the highest percentage of unsuitable care (56 per cent) was among the aged, for whom, moreover, the percentage of unknown home conditions was low (see Table 52); and over half of those receiving unsuitable care were receiving more skilled care than necessary. Among persons between forty and seventy, there was a higher percentage of unknown home conditions and a high percentage (47 per cent) of unsuitable care, of which over a fourth was more skilled care than the patient required. The lowest percentage of unsuitable care (22 per cent) was among the children, and it consisted almost entirely of inadequate care or care in an unsuitable home. Among the younger adults, the percentage of unsuitable care (28.5 per cent) was higher than among the children, although the

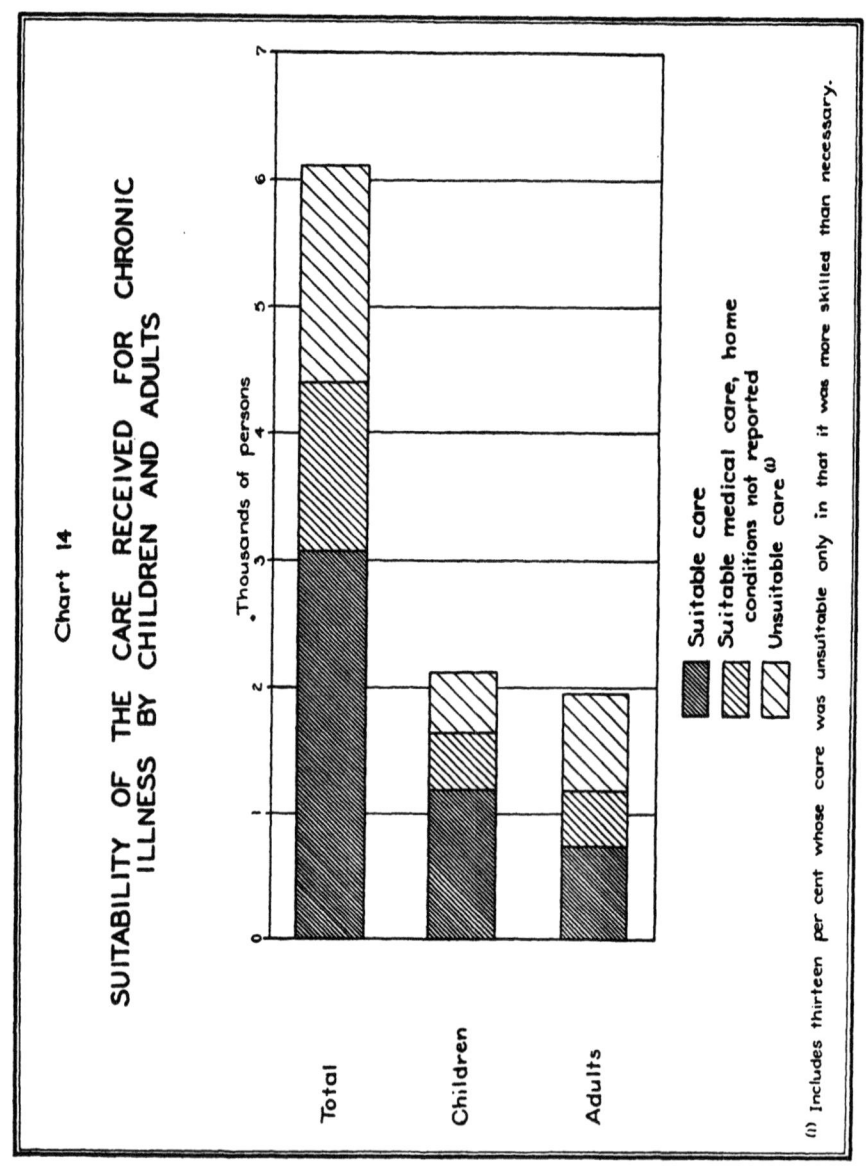

Chart 14

SUITABILITY OF THE CARE RECEIVED FOR CHRONIC
ILLNESS BY CHILDREN AND ADULTS

Thousands of persons

Total

Children

Adults

Suitable care

Suitable medical care, home
conditions not reported

Unsuitable care (l)

(l) Includes thirteen per cent whose care was unsuitable only in that it was more skilled than necessary.

percentage of unknown home conditions was much higher, being highest in this age group.

Of approximately 300 persons, for whom home care through the services of a visiting houseworker or practical nurse was indicated, 4 per cent were children, over a third were aged persons of seventy years or over, and about 60 per cent were adults under seventy. Nearly two thirds of the aged in this group of 300 were persons getting skilled nursing care at home but needing only custodial care. Of the adults under seventy years of age in the group, 69 per cent were persons receiving nursing care but needing only custodial care.

TABLE 53

CHRONIC PATIENTS OF NURSING SERVICES CLASSIFIED BY REASON FOR NOT BEING
IN AN INSTITUTION OR IN A PROPER INSTITUTION

Reason	At home		In institution
	Number	Per cent	
Total	775	. . . . .	6
Total reporting reason	500	100.0	2
Opposition to institutional care . . .	270	54.0	0
Private institution	186	37.2	0
Public institution	84	16.8	0
No vacancy	20	4.0	1
No provision	15	3.0	0
Personal traits	3	0.6	0
Other	192	38.4	1

Nearly 3 per cent of all the patients were temporarily in institutions at the time of the census, all of whom, with the exception of 12 persons, were receiving suitable care.

Lack of Institutional Beds

The nursing services reported 775 persons, or 12.7 per cent of their patients, who needed institutional care but were at home. This was a somewhat smaller proportion than the family agencies reported. The largest percentage of patients of any one nursing service in need of admission to an institution was 41 per cent in the East Harlem Nursing and Health Service, which reported 39 chronically ill patients. In three agencies, with 626 patients, about 29 per cent in each agency needed institutional care. In another agency, reporting over 800 patients, 15 per cent needed institutional care. The two large orthopedic nursing agencies reported less than 10 per cent in need of institutional care.

The reason why the patient was not in an institution or not in a suitable type of institution, as shown in Table 53, for 500 patients, was given as opposition to institutional care for 54 per cent and as lack of provision for 7 per cent. Various unclassified reasons were given for 38 per cent. For several patients, the reason given was "personal traits." If there had been no opposition to institutional care on the part of the patient or his family, it is probable that institutional facilities would have been reported as lacking in a larger percentage of cases.

For the patients for whom nursing services were primarily responsible, over 750 in institutions were needed, in addition to those in use at the time of the census. Eighty-five per cent of these beds were needed for hospital care and the remaining 15 per cent were needed either for custodial care or for custodial care with clinic supervision because the patients' homes were unsuitable for their care.

The different types of institutional care needed for children and adults are shown in Chart 15. Over half of the beds required were for children— slightly over half of the hospital beds, about one fourth of the custodial beds, and more than three fourths of the beds for patients needing clinic supervision in an institution. Only 13 per cent of the additional beds required were for patients sixty years of age or over, and the need for this group was almost entirely for hospital beds. Seventy-five per cent of all the additional institutional beds needed for persons at home who should have been having institutional care were required for the patients of nursing agencies.

In addition to the known institutional needs for this group there were about 1,000 patients unsuitably cared for at home, either from a social or medical standpoint, for whom information was lacking as to whether proper care could be given in the home. Undoubtedly some of these persons needed care in custodial institutions either with or without clinic supervision in addition, but none of them needed hospital care.

SUMMARY

Borough Distribution of Service

Nearly half of the patients reported by nursing agencies lived in Manhattan; nearly a fourth, in the Bronx; about one fifth, in Brooklyn; less than a tenth, in Queens; and less than 1 per cent, in Richmond.

Manhattan's proportion of chronic patients under care by nursing services is nearly one and a half times its proportion of the city's population. The proportion of the chronic patients living in the Bronx is considerably higher than the borough's proportion of the population. Brooklyn's proportion is just half and that of the other two boroughs is less than half of the proportion of the population in each of these boroughs.

Nursing agencies that serve all the boroughs reported nearly 30 per cent of the patients. Agencies serving Manhattan and those limited to Brooklyn reported about the same percentage, 12 per cent. The services in Queens reported 4 per cent.

Amount of Service Received by Chronic Patients

The chronic patients reported had been under care of the nursing agency for periods varying from less than three months for about a tenth to fifteen

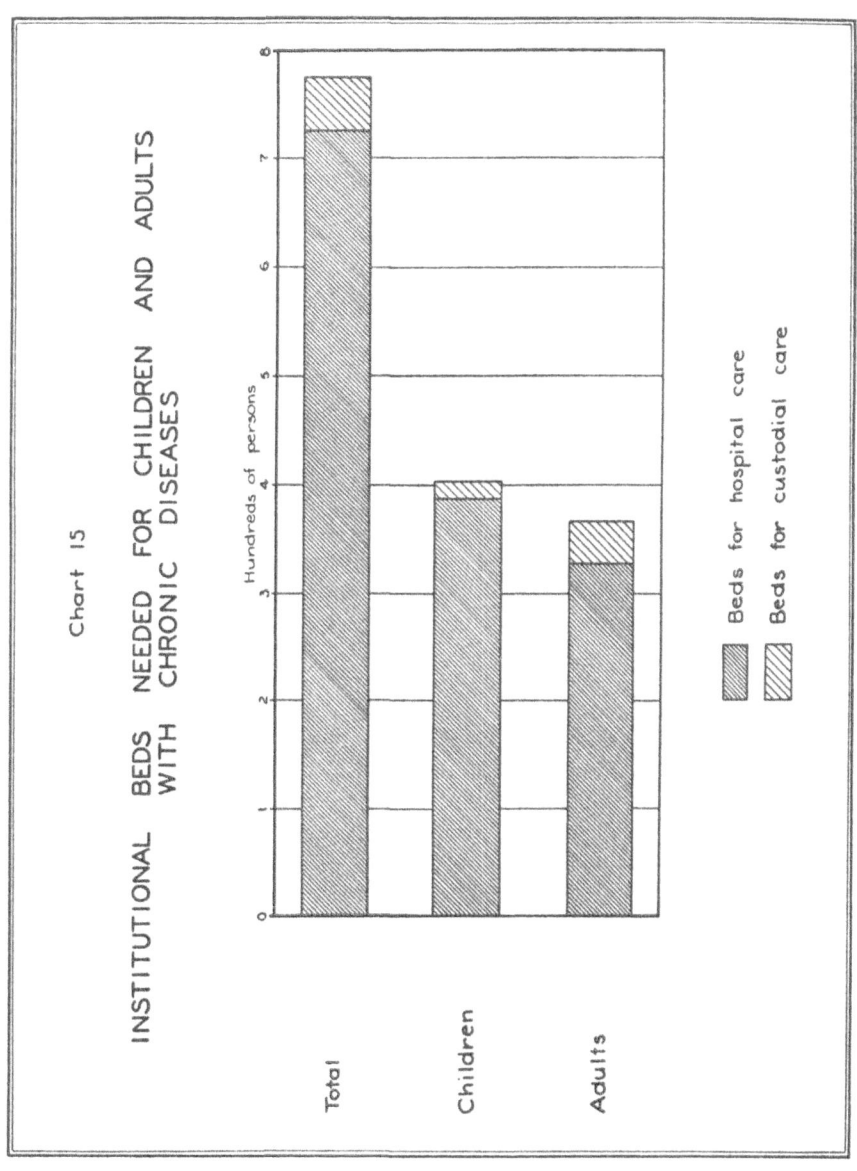

Chart 15

INSTITUTIONAL BEDS NEEDED FOR CHILDREN AND ADULTS
WITH CHRONIC DISEASES

years or longer for 3 per cent. A few persons had been under care twenty years or more. Nearly a fourth had been under care between three months and a year. Less than a fourth had been under care five years or longer.

More persons with long periods of care, at least ten years, were found among those between sixteen and forty years of age than in any other age group.

The number of visits made by a nurse to these patients varied from less than ten visits for more than a fourth to 300 visits or more for slightly over 1 per cent. Six persons had received 500 visits or more.

An equal number (43 per cent) had received less than 20 visits each and between 20 and 100 visits each; and the number who had received 100 visits or more was about one third as many (14 per cent).

The frequency of the nurses' visits was reported for less than two thirds of the patients. Of these, 14 per cent were visited at least once a week, nearly a third of whom were visited three times a week; about half were visited at least once a month; about two fifths at least once in three months but not oftener than once a month; and nearly one tenth were visited at intervals of over three months.

Chronic Patients under Care

Age, Sex, and Marital Status. Nursing services were caring for 6,400 chronic patients or nearly a third of all the chronically ill persons found by the census under the care of the medical and social agencies of the city. Over two thirds of this number were reported by special orthopedic nursing services for children.

Over two thirds of the chronic patients of nursing services were children under sixteen years of age and over three fourths were under twenty-one years of age. About one eighth were forty years of age or over; and 9 per cent were sixty years of age and over. The aged, seventy years of age or over, were only about 4 per cent of the whole number.

Among the adults, females predominated. Among the children, there were a few more boys than girls. The distribution of the sexes among Negroes, who were 5 per cent of the whole number, was about the same as among white persons.

Over two fifths of the adults were married, the remainder being either single, widowed, or divorced. Unmarried women made up the largest percentage of the whole number, married women came next, then unmarried men, and finally married men. Women were nearly twice as numerous as men among the unmarried.

Medical Condition. Diseases found most frequently among the adults were, in the order given, cancer, rheumatism and arthritis, circulatory diseases, paralysis, and fractures.

Nearly a third of all cancer patients and of all patients with fractures were reported by the nursing services, which is the same proportion that all the chronic patients of nursing agencies represent in the whole census.

About a fifth of all patients with diseases of the nervous system and of those with arthritis and rheumatism were reported by these agencies.

Poliomyelitis caused half of the orthopedic disorders among the children and also a third of the illness in the younger adult group. Other causes of illness among children in the order of numerical importance were non-pulmonary tuberculosis, spinal cord diseases, rickets (found in connection with a special preventive campaign that was being conducted at the time of the census), and heart disease. Other diseases appeared in smaller numbers.

The percentage of mentally abnormal persons reported by this group of agencies was smaller than that reported by other agencies. It was 6.4 per cent in contrast to 24.4 per cent among the chronically ill clients of family service agencies. A much higher percentage of persons over forty years than of younger persons were reported to show some mental abnormality.

A favorable prognosis was reported for a fourth of the children, a fifth of the younger adults, and 6 per cent of those forty years or over. No other group of agencies reported as high a percentage of persons with a favorable prognosis.

Social Condition. The homes of more than four fifths of the patients whose home conditions were reported were suitable for their care in respect to physical condition and the make-up and attitudes of the family. The homes of nearly 4 per cent were totally unsatisfactory and those of an additional 15 per cent were unsatisfactory in some respect. For a fourth of the homes, either all conditions were unknown or some unknown conditions were combined with other conditions reported as unsatisfactory.

Seventy per cent of the adults had some financial resources of their own. Six per cent were entirely dependent upon welfare agencies. The remainder were receiving assistance from family and friends, as well as from welfare agencies. Three per cent of all the children were wholly dependent upon welfare agencies and the remainder were dependent upon their families aided by welfare agencies.

Care Needed and Received by Chronic Patients

Half of all the chronic patients of nursing agencies were reported as being suitably cared for both medically and socially—56 per cent of the children and 38 per cent of the adults. Over a fourth were getting unsuitable care from either a medical or social standpoint or both, a small proportion of whom were getting more skilled care than they required. The rest, over a fifth, were getting suitable medical or nursing care but their home conditions were not recorded.

Nearly nine tenths of the persons needing medical or nursing care were found to be receiving it; but less than a fourth of those needing only attendant care were receiving that type of care. Since nursing services are not organized to provide the custodial type of care for the chronic sick in their homes, many patients needing only attendant care were found to be receiving skilled nursing care.

Probably a tenth of the adult chronic patients found in the care of nursing agencies could have been taken care of more adequately by a less skilled personnel than the trained visiting nurse. The indications were that trained attendants or visiting houseworkers would also have been the best means of care for several hundred patients reported by other agencies.

Nearly 800 additional beds in institutions would be required for the care of patients reported by nursing agencies who needed institutional care. Eighty-five per cent, or 675, of the additional beds needed are hospital beds and 15 per cent, or 125, are custodial beds, of which about half should be in institutions that could arrange for clinic care for their patients.

More than half of these additional 800 beds required are needed for children, more than a third for adults under sixty years of age, and 13 per cent for persons over sixty years of age.

THE FACILITIES OF NURSING SERVICES IN RELATION TO THE CARE OF THE CHRONIC SICK

DEVELOPMENT OF VISITING NURSE SERVICE IN NEW YORK CITY

Visiting nurse service, organized as such, was begun in New York City, in 1877, when the Woman's Branch of the New York City Mission Society engaged five trained nurses to go into the homes of the sick poor. Earlier, in 1869, under the auspices of this organization, several members of the Sisterhood of the Good Shepherd were engaged in visiting the sick. It is recorded that they were "much devoted to their undertaking, and abundant in toil, making several hundred visits to those sick or in prison per year."[11] As early as 1846, the Sisters of Mercy, a Roman Catholic religious order, were nursing the sick at home, with a devotion and efficiency that coerced reluctant praise from a bigoted chronicler.[12] In 1893, the Henry Street Visiting Nurse Service was organized by Miss Lillian D. Wald of the Henry Street Settlement. This was the pioneer organization in public health nursing as it is known today.

Nursing service provided by a municipal health department was first known in this country, in 1898, in Los Angeles. The New York City Department of Health first employed nurses in 1902 to care for cases of diphtheria, scarlet fever, and measles. In 1903, a special nurse was employed by the department for tuberculosis work. School nursing, patterned after experiments in England, was started here in 1902, when Miss Wald placed a Henry Street nurse in one of the city schools to demonstrate its value.

The Department of Health now has a Bureau of Public Health Nursing organized in 1928. The functions of its nurses are performed in connection with the work of two other bureaus: the Bureau of Child Hygiene—prenatal work, general instruction in the care of the new born, and health supervision of school children; and the Bureau of Preventable Diseases—district nursing of all reported tuberculosis and contagious diseases, instruction about quarantine, supervision during the period of quarantine, inspection and termination of cases, home visits in cases of tuberculosis and cases of venereal diseases under clinic care.

In 1909, the Metropolitan Life Insurance Company undertook to offer home nursing to its industrial premium policyholders in the United States and Canada. The existing visiting nurse services were asked to furnish this service, payment being based upon the exact cost of the visits made. This practice was followed by other life insurance companies.

Immediately after the organization of the Welfare Council of New York City, the nursing agencies of the city formed the Section on Public Health

[11] Richmond, Rev. J. F., New York and Its Institutions, 1609–1873: The Bright Side of New York. New York, E. B. Treat, 1873, revised edition, p. 342.
[12] *Ibid.*, p. 346.

Nursing of the Health Division, which later, in January, 1930, merged with the Health Administration and Education Section. Twenty-three nursing agencies were represented at that time, including the municipal Bureau of Public Health Nursing and twenty-two nursing services under voluntary auspices. These agencies vary widely in size and function. Some of the smaller services employ only one nurse or several nurses and cover a small area; and the two largest organizations, covering one or more boroughs, employ from 100 to 200 nurses. Some of the services are restricted in func-

TABLE 54

TYPES OF AGENCY OFFERING HOME NURSING SERVICE IN NEW YORK CITY, 1928,
CLASSIFIED BY TYPE OF SERVICE

Type of agency	Total	TYPE OF SERVICE		
		Educational nursing	Bedside nursing	Educational and bedside nursing
Total	25	8	9	8
Nursing organizations	13	1	7	5
Hospitals	3	0	0	3
Health centers	3	3	0	0
Settlements	3	3	0	0
Family welfare agencies	1	1	0	0
Life insurance companies	2	0	2	0

tion to a special form of illness, a special type of preventive health work, or a particular group of clients. Others include in their activities all forms of visiting nurse service.

In addition to the work of the organized nursing services, a large amount of service to the sick in their homes is given by nurses and medical social workers connected with the out-patient clinics of hospitals. Such service consists mainly of advice and assistance intended to make possible adequate medical care. The volume of this work is not known. The amount of such service that chronic patients receive is not known, as clinic facilities were not included in this study. For health service, the Health Inventory showed that approximately 385,000 home visits were made from clinics of voluntary and official agencies in a year.[13]

FACILITIES FOR THE CARE OF THE CHRONIC SICK

Nursing Agencies Included

There were twenty-five voluntary organizations in the city giving nursing care at home to chronic patients as defined in this study. (For a list of these agencies, see Appendix VI.) There is no municipal service of this

[13] Davis, Michael M., and Jarrett, Mary C., A Health Inventory of New York City: A Study of the Volume and Distribution of Health Service in the Five Boroughs. The Welfare Council of New York City, 1929, pp. 18, 301.

kind. The Department of Health through its nursing service gives home supervision in several other types of illness. (See p. 213.) The Department of Hospitals provides for home supervision of clinic patients through the social service departments of the municipal hospitals but has no home nursing service.

The twenty-five nursing services included in the survey were conducted by various types of agency as shown in Table 54.

The types of agency that furnish this service for the different boroughs is shown in Table 55.

TABLE 55

TYPES OF AGENCY OFFERING HOME NURSING SERVICE IN NEW YORK CITY, 1928,
CLASSIFIED BY BOROUGH

Type of agency	Agencies	Manhattan	Bronx	Brooklyn	Queens	Richmond
Total	25[1]	17	9	5	8	4
Nursing organizations . .	13	8	6	2	4	2
Hospitals	3	2	2	3	2	2
Health centers	3	3	0	0	0	0
Settlements	3	3	0	0	0	0
Family welfare agencies .	1	1	1	0	0	0
Life insurance companies[2]	2	0	0	0	2	0

[1] The total of agencies is less than the sum of those serving the separate boroughs because some agencies serve more than one borough.

[2] The life insurance companies actually include all the boroughs in their service; but in the boroughs other than Queens, they gave the service entirely through the community visiting nurse services; and one of them has done so in all boroughs since 1930.

Seventeen of the 25 nursing services of the city are Manhattan agencies, 9 of which extend their activities into other boroughs. The activities of 6 of these extended into two boroughs; of 1, into three boroughs; and 2 services sent their nurses into all the boroughs. One Brooklyn agency served a section of Queens; one Queens agency served a section of Brooklyn. Of the 14 agencies serving but one borough, 8 served Manhattan, 2 Brooklyn, and 4 Queens.[14] The area covered by each organization in its nursing service is shown in Appendix VI. The service offered by the life insurance companies to their policyholders is city-wide; and they maintain their own service in communities where there is no visiting nurse service through which they can obtain it.

In Queens, where there was no public health nursing organization covering the borough,[15] the greater part of the visiting nurse service was being

[14] The Richmond Center of the Henry Street Visiting Nurse Service, in 1929, became a separate organization, the Visiting Nurse Service of Staten Island.

[15] Early in 1930, the Henry Street Visiting Nurse Service extended its service to give nursing care and health teaching to the Sunnyside section of Queens, a small section devoted to a large scale housing development for families of moderate means. In December, 1930, it temporarily extended its service to include all sections of the borough not already covered by such service, and an additional office was opened in Jamaica. By 1932, ten nurses were covering all of the borough except the Flushing district of the North Shore Nursing Service and a small district covered by the Brooklyn Visiting Nurse Association, which has been gradually withdrawing its service from Queens.

given by the Metropolitan Life Insurance Company and the John Hancock Life Insurance Company.[16] In the other boroughs, the insurance companies obtain this service on a paid basis from the Henry Street Visiting Nurse Service and the Visiting Nurse Association of Brooklyn.

There are several social service departments of hospitals that are strictly speaking nursing services—the New York Orthopedic Dispensary and Hospital, the Memorial Hospital for the Treatment of Cancer and Allied Diseases, and the Norwegian Lutheran Deaconesses Home and Hospital. This is especially true of the New York Orthopedic Hospital and Dispensary. The services of the nurses are confined to orthopedic work and they do no social case work. At the Norwegian Lutheran Deaconesses Home and Hospital also no social case work is done. The Memorial Hospital Social Service Department works among dependent patients in both the hospital and the clinic, giving bedside care and home nursing to patients whose admission to the hospital is deferred and to patients whose disease is too advanced to benefit by treatment. It seemed advisable to list these departments as visiting nurse services.

Several organizations offering special forms of home nursing were not included in the survey because they do not give care for chronic illness. The Maternity Center Association and the Brooklyn Maternity Center Association do antepartum, delivery, and postpartum work; and they do no nursing work for chronic patients. The New York Chapter of the American Red Cross sends nurses out for governmental services and for special duty in time of disaster and on special occasions. Nursing groups attached to social service departments of hospitals, clinics, day nurseries, and other social agencies that do not have an organized nursing department are not included in the study.

Two nursing services had recently been discontinued, but efforts were being made to keep one of them in existence. The Williams Institutional Church in the Harlem district discontinued its nursing, in 1925, owing to insufficient funds to carry on the work among the Negro families in the neighborhood. The North Shore Public Health Nursing Association was organized in 1927 with one worker; by the fall of 1928 it had been discontinued; but within a few months it was reorganized. It now has a nursing staff consisting of a supervisor and several assistants.

Several nursing organizations included in the study and listed among available facilities did not furnish records for the census of chronic sick persons. The Jamaica District Nursing and Social Service Committee and the nurse of the John Hancock Mutual Life Insurance Company in the Rockaway district of Queens did not send in records. Christodora House, during the period of rebuilding, had one nurse taking care of old clients but not taking new cases and no chronic patients were listed there at the time of the census. After the new building was completed, two staff nurses were engaged—one, on full time for public health and educational nursing

---

[16] The John Hancock Life Insurance Company gave up its own nurses, in 1930, and now purchases this service from the Henry Street Visiting Nurse Service as in other boroughs.

doing no bedside work. The Little Sisters of the Assumption and the Recreation Rooms and Settlement also reported that they had no chronic patients at the time of the census.

In connection with home nursing service for the chronic sick, two agencies that contribute service in this field should be mentioned. The first is the Fraternity for Friendly Service, which has on its staff in addition to two occupational workers and two friendly visitors four home visitors, who give simple nursing service. Shortly after the study was made, a trained nurse was added to its staff. In the fiscal year 1930, this nurse made nearly 1,000 home visits to disabled patients. As one of the chief objects of this organization is to furnish occupation for homebound invalids, the patients reported by it in the census were included in the section on agencies for sheltered work. The other agency is the New York Chapter of the American Red Cross, which conducted classes for instruction in home hygiene and the care of the sick among housewives and high school girls. Although the main object of these courses was health education, the pupils were also taught the simpler tasks of home nursing. In 1927–1928, 1,584 certificates were issued for completion of the course.[17]

In caring for chronic patients at home, the nurse often finds that her service consists largely of household tasks, which a less skilled worker could do equally well. There is no organized community service in this city to provide attendants or visiting houseworkers. This subject has been referred to above in the discussion of the responsibility of nursing agencies toward the chronic sick. (See pp. 186–188.)

Types of Nursing Service

Among these 25 nursing agencies, three main types of service are found: (1) educational nursing; (2) specialized nursing care for a particular group of clients; and (3) home nursing and bedside care. A list of these agencies, with the type of service they perform, is given in Appendix VI.

There is no sharp dividing line between educational work and nursing, since all nursing agencies are to a greater or less extent engaged in health education and supervision. Not all of them, however, give bedside nursing care. The type of nursing provided by different types of agency is shown in Table 54. Seven of the agencies included in this report do educational work entirely; and one agency combines educational work with physiotherapy for orthopedic cases among children. Nine do chiefly bedside nursing with little educational work. Eight agencies do both bedside nursing and educational work.

The 8 services in the first group of educational nursing services were conducted by three settlements—a health center, an agency for crippled children, and a family welfare agency with three branches of nursing service. Of the 3 services in the second group of specialized services, two are for orthopedic children and the third for cancer patients. The specialized nursing services for maternity cases, contagious diseases, and

[17] The New York Chapter of the American National Red Cross, Annual Report, 1928, p. 14.

tuberculosis are outside the scope of this study. There were 15 services in the third group of community nursing agencies that give bedside care. Of these, 5 were public health nursing organizations; 7, are nursing services under church auspices, of which 1 was supported by a number of Protestant churches and 6 were orders of Catholic Sisters; 1, a home nursing service maintained by a hospital; and 2, services provided by life insurance companies in Queens.

Educational Nursing. Seven nursing groups are interested primarily in educational health work—the Association for Improving the Condition of the Poor with its three divisions of nursing work, the Bowling Green Neighborhood Association, the Judson Health Center, Christodora House, and the Recreation Rooms and Settlement. These agencies carry on constructive health education programs, in which the chief features are baby and preschool hygiene, maternity hygiene, supervision of diet and general instruction in prevention of disease, and supervision of patients with tuberculosis. No bedside care is furnished by these groups except in emergencies. Regular bedside nursing required for their patients is provided by the Henry Street Visiting Nurse Service.

The Association for Improving the Condition of the Poor, with a staff of fifty-six nurses, supervisors, and dietitians at the time of the study, works from three centers, the main office on East 22nd Street, the Columbus Hill Health Center, and the Mulberry Health Center. Its Educational Nursing Bureau was first established for preventive and educational nursing work among families in which there was tuberculosis. The health demonstration at the Mulberry Health Center, in a district inhabited largely by Italians, had been carried on since 1920. The educational home visits were an especially important feature of the campaign. Malnutrition was the chief subject of study there at the time; health education and careful diet supervision were going on hand in hand. The Columbus Hill Health Center is in a district with a large Negro population. In July, 1928, the staff of white nurses was replaced by Negro nurses. Nutrition classes and other branches of an educational program were included in the demonstration; and much of the educational work had been done among patients attending a venereal disease clinic in the district. Nearly a fifth of all the chronically ill Negroes under the care of nursing agencies were reported by this agency. Negroes numbered 5 per cent of all the chronic patients under the care of nursing agencies.

The patients reported by the Association for Improving the Condition of the Poor were in some instances receiving nursing care from the Henry Street nurses. Many of them were receiving financial aid through the family welfare service of the organization.

The Bowling Green Neighborhood Association had four graduate nurses, who visited patients in the neighborhood of the settlement. It also carried on the usual program of health education in this district. In addition, in coöperation with the Department of Health, it was doing an intensive piece of follow-up work with tuberculosis cases in one section of the Corlears district. Part of the time of one nurse was assigned to the tuberculosis clinic and follow-up. The Judson Health Center with its ten nurses had a similar educational health program. It drew its patients largely from the clientele of the settlement. A small number of chronic patients were reported by the Bowling Green Neighborhood Association and a still smaller number by the Judson Health Center. Christodora House and the Recreation Rooms and Settlement employed nurses for health education and supervision among the clientele of the settlement. Neither had any chronic patients to report.

Specialized Nursing Care. The Memorial Hospital for the Treatment of Cancer and Allied Diseases, through its Social Service Department, gives home nursing care to cancer patients only. The other cancer hospitals, the New York Skin and Cancer Hospital[18] and the New York City Cancer Institute, do not have a home nursing service. All of the nursing groups that give bedside care may have cancer patients. In the census, 250 patients with cancer were found to be receiving home nursing care, of which nearly three fourths were reported by Memorial Hospital and the remainder by other nursing agencies giving bedside care.

Memorial Hospital had a supervisor and five assistant nurses for its visiting nurse service. Some of the patients receiving home nursing are able to attend the out-patient clinic, and others are bedridden and incurable. The nurses bathe the patients, give dressings, and make beds. The hospital does not keep hopeless cases for treatment in the wards; and families are advised to keep incurable patients at home with the assistance of the visiting nurses.

The nursing and supervision of orthopedic patients in New York City is done by three agencies: the Association for the Aid of Crippled Children reported over 2,500 patients; the New York Orthopedic Hospital reported over 1,600 patients; and the Brooklyn Visiting Nurse Association, which has a special department for orthopedic children, reported over 600 orthopedic patients. The majority in each group were children.

The first organization covers Manhattan and the Bronx; and the second, through its social service department, which is essentially a nursing service, covers all of Greater New York and its suburbs, following up patients after operative treatment and those awaiting admission for treatment. The Brooklyn Visiting Nurse Association gives this service in Brooklyn and at the time of the study gave it also in the Woodhaven, Glendale, and Richmond Hill districts of Queens; but it has gradually reduced its service in Queens, which is now limited to one small district. Otherwise the borough of Queens is without a special orthopedic service; and the Henry Street Visiting Nurse Service endeavors to cover this work as far as possible. There is no special service of this kind in the borough of Richmond. A large number of patients from Queens visit the Manhattan clinics; and in a great

---

[18] Now the Stuyvesant Square Hospital.

many instances, no continuous treatment is followed due to lack of supervision. The development of clinic service in orthopedic work in Queens is as important as an expansion of the orthopedic nursing service.

Hospital facilities for crippled patients were found to be adequate when Henry C. Wright made his survey of cripples in 1920 in New York City.[19] In 1928, the New York Orthopedic Hospital, the Hospital for the Ruptured and Crippled, and the House of St. Giles the Cripple were used to 88, 84, and 96 per cent respectively of their capacity. The Hospital for Joint Diseases was used to 75 per cent of its capacity; only half of its 250 ward beds, however, are reserved for orthopedic patients.

The facilities for convalescent care for crippled children are probably sufficient in respect to the total number of beds available, but there is a deficiency in the number of beds used for children of certain ages, both for crippled children and others. (See also Chapter 4, dealing with convalescent homes.)

The organization of facilities during epidemics of poliomyelitis has been discussed in a section of this report that deals with the special problems of orthopedic patients.[20]

An outstanding contribution of this group of orthopedic nurses is the educational influence of their service. Persistent efforts are needed to make parents realize the importance of regular treatments in nearly all cases of children with orthopedic difficulties. Moving from one district to another constantly necessitates a search for delinquents.

There is splendid coöperation between the voluntary agencies and the Board of Education in regard to crippled children in the public schools. Since 1928, physiotherapists have been giving treatments in the public schools in Manhattan and the Bronx. This service, supported by contributions from several voluntary organizations[21] since 1926, was undertaken to give the benefit of treatment to children whose parents would not allow them to be absent from school to attend the clinics. A doctor's and parent's consent are needed to permit a child to receive this attention. In addition, the permit for treatment must also be signed by the Assistant Director of Health Education, who is in charge of the Division of Physically Handicapped Children of the Department of Education. In Brooklyn, the Visiting Nurse Association cared for a number of school children treated in the school building usually once a week, except in Public School 219, where two treatments a week were given. These orthopedic patients received massage, muscle training, and corrective exercises. The service was paid for by the child's family.

The Association for the Aid of Crippled Children employed one physio-

---

[19] Wright, Henry C., Survey of Cripples in New York City, made under the auspices of a Special Committee on Survey of Cripples. Published by the Committee on After Care of Infantile Paralysis Cases, 1920, p. 14.

[20] See vol. 1, Chapter 3, The Special Problems of Some Main Groups of Chronic Diseases, pp. 137-139.

[21] Through the Association for the Aid of Crippled Children, the Morris Aaron Organization for Crippled Children pays for physiotherapy in the schools in Manhattan and the New York Philanthropic League in the Bronx.

therapist on half time to give home treatments to children living in the outlying districts of the Bronx. Eight children were receiving this care. Before the treatment was given, a written statement from the physician in charge of each child must be secured and in addition, a statement of consent by the parents. This service in the home saves the patient all tedious transportation, waiting in the clinic until his turn comes, and waiting again to be taken home until all other children in the district are ready to go. For these reasons, the Association considered creating a staff of physiotherapists for home treatments but found that in the majority of cases the doctors preferred to have the children come to the hospital for their treatments. If the treatment is given in the home, it is more difficult to secure the necessary medical supervision. The parents are apt to consider the home treatment sufficient and to fail therefore to take the child to the clinic to be seen by the doctor. Close medical supervision of every child probably cannot be carried on successfully in the home without outdoor medical service.

The Association for the Aid of Crippled Children carries on its work from a central office and ten district offices distributed throughout the two boroughs, Manhattan and the Bronx. It has a plan under consideration for extending its service to Queens. All crippled children attending public schools in Manhattan and the Bronx are registered with this Association. In the Rhinelander School for Crippled Children, educational and follow-up nursing service was given by the Children's Aid Society.[22] About 4,000 children were cared for annually by the Association.

The nurses of the New York Orthopedic Dispensary and Hospital care for patients of the hospital, both children and adults. When a patient gets instruction for exercises in the clinic the nurse responsible for his care is present. Every patient upon discharge from the hospital is visited by a nurse to see that casts or braces are properly adjusted. Her services are restricted to the orthopedic needs of the patient; and other organizations are called upon for assistance, if the clinic patients require adjustment of other health and social conditions.

The Brooklyn Visiting Nurse Association had a special nurse for orthopedic cases among children in each of its eight nursing districts. The nurse visits the home in order to give the treatment. In the Main district of Brooklyn, however, in the neighborhood of the Long Island College Hospital, patients are asked to come to the orthopedic department of Polhemus Clinic, which is the out-patient department of the Hospital, for treatment. Exceptions are made only in the case of a helpless patient, who is treated at home. The Association provides the nursing service for this clinic of the Long Island College Hospital. This service, established in 1919, has led to an increase in the number of patients treated and has also proved to be a great saving of the nurses' time. About 1,200 children are supervised in a year.

[22] This school was closed in July, 1931, because the demand for its services decreased as special classes for crippled children were organized in the regular public schools when needed.

Home Nursing and Bedside Care. Fifteen nursing agencies furnished bedside care to patients ill at home. Henry Street Visiting Nurse Service, the Visiting Nurse Association of Brooklyn, Jamaica District Nursing and Social Service Committee,[23] and the North Shore Public Health Nursing Association are public health nursing organizations organized independently.

The Norwegian Lutheran Deaconesses Home and Hospital has lately developed a visiting nursing service in connection with its hospital and nurses training school.

There are six groups of Catholic nursing Sisters—the Dominican Sisters of the Sick Poor, the Little Sisters of the Assumption, the Missionaries of St. Augustine, the Sisters of the Bon Secours, the Nursing Sisters of the Sick Poor in Brooklyn and in Queens.

The East Harlem Nursing and Health Service began its nursing work in connection with the health demonstration carried on in that district over a period of years under the auspices of various welfare groups. After the demonstration period, the organization continued to carry on a generalized intensive nursing program for its own district. Within this district it functions for the Henry Street Visiting Nurse Service, the Association for Improving the Condition of the Poor, and the Maternity Center Association.

The New York City Mission Society, Woman's Branch, gives nursing service to the needy among the seven mission churches of the society. All but one of these churches are below 14th Street. The seventh is in a Spanish section on West 115th Street. The Society accepts all calls, referring to other nursing agencies patients who fail to coöperate. The work is supervised by the pastors of the Missions. It includes not only actual nursing but also household duties, when necessary. Its nursing staff of twelve includes one practical nurse.

The Metropolitan Life Insurance Company and the John Hancock Mutual Life Insurance Company furnish bedside nursing service to their policyholders through the organized visiting nurse services except in Queens.[24]

Personnel

The number of persons of different grades of training employed in nursing services under different auspices is shown in Table 56.

Not included in this study, because they do not directly take part in the care of chronic patients, are the staff of the Bureau of Public Health Nursing in the Department of Health, which numbered 574 graduate nurses and supervisors and 72 practical nurses at the time of the study; nurses in the field of tuberculosis service; and nurses attending maternity cases exclusively. It should not be forgotten in considering the problems of chronic illness, that the Health Department nurses have an important

[23] Early in 1929, this organization gave up its nursing services because of lack of funds. It now refers all nursing calls to the Henry Street Visiting Nurse Service.
[24] The latter company has since adopted this policy in Queens also.

relation to the prevention of chronic disease and disability through their follow-up and educational work in connection with acute conditions that may become chronic if neglected or that predispose the patient to acquire a chronic disease. This is especially true in regard to their work with school children in the correction of physical defects and in follow-up of children recovering from contagious disease. When the number of nursing staff is not sufficient to perform these duties adequately, the result must inevitably be much chronic illness that could have been prevented. The Health Department's Committee on Neighborhood Health Development studied the public health nursing requirements of the city and reported,

TABLE 56

PERSONNEL ENGAGED IN NURSING SERVICE IN NEW YORK CITY OUTSIDE
THE DEPARTMENT OF HEALTH, BY TYPE OF AGENCY, 1928

Type of agency	Agencies	PERSONNEL				
		Total	Graduate nurses	Student nurses	Practical nurses	Others
Total	25	667	531	35	88	13
Nursing organizations	13	529	403	35	88	3
Hospitals	3	27	19	0	0	8
Health centers	3	30	28	0	0	2
Settlements	3	9	9	0	0	0
Family welfare agencies	1	39	39	0	0	0
Life insurance companies . . .	2	33	33	0	0	0

in 1931, that 800 additional nurses were needed for adequate care in the fields covered by the department's nursing service, or about twice the number then available, including those employed by private agencies.[25]

Four hundred and eighteen registered nurses and supervisors furnished home nursing and bedside care. The Henry Street Visiting Nurse Service had 216 nurses and supervisors and 20 to 30 nurses as students on its staff; the Brooklyn Visiting Nurse Association had 109 nurses besides the specially trained orthopedic nurses discussed below. At the time of the survey, the Metropolitan Life Insurance Company in Queens had 30 nurses; the East Harlem Nursing and Health Service, 24; the New York City Mission Society, Woman's Branch, 11; the Little Sisters of the Assumption, 9; the John Hancock Mutual Life Insurance Company, the Missionaries of St. Augustine, and the Norwegian Lutheran Deaconesses Home and Hospital, 3 each; the Recreation Rooms and Settlement, the Dominican Sisters of the Sick Poor, 2 each; the Nursing Sisters of Brooklyn and of Queens, the Jamaica District Nursing and Social Service Committee, the North Shore Public Health Nursing Association, the Christodora House, and the Sisters of the Bon Secours, 1 registered nurse each.

[25] City of New York Department of Health, *Weekly Bulletin*, vol. 20, No. 18, May 9, 1931, pp. 138-139.

Eighty-eight nursing Sisters and practical nurses did bedside nursing and gave other services needed in the home. They were attached to the following nursing services: Nursing Sisters of the Sick Poor of Brooklyn, 29; Dominican Sisters of the Sick Poor, 20; Sisters of the Assumption, 15; Sisters of Bon Secours, 10; Nursing Sisters of the Sick Poor in Queens, 7; Missionaries of St. Augustine, 6; and the New York City Mission Society, Woman's Branch, 1 practical nurse, a Russian woman doing special work among the Russians. The Jamaica District Nursing and Social Service Committee at the time of the study had practical nurses on call.

The 9 nurses and supervisors of the Brooklyn Visiting Nurse Association's orthopedic service and the 8 nurses and 2 supervisors of the New York Orthopedic Hospital and Dispensary had received specialized hospital training in orthopedic work. The 17 nurses and supervisors of the Association for the Aid of Crippled Children had received besides their nurse's training some training in social work and acquaintance with orthopedic care.

The Henry Street Visiting Nurse Service was giving field experience and instruction in public health nursing to 30 student nurses. This group under careful supervision perform the same duties as the graduate nurse. The East Harlem Nursing and Health Service employed two nurses' aides to assist the nurses in maternity work.

The insufficient number of visiting nurses in Queens was considered at a meeting of representative citizens of that borough in 1928. In figures presented by the Public Health Nursing Section of the Welfare Council, it was estimated that Queens needed 420 public health nurses or ten times as many as it had. The Henry Street Visiting Nurse Service has since extended its work to Queens, with 10 nurses in the field.

The Metropolitan Life Insurance Company had 30 nurses in Queens and expected to add 4 more; the John Hancock Life Insurance Company had 3 and expected to add 1 in the Jamaica district;[26] the other 3 nursing agencies employed altogether 10 nurses. The North Shore Public Health Nursing Association, which had one nurse at the time of the study, added a second in January, 1930.

Clientele Served

None of the general community nursing agencies discriminate in their intake policies against any patient on account of age, race, or creed or refuse any type of non-contagious illness. The three specialized services are limited to a particular class of patients.

Contagious diseases, as mentioned above are the responsibility of the Department of Health. The Henry Street Visiting Nurse Service and the Visiting Nurse Association of Brooklyn are the only other nursing groups that attend contagious cases at home. The nursing services work in close coöperation with the Department of Health.

Every child discharged from the municipal contagious hospitals with

[26] The John Hancock Life Insurance Company now purchases nursing service from the Henry Street Visiting Nurse Service in Queens as in the other boroughs.

a diagnosis of poliomyelitis is referred to the Children's Welfare Federation, which refers the child to the nursing agency specializing in that particular type of case. Patients from Manhattan and the Bronx are reported to the Association for the Aid of Crippled Children and from Brooklyn and parts of Queens to the Visiting Nurse Association of Brooklyn. A daily report is posted at the Department of Health offices in each borough and the agencies concerned get the names and addresses of such patients. A home visit is made during the patient's quarantine at the contagious hospital and regular visits to the home are made immediately after quarantine restrictions are raised. This assures a fairly adequate supervision over this type of crippling disease.

Coöperation with hospitals having orthopedic service has been established, by which the Association for the Aid of Crippled Children does the follow-up work for such institutions in Manhattan and the Bronx with the exception of the New York Orthopedic Hospital, which has its own follow-up service. Crippled children in Manhattan and Bronx public schools are also reported to the Association, as mentioned above. For these boroughs fairly close supervision of patients crippled through infectious diseases has been established; and instances should no longer occur, in which treatment was not given until crippling conditions had advanced so far that little improvement could be expected. Control over congenitally crippled children will probably be more difficult to achieve. The family is usually anxious to keep such a condition secret and do not realize the harm done to the child by not seeking assistance for early treatment.

The six Catholic Sisterhoods do all forms of nursing except prenatal and postpartum work and nursing of contagious cases. The Mother Superior of one Order said that their service was intended to help patients with acute illnesses and they did not as a rule receive chronic patients, although they continue their service if a chronic condition develops while the patient is under their care. From the four Catholic nursing services that furnished records for the census, 63 chronic patients were reported.

Insurance companies limit their services to policyholders. The Metropolitan Life Insurance Company furnishes nursing care to acutely ill industrial and intermediate policyholders and group certificate holders. The John Hancock Mutual Life Insurance Company extends its nursing service to small policyholders. Cases of illness among such policyholders of the former company resident in all boroughs except Queens are reported to either the Henry Street Visiting Nurse Service or the Visiting Nurse Association of Brooklyn; and those in Queens are cared for by the company's own nurses. The latter company followed the same practice until 1930, when it adopted the same system in Queens as in the other boroughs.

Length of Nursing Care

The nursing organizations giving bedside care have no rules governing the length of time a patient may be kept under care or the number of visits that may be made to one patient. Many patients are visited over a period of years. A patient with chronic disease under the care of the Henry Street Visiting Nurse Service or the Visiting Nurse Association of Brooklyn must be seen at least every three months by a doctor.

The average length of a visit in the Henry Street Visiting Nurse Service is 28 minutes, except in maternity cases, in which the average time required per visit is from 30 minutes for prenatal care to 59 minutes for care of the mother and new-born baby. The average time for the care of a chronic patient is 40 minutes.[27] A study made in 1925 showed an average of 53 minutes for chronic patients. The Henry Street Visiting Nurse Service has found that its increased emphasis on health service and mental hygiene in recent years has resulted in an increase in the average length of the nursing visit for all purposes.

The Mother Superior of the Sisters of Bon Secours told of a patient who had been visited every second day over a period of ten years; another who received two visits a week over a period of six years, and a third patient suffering from hemiplegia, who had been visited daily for four years by the nursing Sister, who also took care of the house and did some cooking.

The New York Orthopedic Dispensary and Hospital, as far as is possible with its staff of eight nurses in the field, attempts to follow up post-operative cases in all the boroughs for three years after discharge from the hospital or from its Convalescent Home in White Plains. In some instances, the Board of Education calls upon the Association for the Aid of Crippled Children to follow up and supervise the clinic attendance of patients who have previously attended the New York Orthopedic Dispensary and Hospital.

The two other groups caring for orthopedic patients have no rule in regard to the period for which treatments are given. In the orthopedic field service may be extended over a period of years. The accepted rule for a minimum of care, if so ordered by the physician, is three treatments a week in the first year after the onset of poliomyelitis, two treatments a week in the second year, and one treatment a week in the third or subsequent years. Most children with bone tuberculosis or rickets need careful supervision over long periods.

The Association for the Aid of Crippled Children cares for children from birth to sixteen years of age. In some instances this age limit is extended if the patient's condition warrants further supervision.

The Brooklyn Visiting Nurse Association does not place on its inactive list the name of any crippled child needing treatment and supervision unless there is a complete refusal on the part of the family to accept the service. In some cases of children needing operative treatment, an occasional visit is made over a period of eight or nine months in the attempt to gain the parents' consent.

The Metropolitan Life Insurance Company considers that in chronic cases the instruction of the family in the care of the patient is the chief

[27] Wales, Marguerite A. and De Bonneval, Mabel C., The Value of Measuring Rods in a Visiting Nurse Service. *Public Health Nurse*, vol. 19, No. 3, March, 1927, p. 119.

object of the nurse's visits, and that such patients will usually require six to eight visits. In cases of prolonged illness, the decision for an extension of the service is made at the main office of the company and a special permit is issued for each period of extension. In Queens, where the Company employed its own nurses, it was lenient toward the chronic patient in the application of its general policy because there was then no other nursing agency in the borough. Its maximum visit policy for chronic patients seemed to be more strictly enforced with the community nursing agencies, since each separate visit had to be paid for by the Company. The John Hancock Mutual Life Insurance Company allowed eight visits per patient; and its regulations governing the extension of the service were similar to those of the Metropolitan Life Insurance Company.

Discharge of Patients

The Visiting Nurse Association of Brooklyn, the Metropolitan Life Insurance Company, the John Hancock Mutual Life Insurance Company, and the Memorial Hospital for Cancer and Allied Diseases are the only nursing groups that have a definite policy of referring patients whom they cannot continue to visit.

The Visiting Nurse Association of Brooklyn has an understanding with the Sisters of the Sick Poor in Brooklyn that patients requiring more than the customary allowance of time per visit or needing household help and often other assistance, shall be taken care of by the Sisters. The Visiting Nurse Association in return looks after patients in distant parts of the city, which are within easier reach of the district centers of the Visiting Nursing Association than of the convent.

The Metropolitan Life Insurance Company states that it often has difficulty in referring patients for whom it cannot continue to care. The Little Sisters of the Sick Poor in Queens refuse to take patients if they are too far away from the convent. The same statement was made at the John Hancock Mutual Life Insurance Company.

The Little Sisters of the Sick Poor in Brooklyn and in Queens on the other hand spoke of a practice of other nursing agencies of unloading cases on them. The patients referred to them are often so ill that a day and night service is needed, which is very hard on the Sisters. "They know that we cannot refuse them or refer them elsewhere after having been called in," said the Mother Superior of the Little Sisters of the Sick Poor in Queens.

The Memorial Hospital for Cancer refers patients to the Henry Street Visiting Nurse·Service, the Catholic nursing homes, and the institutions for the chronic sick. At times, after a cancer patient has been referred to the Henry Street Service, the social service department of the hospital is still called on for further visiting, because of the pressure due to the demands on the Henry Street nurses for care of the acutely ill. These patients may then have to be placed in homes for incurables or sent to the Cancer Institute on Welfare Island. Transfer of such patients to the Cancer

Institute, however, is found to be unsatisfactory, as about 25 per cent of these referred patients leave dissatisfied within a week.

In all other nursing services giving bedside care, inquiries in regard to the referring of cases that could not be carried any longer brought no information other than, "We refer them elsewhere." This usually means that, unless arrangements are made for institutional care, the patient is referred to the Catholic nursing Sisters.

Charges for Service

Charges for nursing service are always adjusted to the patient's ability to pay. All of the nursing agencies care for a large number of patients free of charge. Charges for services were made on a per visit basis, the cost having been estimated on the actual cost of the average visit. The Henry Street Visiting Nurse Service and the East Harlem Nursing and Health Service charged $1.15 per visit. The Visiting Nurse Association of Brooklyn charged $1.10 per visit. The Norwegian Lutheran Deaconesses Home and Hospital, the Jamaica District Nursing and Social Service Committee, and the North Shore Public Health Nursing Association each charged $1.00 per visit. For high colonic irrigation a special charge of $2.00 was made, by the Jamaica District Nursing and Social Service Committee and of $3.00 by the Norwegian Lutheran Hospital.

No fees are charged by the Catholic nursing groups with the exception of the Sisters of Bon Secours. Voluntary contributions towards the support of the work are accepted. The patient pays the Sister's carfare to and from the convent. These organizations state that they do not take patients who are able to pay for service elsewhere.

The nursing service of the Memorial Hospital Social Service Department is free of charge, and only patients who cannot afford to pay are given this service. Medication and dressings are supplied to patients at home.

Cancer patients of the Cancer Institute, who were taken care of by the Henry Street Visiting Nurse Service, received dressings supplied by the local branch of the American Red Cross through the Social Service Department of the Cancer Institute. Medication was supplied from the Cancer Institute. Service to these cancer patients was free of charge.

Henry Street Visiting Nurse Service established an hourly nursing service several years ago to provide nursing for the patients who are able to pay a reasonable fee and who do not need an all-day service. Calls are made as near the time the service is desired as possible. Charges are made at the rate of $2.00 a visit. If the visit requires more than an hour it is charged for at the rate of 50 cents for each additional twenty minutes of service. The service must not exceed three hours per day. In 1929, 990 appointment service visits were made. The service has not been widely advertised. The Brooklyn Visiting Nurse Association also has an appointment service with a charge of $1.50 an hour.

The service of a graduate nurse for the whole day is too expensive a luxury for the group of business and salaried persons; only the wealthier group can afford it. The visiting nurse service has filled the need for the poorer classes. The largest group, the self-supporting middle class, cannot afford private nursing service and do not wish to accept services subsidized for charitable purposes. It is a well-known fact that a great many people avail themselves of services from charitable institutions, although they could afford to pay a reasonable fee. There is an excuse for this in the fact that service at a reasonable rate is not generally available.

ADDITIONAL SPECIAL FACILITIES FOR CRIPPLED CHILDREN

Nutrition

The nurses of the Association for the Aid of Crippled Children are supervising diets in connection with the general health of the patient. The Brooklyn Visiting Nurse Association also gives this service to its orthopedic patients, as well as to others who need it. It is the only nursing agency with a nutritionist on its staff whose sole duty is to supervise the diet as ordered by the physician in charge. The New York Orthopedic Dispensary and Hospital nurses do not supervise diets but limit their services exclusively to orthopedic work.

Appliances and Artificial Limbs

The Association for the Aid of Crippled Children has a fund for supplying shoes, braces, crutches, and other apparatus to needy patients. In many instances such expenditures are reimbursed by parents on an installment basis. Repairs on such appliances are likewise taken care of by the organization. The New York Orthopedic Hospital and Dispensary also supplies necessary apparatus when necessary. The Walter Scott Industrial School for Crippled Children, the New York Philanthropic League, the House of the Annunciation, and the Rhinelander School for Crippled Children provide appliances free of charge for patients recommended by the Visiting Nurse Association or the Brooklyn hospitals. The Philanthropic League of Jamaica and a small auxiliary committee connected with the Jamaica Hospital sometimes furnish braces or other apparatus for needy patients.

Transportation

Transportation to and from the hospital or clinic is supplied by the Association for the Aid of Crippled Children in Manhattan and the Bronx for children under the organization's care. A bus accompanied by an attendant in addition to the chauffeur calls at stated hours at the different hospitals with orthopedic services. Additional service for three afternoons a week was provided during most of the year of this study, 1928–1929. Taxi service is also supplied as needed from a special fund for the purpose.

The transportation of crippled children to clinics is a complicated and expensive service, for since the hospitals receive patients from all parts of the city, it may be necessary to carry the child upon discharge to a clinic far distant from his home. Continuity of treatment is especially important in orthopedic cases, as the individual interest of the physician in the particular child and the confidence of the parents in the physician play a large part in successful treatment. If a child living at a great distance is once admitted to a hospital in Manhattan, transportation to the clinic must later be provided for him over the long distance possibly for a period of years.

Most of the necessary treatments for children in Brooklyn were given in the patient's home, except in the Main district, in the neighborhood of the Long Island College Hospital. When necessary, the Brooklyn Bureau of Charities provided transportation for Brooklyn children. In Queens, members of the Philanthropic League took patients to and from clinics.

Transportation of helpless children to and from school has been supplied by the Board of Education since 1913. This service was taken over in that year from the Association for the Aid of Crippled Children. The number of crippled children given transportation in 1926 was 2,550. Later reports of the Board of Education do not give the number of children carried, but give the cost of the service as $405,000 in 1926; $435,000 in 1927; and $490,000 in 1928.[28] At the close of the school year in 1928, there were 2,665 children registered in the crippled classes of the elementary schools.[29] The transportation facilities seemed to be adequate in relation to the number of children needing the service. Additional transportation needed for high school children has since been provided.

SUMMARY

1. Home nursing service for chronic patients as defined in this study, is furnished entirely by voluntary agencies. The Department of Hospitals has no visiting nurse service, although the social workers of the municipal hospitals make home visits. The Department of Health in its Bureau of Nursing is not concerned with chronic diseases other than the contagious forms, such as tuberculosis and venereal diseases.

2. Twenty-five nursing services were maintained by voluntary agencies of different kinds at the time of the survey. These services were of three main types—7 agencies doing almost entirely educational work; 3 specialized agencies, one for cancer and two for orthopedic cases; and 15 community nursing services for the care of the sick, varying in scope from 5 services employing one nurse each to 2 services with a staff of 100 and 200 nurses respectively.

3. Nearly 670 persons were employed in home nursing service in the agencies studied, of whom over 500 were graduate nurses and 100 were practical nurses or attendants, the rest being student nurses. Four fifths

[28] Superintendent of Schools, City of New York, Annual Report, 1925–1926, p. 492; 1926–1927, p. 489; 1927–1928, p. 351.
[29] Ibid., 1927–1928, p. 503.

of the entire number were attached to nursing agencies and a fifth were engaged in nursing services conducted by health centers, hospitals, family welfare agencies, settlements, or life insurance companies.

4. The agencies doing mainly educational work had 78 nurses; the specialized services had 42 nurses; and the community nursing services had 547 nurses, a fourth of whom were either student or practical nurses.

5. Medical social workers from hospitals and clinics also care for many chronic sick patients in their homes who are in need of service and assistance in maintaining a suitable régime but who do not require nursing. The share of the home care of the chronic sick that the medical social workers may be expected to bear has not yet been studied.

6. In relation to chronic illness, the responsibility of public health nursing organizations extends to both prevention of chronic disease and disability through educational work and care of the chronic sick through home nursing.

CHAPTER 7

Visiting Doctor Service in Relation to the Care of the Chronic Sick

VISITING DOCTOR SERVICE FOR CHRONIC PATIENTS

WHERE a general outdoor medical service is found, other, that is, than outdoor service for obstetrical care, it is usually intended primarily to serve the acutely ill patient who can be cared for in his own home through one or two visits from a physician and as a rule it serves children more frequently than adults. Such a service helps to keep hospital beds free for patients who need the elaborate diagnostic and laboratory facilities of a hospital. It has been used less frequently for chronic than for acute patients, partly no doubt because it is more difficult to organize the home over a long period for the care of a sick person, especially an adult, than for the short period of care ordinarily required for acute minor illnesses.

There seems to be, however, a growing conviction that chronic illness as well as acute illness could often be cared for advantageously by visiting doctor service, if nursing facilities were also made available. Many believe that home care has advantages both for the patient, when he would be happier at home, and also for the community, since it is apt to be more economical than institutional care. In families with sufficient means, it is customary to keep chronic invalids at home with a private physician in attendance and a nurse if necessary; and under these conditions the sick person, if well cared for, is usually much happier than he would be in an institution. If it is practicable for the community to provide such care for dependent patients whose home conditions permit it and if it can be given as economically as institutional care, it would seem that home care should be made available for these patients as well as for those financially more fortunate.

In a recent survey of the hospital needs for treatment of contagious diseases in the Bronx, the conclusion was reached that a system of home medical care with the requisite nursing service was desirable in certain cases of contagious disease. "The adoption by the City of the policy of home nursing care for suitable cases, in addition to hospital care, should result in material improvement in the control of contagion within the home and in lowered mortality, and, for those patients who would otherwise be hospitalized, in a substantial reduction in the cost of care. . . . The City could with advantage provide home nursing care, particularly for children under five years of age, utilizing organized competent visiting nurse services, under the supervision of externes or physicians from the staffs of the communicable disease hospitals, or of other qualified physicians."[1] It

---

[1] Phillips, Anna C., A Survey of the Communicable Disease Hospital Needs of the Borough of the Bronx, City of New York. The New York City Visiting Committee of the New York State Charities Aid Association, 1932, p. 58.

seems probable that similar provision for home nursing care under medical supervision would be an advantageous method of care for certain chronic patients. Centralized direction of the medical service as well as of the nursing service would be essential to the success of this method.

The special report on cancer in Massachusetts[2] recommended that "efforts be directed toward the extension of local district nursing service, to the end that through better care of terminal cases at home the volume needing hospitalization may be diminished and the comfort of the patient during his last days may be enhanced through being able to remain in the home environment." Such a service must necessarily be under medical supervision. Memorial Hospital, in providing nursing service in inoperable patients in their own homes also takes the attitude that institutionalization is a less desirable form of care for this type of chronic patient than care at home.

The development of a visiting doctor service caring for chronic invalids depends upon the availability of other services such as visiting nurse service and provision for housekeepers or attendants to go into families unable to manage without such assistance. Cancer patients in the terminal stages of the disease can be taken care of as comfortably at home as in a hospital, with occasional visits from a doctor if the family either has visiting nurse service or has learned how to care for the patient. Many of the less severe paralyses of the aged are also suitable for home care with occasional medical oversight. Certain patients with chronic cardiac conditions may remain at home if medical oversight is available at times when they need bed care for a few days. Children with heart disease under treatment at the Massachusetts General Hospital in Boston are kept at home when confined to bed, if suitable conditions can be arranged, and visited by a physician from the clinic staff as well as by a social worker.[3]

New York City has never had organized outdoor medical service for the entire city nor for any one borough; and the possibilities of home care for the sick through visiting doctor service have not been considered on any large scale in this city. Seven hospitals as part of their maternity service send physicians into the patients' homes for deliveries. A number of general and special hospitals send a physician to a patient's home in certain situations. Two unattached dispensaries maintain a visiting doctor service with one physician each. A third dispensary discontinued a service of this kind in 1928; and now its staff physicians make home visits if a special need arises. Social agencies occasionally call upon individual doctors to visit patients in their care, but as organized medical services in hospitals and clinics have increased, this kind of informally arranged visiting has become rare.

The various small and unrelated services of this kind in New York and

[2] Special Report of the Departments of Public Health and Public Welfare Relative to the Prevalence of the Disease of Cancer throughout the Commonwealth, and particularly of the Disease in its Inoperable Stage or Form. The Commonwealth of Massachusetts, House Document No. 1200, December, 1925, p. 98.
[3] See also vol. 1, Chapter 3, The Special Problems of Some Main Groups of Chronic Diseases, p. 152.

the organized services of a more general character in a number of other communities suggest that the feasibility of this type of service should be given consideration in a program for the care of the chronic sick. Possibly in this city it could not be used as extensively as in a smaller city, because in a community where space is at a high premium, families with low incomes are less likely to have living quarters adapted to the care of a sick person, particularly a chronic invalid. In addition to overcrowding, such factors as noise, lack of outlook on open spaces, and lack of privacy in small apartments contribute to the necessity for institutionalization of chronic patients even when they are ambulant and still more frequently when they are confined to bed or wheelchair. However, there are many instances in which a chronic patient could remain at home if he could have the services of a physician when unable to attend a clinic.

In the administration of the city's home relief for the unemployed, provision was made for employing private physicians and obtaining nursing service from the community nursing organizations in cases of acute illness requiring home care. For a time little use could be made of this provision, because the funds appropriated were not sufficient to relieve the most pressing needs for food and shelter; but an appropriation for this purpose from the State Temporary Emergency Relief Administration has made it possible to put this plan into operation. The policies in regard to medical care for those receiving aid under the old age security law are not yet defined; but hospital and clinic care are relied upon as much as possible and there is no provision for home medical care.[4]

The organization of a visiting doctor service for a large city presents many administrative difficulties. The most advantageous auspices must first be determined. The selection and supervision of the medical personnel must then be carefully safeguarded. The efficient functioning of other necessary services in relation to the medical service must be provided for. Definition of standards of practice is essential in any organization of home medical care. Medical standards must be maintained through centralized responsibility and supervision; and it is as important that visiting physicians should utilize other services such as nursing service and social service as that physicians in hospitals and clinics should do so. Adequate medical records are a further requirement. It is also necessary to have definite policies for the hospitalization of patients who need the laboratory and other diagnostic facilities of a hospital.

The question naturally arises whether home medical care should be a municipal service. It is generally conceded that it would be more economical for the city to care for many of the dependent sick in this way than in hospitals. In New York, a change in the City Charter would be required before such a service could be undertaken; for relief of any kind given in the home is strictly limited to certain groups. The state public welfare law authorizes any measures that seem desirable for the health and welfare of dependent persons; but the provisions of this law do not apply in New York City.[5]

---

[4] See also vol. 1, Chapter 4, The Care of the Chronic Sick in Municipal Institutions, pp. 230–231.
[5] Ibid., p. 230.

No method has been developed for giving medical care to the aged receiving assistance under the old age security law when they are not able to attend a clinic but do not need to be in a hospital. The temporary measure for home medical care authorized as a part of the emergency program for relief of the unemployed will afford some experience upon which to base further consideration of the question whether some form of home medical care for the dependent under municipal or voluntary auspices is practicable and desirable in this city.

In various communities some provision is made by official or voluntary agencies for medical service to the sick in their homes. In some instances, a city physician engaged in private practice makes one visit on request and refers the patient to the appropriate medical agency. In rarer instances, the service is organized for home medical care and physicians connected with a medical institution, whenever it is necessary, treat the patients in their homes. Some examples are given below of the different auspices under which services of this kind are conducted and of the different ways in which they are organized.

Boston. Boston probably has the most completely organized district doctor service in the country. Two voluntary institutions, the Boston Dispensary and the Massachusetts Memorial Hospital, have given service of this kind in certain districts for many years; and since 1931, the entire city has been districted and covered by one or the other. The Boston Dispensary reorganized its service in that year and extended it to cover all districts of Boston not served by the Massachusetts Memorial Hospital. This action followed a recommendation of the Boston Health League, which had studied the situation and concluded that district medical service was much needed in some sections of Boston in which it had never been provided.

The medical work is carried on by district units consisting of a physican in charge and four senior medical students from Tufts Medical School. The visiting nurse service is given in all districts by the Community Health Association. In 1930, nearly 5,000 patients received over 13,000 visits; and the director of the Boston Dispensary estimated that between 300 and 500 of these patients were adults with chronic illness. Such conditions as heart disease, cancer, varicose ulcers, and arthritis have been treated by this service.

The Massachusetts Memorial Hospital for many years has had a district service for obstetrical cases as well as for general medical and surgical cases. This service is supplied both from the hospital's out-patient department and also from a medical dispensary conducted by the dispensary in another district; and it is under the direction of the physician in charge in each place. Physicians respond to calls at any hour of the day or night.

Nursing care is given by the nurses of the Community Health Association in both districts, and in addition by a staff of nurses connected with the dispensary. Over 10,000 visits a year are made by physicians in the two districts.

Chicago. In Chicago, outdoor medical service for the needy poor is given through the Cook County Bureau of Public Welfare. It has a staff of thirty physicians in private practice to whom it assigns the patients from the various districts of the county. The Visiting Nurse Association receives a list of all calls placed and visits for nursing care within a few hours after the physician has seen the patient. In 1928, nearly 21,000 doctor's visits were made through this system. No figures have been published that show the extent to which chronic patients are served.

Indianapolis. Indianapolis has a visiting doctor service in connection with the Indianapolis City Hospital. The doctors are internes in the hospital serving a month at a time. One social worker is assigned to the service.

Minneapolis. Since 1931, home visiting service has been conducted by the Minneapolis General Hospital through a system of fellowships financed by the hospital in the Graduate School of Medicine at the University of Minnesota. Previously, the city has employed four physicians engaged in regular private practice to respond to calls for a physician from the homes of indigent persons. Under the present arrangement there are three medical fellows doing home visiting and one in the hospital to answer calls for this service. The fellows are attached to the medical division of the hospital; and they are under the direction and control of the chief of the medical service who is a full professor in the Medical School. They call on him for advice and if necessary he accompanies them on a visit to the home.

The following evaluation of this service has been made by the superintendent of the hospital: "We think that we have accomplished several things by entering into this arrangement. In the first place we have co-operated with the Graduate School of Medicine and provided four additional fellowships—four postgraduates in the school. Second, we have provided for our medical fellows a service which corresponds very closely indeed to the service which they will enter on when they go out into independent practice themselves. We have provided that these men may get their first experience, in what corresponds to private practice, under the direction and guidance of a capable internist. Fourth, we are enabled to care for many patients in the home for long periods of time who would otherwise be occupying beds in the hospital and producing a certain stasis in the hospital ward services. Lastly, we believe that we are giving much more prompt and efficient service to the indigent citizens of the community than it is ever possible to provide through the medium of part-time service of practicing physicians whose foremost interest must necessarily be in the establishment of their own private practice. It may be mentioned as an interesting fact that, the first month this service was established, the number of calls made jumped to better than eight hundred for the month, as compared with three hundred and eighty-five for the preceding month. Since the first of July the home calls made have continued to increase, and at the present time our home visits number better than nine hundred a month."[6]

Through this service, it is possible not only to keep out of the hospital patients who can be taken care of adequately at home but also to discharge many patients from the hospital earlier than otherwise, because an occasional visit from a physician is all the medical attention they need. The majority of the calls received are for patients with acute diseases, but many chronic patients are also cared for at home.

The service covers the city which is divided into as many districts as there are medical fellows on duty. The hospital is the receiving station for all calls, which come from many sources and are received at any hour of the day or night. Obstetrical service for deliveries in the home is not included. "The average period under the care of the visiting physician is one call only. In other instances two or three calls may be made and the patient then referred to the Hospital Out-Patient Department. Certain cases, however, such as cardiacs, may be under the care of visiting physicians throughout the year continuously. These patients can be taken care of ordinarily just as well in the home as in the hospital."[7]

Philadelphia. There are twenty physicians connected with the Department of Public Health, covering the entire city, who answer calls from their private offices for the treatment of persons unable to pay a private physician. The seriously ill are referred to the city hospital and those able to attend a clinic to the nearest out-patient department. This is not a service for outdoor medical care and the visiting physician has no further responsibility for treatment after the first visit.

Saskatchewan, Canada. An example of visiting doctor service for rural communities is the "municipal doctor system" in the province of Saskatchewan, which was studied by the Committee on the Costs of Medical Care.[8] Here rural communities have levied taxes to engage the services of full-time or part-time physicians to meet the shortage of doctors in rural communities. The system is regarded favorably by both physicians and communities participating. Chronic patients are served as well as the acutely ill.

[6] Remy, Charles E., M.D., Superintendent, Minneapolis General Hospital, New Ideals in Clinical Fellowships. Reprinted from *The Proceedings, Congress on Medical Education, Medical Licensure and Hospitals,* Chicago, February 15 and 16, 1932, p. 2.

[7] Letter received from Charles E. Remy, M.D., Superintendent of the Minneapolis General Hospital, November 25, 1932.

[8] Rorem, Rufus C., The "Municipal Doctor" System in Rural Saskatchewan. Publications of The Committee on the Costs of Medical Care: No. 11. Washington, April, 1931.

Facilities for visiting doctor service in New York City are chiefly for obstetrical care. From the Lying-In Hospital over 6,000 visits were made in the homes of patients by staff physicians in 1931. Two institutions recently merged with the Lying-In Hospital in the Medical Center of the New York Hospital-Cornell Medical College Association, the Manhattan Maternity Hospital and the Berwind Maternity Clinic, also conducted outdoor medical services.

Other institutions with outdoor medical service for obstetrical care are Long Island College Hospital, the New York Nursery and Childs Hospital, Bellevue School for Midwives, and Flower Hospital. In addition to these services which are not included in this study, outdoor medical service is furnished by three dispensaries and seven hospitals in various ways described below.

The New York Dispensary. The New York Dispensary used to have an extensive visiting doctor service, which was discontinued in May, 1928. Late in 1931, it was reëstablished on a less extensive scale. Staff doctors now visit only the dispensary patients who are too ill to attend clinic and who are unable to afford the services of a private physician. At present about fifteen to twenty calls a month for this service are received. It serves children more largely than adults but an occasional chronic patient is cared for. Cardiac patients needing bed care for a week or two are often cared for.

Northern Dispensary. The Northern Dispensary, with an active clinic serving about 6,000 patients annually, also has a district doctor service for clinic patients who are too ill for the time being to attend the clinic. It serves the district between 23rd and Spring Streets and Broadway and the North River. All patients needing nursing service are referred to the Henry Street Visiting Nurse Service for care. In 1930, 600 patients received nearly 700 visits from the staff physician assigned to this service. At the time of the census, 31 chronic patients were reported by the dispensary.

Northeastern Dispensary. The Northeastern Dispensary has an outdoor district service between 40th and 90th Streets and Fifth Avenue and the East River. It is intended for those without the means to employ a regular physician but "a nominal fee is always charged, except where an applicant for help claims and demonstrates his inability to pay." The usual charge for the doctor's visit is fifty cents. There is one visiting physician on the staff for this service. The annual report of the dispensary for 1930 reports over 4,000 patients treated in this department during the year. Among the patients under care at the time of the census, there were 37 chronic patients of the types studied. The dispensary has no visiting nurse service and does not report its patients under care at home to the Henry Street Visiting Nurse Service as a routine practice, although a patient considered to be in special need of nursing service may be referred.

The Northern Dispensary and the Northeastern Dispensary are the only agencies that have a visiting doctor service within the scope of this study. They reported 31 and 37 chronic patients respectively. Their 68 patients

TABLE 57

CHRONIC PATIENTS UNDER THE CARE OF TWO VISITING DOCTOR SERVICES CLASSIFIED BY DIAGNOSIS, EACH AGE GROUP

Diagnosis	Total	AGE GROUP					
		Under 16	16-39	40-59	60-69	70 and over	Not reported
Total	68	11	13	20	14	8	2
Epidemic diseases, syphilis	2	0	0	2	0	0	0
General diseases	12	2	4	2	4	0	0
Rheumatism	6	0	1	1	4	0	0
Diabetes	3	0	2	1	0	0	0
Other	3	2	1	0	0	0	0
Diseases of the nervous system . .	6	1	1	2	1	0	1
Paralysis agitans	3	0	0	1	1	0	1
Other	3	1	1	1	0	0	0
Diseases of the circulatory system .	17	3	3	5	3	3	0
Diseases of the heart	14	3	3	5	0	3	0
Other	3	0	0	0	3	0	0
Diseases of the respiratory system .	7	2	1	1	2	1	0
Diseases of the digestive system, hernia	5	3	0	1	1	0	0
Non-venereal diseases of the genito-urinary system	6	0	3	2	0	0	1
Diseases of the skin and cellular tissue	9	0	1	3	3	2	0
Old age	2	0	0	0	0	2	0
External causes, fracture	1	0	0	1	0	0	0
Ill-defined diseases	1	0	0	1	0	0	0

were of all ages. Their diagnoses show a variety of chronic conditions, among which heart disease predominated. (See Table 57.) Nearly two fifths of these 68 patients had been under care for a year or longer and more than a fourth for less than three months. For about a fourth of these patients, the care received was unsuitable in some respect—2 patients needed to be in an institution; the homes of 10 were unsuitable for their care; and 6 needed a different type of care and too little was reported about their home conditions to indicate whether they could receive it suitably at home. These findings suggest that a visiting doctor service as well as a clinic or hospital should have the required personnel not only for nursing service but also for social service in order that the medical care may be adequately carried out.

New York City Cancer Institute. The Social Service Department of the New York City Cancer Institute has an informal arrangement for calling upon staff doctors to go into the homes of cancer patients who have been examined and diagnosed as inoperable in the clinic but who refuse to enter either the Cancer Hospital on Welfare Island or some other institution. The service is paid for by a special fund raised by the Social Service Department, nursing service is furnished by the Henry Street Visiting Nurse Service, and sterile dressings by the New York County Chapter of the American Red Cross. Only a small number of patients are cared for in this way but there are always some under care. It represents a recognition on the part of the Institute that there are instances in which a cancer patient may spend the last days of his life more happily at home than in an institution and it provides with medical supervision for a group who might otherwise have no medical care. Because this service is informal and little advertised, it was not included in the census of the chronic sick.

Beth Israel Hospital. Beth Israel Hospital visits patients in their homes but does not, strictly speaking, have a district visiting doctor service. Two classes of patients are visited by this service. Patients who have been in the hospital and have an unfavorable reaction are visited by the house doctor; and if they require further treatment they are readmitted to the hospital. The second group are patients referred by private physicians or social agencies for admission to the hospital in whose cases the diagnosis as stated makes it seem doubtful whether the patient will be accepted by the hospital. In such cases a staff doctor visits to determine whether the patient shall be admitted.

Mt. Sinai Hospital. Mt. Sinai Hospital has no visiting doctor service as such. It has several district doctors. When an application is made for admission to the hospital in a case in which there is doubt as to its eligibility for hospital care, one of the district doctors goes to the home to diagnose and pass on the question of admission. Certain classes of patients are not received in the hospital, such as, alcoholism, chronic conditions, and mental diseases; and the district doctor merely determines whether the person visited comes within one of these classes. He does not continue his visits.

In addition to this type of service, the social service department is given the services of a physician for a very limited number of visits a month to the homes of patients who have formerly been under its care. Separate records were not kept for patients visited in this way; but it is likely that a few chronic patients who were originally in the hospital in an acute condition are included in this service. In 1929, a total of 435 visits were made to 402 patients for both of these types of service.

New York Infirmary for Women and Children. The New York Infirmary for Women and Children has maintained an out-practice service since 1850. It serves acutely ill persons who are unable to attend the clinic and cannot afford private physician's fees. Nearly all patients who are cared for by this service live in the neighborhood of the hospital, although the service is not limited to that district. The service, furnished free to patients, is given by a physician who is full time on the hospital staff for that purpose. In 1929, 3,560 visits were made to 554 patients, of whom three fourths were children. Since the physician in charge of the service reported that only an occasional chronic patient was cared for through this service, it was decided not to include it in the census of the chronically ill.

Lenox Hill Hospital. The Lenox Hill Hospital, formerly the German Hospital, by arrangement with the German Society, sends its staff doctors to the homes of the members of the Society for illnesses that do not require hospitalization. In 1930, 2,784 doctors' visits to patients in their own homes were made under this arrangement. Since this service is open, however, only to members of the benevolent society, it was not considered as properly belonging in the census of the chronic sick.

French Hospital. The French Hospital has a similar arrangement with the French Benevolent Society but the service is much smaller. Here staff doctors go to the patient's home only to ascertain whether he should be hospitalized. If he continues to need medical care in his home, the care is transferred to a private physician. Only 121 such visits were made in 1929.

Hospital for Joint Diseases. The Hospital for Joint Diseases has a plan for monthly visits as long as necessary to patients in plaster casts who have been discharged from the hospital but need medical oversight. This is a very small service, only 77 visits having been made by physicians in 1929.

SUMMARY

A number of cities have some provision for home medical care for the indigent under either official or voluntary auspices. Outdoor medical service for obstetrical care is an established practice.

1. Some of the municipal services for general medical care at home are not strictly speaking visiting doctor services, since the responsibility of the city physician is limited to one visit for the purpose of referring the patient to the appropriate hospital or clinic.

2. The visiting doctor service that assumes responsibility for home treatment and secures the necessary nursing care is usually a department of a medical institution.

3. In some instances, the service is organized for the purpose of affording medical students and fellows opportunities for treatment of the sick at home as part of their medical education.

4. Where visiting doctor service exists, the large majority of the calls upon it are for acute illness; but many chronic patients are also cared for by this means.

5. The possibility of caring for chronic patients in their homes through visiting doctor service is beginning to receive attention. A great many patients who could be taken care of at home equally well or possibly better occupy hospital beds for long periods. The resulting expense to the community is probably much greater than the cost of well-organized home care.

6. New York has no service for home medical care covering the city or any one borough. Two medical dispensaries have each a visiting physician on the staff for home care of patients in their districts. From a third dispensary, staff physicians visit patients too ill to attend clinics. Seven hospitals also make a practice of sending a physician to visit a patient at home when necessary.

7. Physicians from all ten institutions make approximately 12,000 visits a year. The two medical dispensaries that offer the service regularly together recorded about 4,700 visits in 1930. They reported 68 chronic patients receiving this care in the census of the chronic sick.

8. There seems to be a trend toward home care for the sick rather than institutional care, whenever it is possible, both for acute and contagious diseases and for chronic diseases. There are certain conditions in both types of disease that can be adequately treated at home.

9. The experiment in home care of the sick that is being undertaken in this city by the temporary emergency relief agencies of the state and city will tend to focus attention upon this method of care.

10. Since public home relief in New York City is strictly limited to certain classes, a revision of the Charter would be necessary before a visiting doctor service could be provided by the city beyond the present emergency due to unemployment.

11. An adequate service for home medical care requires centralized responsibility and supervision in order to maintain medical standards; careful selection of personnel; definition of standards of practice; definite policies in regard to integration of hospital and home care; efficient records; and provision for the efficient functioning of other required services, namely, nursing service and social service.

12. The experience of other communities in caring for the indigent sick through visiting doctor service seems to indicate that such a service functions most adequately when it is a department of a medical institution.

CHAPTER 8

The Care of the Chronic Sick by Family Service Agencies

SECTION A

THE PROBLEM OF CHRONIC ILLNESS IN RELATION TO THE WORK OF THESE AGENCIES

THE clients of a family service agency come to its attention as a rule because of financial need. The responsibility of the agency, however, goes beyond the relief of this condition. It endeavors to uncover the causes that led to the need and to assist the members of the family to organize their lives in order to become as far as possible a self-supporting and harmonious unit. If resources for self-support cannot be developed within the family, the agency must obtain financial assistance, from its own funds or through other agencies, in the form of monetary relief at home or of care provided by an institution.

At all points in the work of family agencies, chronic illness is a factor of outstanding prominence. It appears as a leading cause of dependency, which brings applicants for assistance. It decreases the earning capacity of some members of families and demands the services of others for the care of the sick. When it causes the death of the bread winner, it leaves families destitute. It creates the need for providing financial support or obtaining institutional care for persons totally incapacitated.

In the interests of the clients' mental and physical well-being as well as of their economic support, the agency seeks to learn their state of health through medical examination and to correct their physical defects. The services looking toward prevention of chronic disease are, therefore, of great concern to family agencies, as well as the problems of assistance and care in chronic illness.

Chronic disease is always a social as well as a medical problem. Even when the financial resources are sufficient, a protracted illness invariably involves a readjustment of habits of life on the part of the patient and usually of other members of the family as well. Securing the necessary medical services is of course the first consideration, but the economic and vocational problems connected with chronic illness are no less pressing. Often the problem of vocational training for a child crippled by poliomyelitis or of vocational retraining of an adult partially incapacitated by chronic illness is more difficult than the problem of obtaining medical care. Readjustment of the family budget may be necessary when expensive treatments, such as insulin injections, are required. A change of living quarters may be necessary for the family in which there is a sufferer from chronic cardiac disease. Assistance with the housework may enable a mother with some severe physical disability to have satisfactory care at home and so prevent the breaking-up of the family.

Among families on the border line of poverty or those of small means, chronic illness with consequent loss of income and extra expenses may soon lead to destitution, especially if the invalid is the chief wage earner. Of the total amount of relief given to 458 families in regular allowances by the Charity Organization Society, in 1928–1929, 54.3 per cent went to families in which physical or mental illness of the chief wage earner was the main cause of the financial need.[1] The greater part of this illness presumably was of long duration. Another 9.7 per cent went to persons whose chief cause of need was classified as "old age," and the disability of some of these persons was probably due to chronic illness.

Physical disease, either as the main cause of the need or as a contributing cause, appears in a large majority of the families that come to family service agencies for help. The New York Charity Organization Society, in 1926–1927, found physical problems in 76 per cent of its families.[2] Among 14,000 families under the care of three family agencies of Manhattan, in 1925, 87 per cent presented a health problem, either physical or mental.[3]

In addition to the cost of service for health education and supervision by the agency's staff and the cost of medical examination and treatment furnished by the family society or by medical agencies, a large part of the expenditures for financial relief by family agencies goes to families made destitute through illness. In a study of family relief in Philadelphia, made in 1926, it is stated that " 56 per cent of the relief disbursements of the Jewish Welfare Society and 44.4 per cent of those of the Family Society were made to families in which illness was the main cause of distress."[4]

It is not always possible to distinguish between acute and chronic illness in the available statistics on the subject. In the figures given below, an attempt has been made to show the proportion of physical problems occurring in the work of several family agencies of New York due to the chronic diseases included in this study.

In a study of clients of four large family service agencies of New York, in 1927, which included 14,000 families with over 67,000 members, chronic diseases of the types included in this study were found in more than one third of the families.[3]

The Charity Organization Society for the year 1927–1928 reported 7,677 physical disease problems among 4,666 families. This figure represents the minimum number of physical problems, for if tuberculosis were a problem in a family and several members of the family were tuberculous, the prob-

---

[1] The Charity Organization Society of the City of New York, Annual Report, Forty-seventh Year, October 1, 1928, to September 30, 1929, p. 21.

[2] White, Helen C., The Relation of the Family Case Work Agency to the Clinic. *Hospital Social Service*, vol. 18, No. 1, July, 1928, p. 10.

[3] Bryant, Louise Stevens, Better Doctoring—Less Dependency: A Study of the Relations Between Medical and Non-Medical Agencies, with Special Reference to Clinic and Family Services. Committee on Dispensary Development of the United Hospital Fund of New York, 1927, pp. 8–10.

[4] The Philadelphia Relief Study: A Study of the Family Relief Needs and Resources of Philadelphia, Committee on the Philadelphia Relief Study, 1926, p. 10.

lem would be listed only once. Nearly 50 per cent of these 7,677 physical problems were problems of chronic diseases, such as are included in the present study.[5]

The Association for Improving the Condition of the Poor, during the year 1926–1927, found 13,587 health problems among the 5,681 families under its care, of which 29.2 per cent were caused by chronic diseases of the forms included in this study.[6]

The Brooklyn Bureau of Charities, during the year 1926–1927, had 3,540 families under care presenting 6,327 physical disability problems, of which 32.6 per cent were problems of chronic disease.[7]

The annual report of the Jewish Social Service Association, 1927, shows that 97.4 per cent of its 3,248 families receiving major care presented health problems and 64.3 per cent had chronic disease problems.[8]

The United Jewish Aid Societies of Brooklyn in its annual report of 1927 states that 93 per cent of its families receiving major care had health problems. In 49 per cent of its families, there was a problem of chronic disease.

It would seem that the conclusion might be drawn from these figures that there is a problem of chronic illness of the type, but not the degree, with which this study deals in fully half, and probably a larger proportion, of the families with which the family service agencies deal and that from one fourth to one half of all the health work of these agencies is concerned with chronic illness.

Six of the family welfare societies represented in the census, having 92 per cent of all the patients reported by such agencies, were reporting their case loads by number of families monthly to the Department of Statistics of the Russell Sage Foundation.[9] From these reports, the total case load was obtained for the month the census was taken. The average percentage of families in which there was a chronically ill person incapacitated by illness among all the families under care by the six agencies reporting was 15.3 per cent. The proportion of families with members incapacitated by chronic illness in the different agencies varied from 10.6 per cent to 22.7 per cent. In addition to those who were disabled by illness, it would appear from the figures above on the frequency of chronic illness that the number of clients

[5] The Charity Organization Society of the City of New York, Annual Report, Forty-sixth Year, October 1, 1927, to September 30, 1928, pp. 13, 21.

[6] New York Association for Improving the Condition of the Poor, Report of Problems and Services in Health and Social Work During the Fiscal Year 1926–1927, Statistics Bureau, 1928, pp. 1, 10.

[7] Brooklyn Bureau of Charities, Department of Service and Relief, Annual Statistical Report, 1926, 1927, p. 1.

[8] Jewish Social Service Association, Annual Report, New York, 1927, p. 4.

[9] This department has been collecting and compiling monthly statistics of family welfare agencies since January, 1926. Its first emphasis was "upon the problem of obtaining comparable and adequate statistics of the operation of these agencies for comparison and combination." By May, 1928, the department believed that a "common scheme of statistics is now in use in a considerable number of agencies and is producing reasonably comparable data." See Hurlin, Ralph G., Some Results of Two Years' Study of Family Case Work Statistics, Reprinted from Proceedings of the National Conference of Social Work, 1928. In July, 1928, the Welfare Council undertook the collection and analysis of monthly statistics of family service agencies in New York City as part of the Central Reporting Service of its Research Bureau.

suffering from chronic disease but not incapacitated by it is even larger than the number disabled by it.

It is difficult to estimate what percentage of the case load of all of the family service agencies were cases of chronic illness at the time of the census. The total case load was not taken at that time in every agency and the annual reports of the agencies give the total number of families known during the year and cared for throughout the year but not the number of persons under care in a particular month.

The data obtained in the census related to individuals who have been or probably will be incapacitated by chronic illness for at least three months. Therefore the discussion of this group of persons leaves largely out of consideration the subject of prevention of chronic disorders through physical and mental hygiene, health examination, and early medical treatment. The discussion that follows is confined to the problems of care for persons chronically ill and unable to carry on their ordinary activities.

CHRONICALLY ILL PERSONS UNDER CARE

Records of 2,052 persons were obtained from eleven family service agencies. These are all of the agencies of this type in the five boroughs with the exception of one agency in Richmond and four chapters of the American Red Cross, three in Queens and one in Richmond, each of which has a comparatively small case load.

There were 484 persons who were receiving some form of assistance from another type of agency at the same time that they were under the care of family service agencies. Most of them were persons reported by both the nursing and family service departments of the Association for Improving the Condition of the Poor. In eliminating duplicates for tabulation of the census totals, nursing service was regarded as taking precedence over family service from the standpoint of care in illness, so that the total number of patients in the care of family agencies appearing in tabulations of the total census is 1,568. In this section of the report, however, the full number of 2,052 persons have been described.

The 2,052 chronically ill persons in the care of family agencies are nearly 10 per cent of the whole number of persons in the census. Five family service agencies in Manhattan serving also, with one exception, the Bronx reported 74.6 per cent of the patients. Four agencies in Brooklyn reported 23.1 per cent. Two agencies in Queens reported 2.3 per cent.

The proportion of patients of Queens agencies is small because the one agency that attempts to cover the work of the entire borough, the Family Welfare Society of Queens, had not received sufficient financial support to permit a complete program for the borough. It had only three district offices and a staff of nine case workers. With this staff, it was impossible to cover the borough, which is made up of twenty or thirty communities scattered over a great area.

The relatively small proportion of patients reported by the Brooklyn agencies is partly explained by the fact that the total staff of social case workers of the four Brooklyn agencies was less than half as large as that of the five Manhattan agencies. It is probably also to some extent due to the relative scarcity of health agencies in Brooklyn in comparison with such resources in Manhattan. Brooklyn evidently has a smaller proportion of its chronic sick under the care of welfare agencies than Manhattan or the Bronx. In the whole census, half of all the patients who were city residents came from Manhattan, with 29 per cent of the city's population, about a fourth from Brooklyn, with 37 per cent of the population; and 17 per cent from the Bronx, with 17 per cent of the population.[10]

Age and Sex

Less than 10 per cent of the patients reported by family service agencies were children under sixteen years of age, although children were 31 per cent of all persons found in the census. The high percentage of children in the total census is due to three groups of agencies that specialize in children's services and reported three fourths of all the children in the census—orthopedic nursing services, convalescent homes, and agencies for the after-care supervision of cardiac children.

About 40 per cent of the chronically ill clients of the family service agencies were in the years forty to sixty. Twenty-nine per cent were in the younger adult period of life. Twenty-two per cent were older persons sixty years of age and over, about half of whom were seventy years of age or over. The percentage of persons of different ages reported by family service agencies is shown in Table 58 below. (See also Chart 16.)

TABLE 58

CHRONICALLY ILL CLIENTS OF FAMILY SERVICE AGENCIES
CLASSIFIED BY SEX, EACH AGE GROUP

Age group	Total		Male		Female	
	Number	Per cent	Number	Per cent	Number	Per cent
Total	2,052	100.0	1,162	100.0	890	100.0
Under 16 years	193	9.4	83	7.1	110	12.4
16–39 years	586	28.7	332	28.6	254	28.6
40–59 years	809	39.6	541	46.7	268	30.1
60–69 years	237	11.6	106	9.1	131	14.7
70 years and over	218	10.7	91	7.8	127	14.2
Not reported	9	. . . . .	9	. . . . .	0	. . .

There were more males (56.6 per cent) than females (43.4 per cent), particularly among the older adults up to sixty years. Among those seventy years of age and over, women were in the majority. Among Negroes, who numbered only 96 persons, there were more females.

[10] Population estimated by the United States Bureau of the Census for July 1, 1928, based upon the Census of 1930.

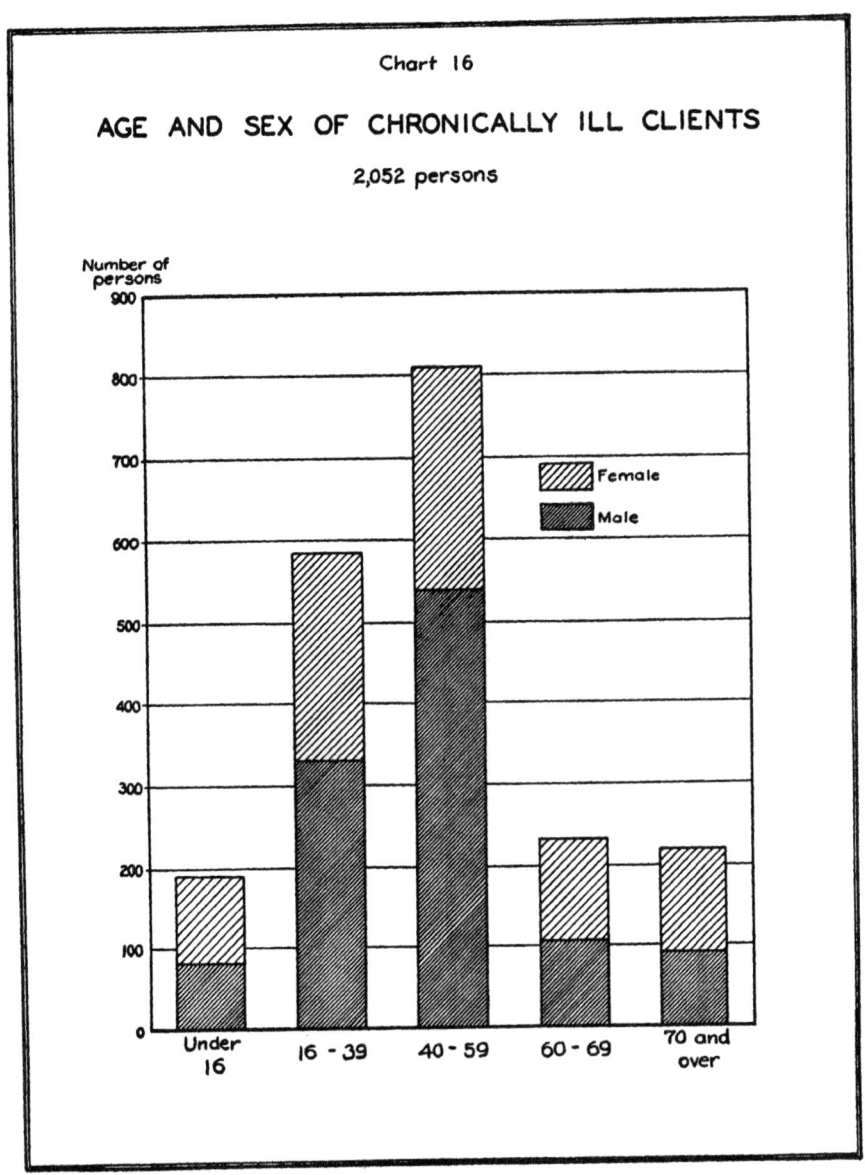

Chart 16

AGE AND SEX OF CHRONICALLY ILL CLIENTS

2,052 persons

Diseases

The diagnoses of the chronically ill persons under the care of the family service agencies are shown in Appendix Table 8. Heart disease caused the illness of more persons (15 per cent) in this group than any other condition. Diseases of the nervous system came next with 14 per cent. Rheumatism came next with 8.5 per cent. Diseases of the respiratory system were next with 7.3 per cent. Syphilis, diseases of the digestive system, and old age came next, each with about the same number of patients, 6 per cent. There were 99 patients with asthma, 89 with diabetes, and 63 with cancer. All of the degenerative diseases that are commonly thought of as occurring in old age were found not only in persons of forty years of age and over but also among the younger adults.

A secondary diagnosis was reported for 27 per cent of the patients and a tertiary diagnosis for 4.3 per cent. No doubt, other persons were suffering from complicating diseases that were not recorded. The diagnoses most frequently given as subsidiary to the primary cause of the chronic illness were heart disease, 93 persons; diseases of the digestive system, 67 persons; syphilis, 44 persons; and rheumatism, 38 persons.

Heart disease was the most important single disease for every age group except persons sixteen to thirty-nine years of age and the aged, seventy years and over. Among the aged, more than half were suffering from the infirmities of old age. Heart disease and rheumatism were next, with 7.4 per cent of the total. Nearly a fourth of the 193 children had heart disease and 10 per cent had syphilis. Among the younger adults, 16 per cent were suffering from diseases of the nervous system and 14 per cent from diseases of the heart. Among persons forty to fifty-nine years of age, 15 per cent had heart disease and 13 per cent diseases of the nervous system. Of all patients suffering from rheumatism and arthritis, 4.4 per cent were in this age group. Among those sixty to sixty-nine years of age, heart diseases were most frequent, occurring in over 14 per cent of all persons in this group. In this age group, nearly 14 per cent had diseases of the nervous system and 11 per cent rheumatism. The diagnosis of 11 per cent of this group was "ill-defined diseases."

Disease conditions found in a larger percentage of the chronically ill clients of the family service agencies than of all the persons in the census were rheumatism, syphilis, diabetes, bronchial disorders, and digestive diseases. The family service agencies reported 50 of the 86 patients in the whole census suffering from chronic alcoholism.

Mental Abnormality

There were 642 persons among the chronically ill clients of family service agencies who were reported to have habits and mental peculiarities that complicated their care. Over 250 were suffering from a definite mental disorder. The question whether any mental abnormality in the patient had been diagnosed or suspected was answered less frequently on the records from family service agencies (78 per cent) than on those from any group of agencies. On the other hand, the percentage of mentally abnormal persons reported was much higher than in other agencies. Some mental abnormality was found in 24.4 per cent of their chronically ill clients. (See Table 59 below.) In 8 per cent, it had been diagnosed and in 16.4 per cent, it was suspected by the social worker responsible for the patient.

That the family agencies found a higher percentage of mental problems than other agencies is probably due to the fact that they must of necessity study the personality of the client in order to assist him. The practice of securing mental as well as physical examinations for clients is growing

TABLE 59

CHRONICALLY ILL CLIENTS OF FAMILY SERVICE AGENCIES
CLASSIFIED BY MENTAL ABNORMALITY, EACH AGE GROUP

Age group	Per cent reported	MENTAL ABNORMALITY			
		Total	None	Diagnosed	Suspected
Total	71.3	1,595	75.6	8.0	16.4
Under 16 years	74.6	144	82.6	4.9	12.5
16–39 years	75.4	442	73.5	11.1	15.4
40–59 years	78.2	633	72.2	8.5	19.3
60–69 years	78.5	186	79.6	5.9	14.5
70 years and over . . .	83.9	183	84.2	2.1	13.7
Not reported	2	7	3	2	2

among family agencies. The percentage of patients with diagnosed mental disorder was considerably higher in the family agencies than in the medical and nursing agencies.

Among those in the middle years of life, there were a larger proportion with mental problems, both diagnosed and suspected, than among the children and older persons. It is in these years, when the adult is expected to be self-supporting, that it is most important for the agency to understand the client's mental condition. The highest percentage of diagnosed cases was in the age group sixteen to thirty-nine years.

An attempt to obtain data on the extent to which chronic disease is influenced by the emotional life is being made by the Division of Adult Hygiene of the Massachusetts Department of Health. In the house-to-house surveys of chronic illness, which this department made in certain cities and rural districts of Massachusetts, information was obtained from the chronically ill aged in regard to their habits throughout life. It is hoped that these data may throw some light on the importance of failures in both physical and mental hygiene as factors in causing chronic disease.[11]

Duration of Illness and Disability

The length of time since the beginning of the illness, recorded for 70 per cent of the patients, is shown below in Table 60.

[11] Lombard, Herbert L., M.D., The Chronic Disease Problem in Massachusetts. *Hospital Social Service*, vol. 22, No. 5, 1930, p. 397. Read before the National Conference of Social Work, November, 1930.

Only about one tenth had been ill less than a year. Nearly a tenth had been ill fifteen years or more. There were 72 patients reported as having been ill for twenty years or more. The illness of nearly half, 46 per cent, had lasted as long as five years; and of two thirds, as long as three years.

TABLE 60

CHRONICALLY ILL CLIENTS OF FAMILY SERVICE AGENCIES
CLASSIFIED BY DURATION OF ILLNESS

Duration of illness	Number	Per cent
Total	1,441[1]	100.0
Under 3 months	15	1.0
Three months and under 1 year	119	8.4
One year and under 2 years	187	13.0
2 years and under 3 years	162	11.2
3 years and under 4 years	162	11.2
4 years and under 5 years	125	8.7
5 years and under 10 years	379	26.3
10 years and under 15 years	159	11.0
15 years and under 20 years	61	4.2
20 years and over	72	5.0

[1] Time since onset not reported for 611 persons.

The length of time that the illness had caused the patient to be incapacitated was recorded but was not tabulated for separate agency groups. In the total census, the duration of the disability and the onset of the disease were reported to have occurred within the same period of years in a large

TABLE 61

CHRONICALLY ILL CLIENTS OF FAMILY SERVICE AGENCIES CLASSIFIED BY
DEGREE OF DISABILITY, EACH AGE GROUP

Degree of disability	Total	AGE GROUP					
		Under 16	16-39	40-59	60-69	70 and over	Not reported
Total	2,052	193	586	809	237	218	9
Bedridden	159	17	37	71	20	14	0
Ambulant	1,601	144	467	616	188	178	8
Wheelchair	61	5	15	20	8	13	0
Semi-ambulant . . .	36	5	12	17	1	1	0
Not reported	195	22	55	85	20	12	1

majority of cases, indicating that the disability usually followed quickly upon the beginning of the disease. Possible inaccuracies, however, in information of this kind given in the agencies' records should be taken into consideration.

The degree of disability, indicated by the fact that the patient was bedridden, ambulant, or semi-ambulant, was reported for 90 per cent of the whole number. (See Table 61 above.) With few exceptions, the chronic sick under the care of family service agencies would naturally be ambulant patients. Nearly 75 per cent were attending clinics for medical care. However, over a tenth of those for whom the information was reported were either bedridden or confined to a wheelchair; and in addition a small percentage were able to walk about during only a part of the day. Patients with these degrees of incapacity were found among persons of all ages about equally.

TABLE 62

CHRONICALLY ILL CLIENTS OF FAMILY SERVICE AGENCIES CLASSIFIED BY
PERIODS OF CARE RECEIVED FOR CHRONIC ILLNESS, EACH AGE GROUP

Period of care received	Total	AGE GROUP					Not reported
		Under 16	16–39	40–59	60–69	70 and over	
Total	1,822[1]	167	516	720	212	199	8
Under 3 months	12.1	15.5	12.0	10.7	15.1	12.1	0
3 months under 1 year	29.2	28.6	30.2	28.9	34.4	23.1	2
One year under 2 years	19.6	19.1	18.6	21.7	16.0	19.6	0
2 years under 3 years	11.3	10.7	11.9	11.9	13.2	11.6	2
3 years under 4 years	9.2	9.0	9.1	9.0	9.0	9.0	3
4 years under 5 years	5.1	4.7	5.0	5.0	6.1	4.5	1
5 years under 10 years	9.7	10.7	10.3	10.0	4.7	12.1	0
10 years under 15 years	3.1	1.7	2.5	3.6	0.6	6.5	0
15 years under 20 years	0.5	0.0	0.2	0.7	1.0	0.5	0
20 years and over	0.2	0.0	0.2	0.1	0.0	1.0	0

[1] Time under care not reported for 230 persons.

The prognosis was considered favorable for more than a third of the children, about 15 per cent of those between sixteen and forty years of age, for 8 per cent of those between forty and seventy years of age, and for 1 per cent of those seventy years of age or over.

Length of Care

The periods of care given to patients of different ages by the agency reporting them, as shown above in Table 62, vary from less than three months for 12 per cent of the whole number to fifteen years or longer for nearly 1 per cent. It is possible that the same patient may also have been under the care of the agency at some previous time. The time reported here is the period during which the agency has had the patient continuously under care for chronic illness.

The length of care up to ten years is approximately the same for all age groups. Some who have been under care for ten years or more are found in every age group, although a larger percentage is found among the aged. About two fifths had been under the care of the agency for less than a year, and another one fifth between one and two years. A fifth had received between two and five years of care from the agency. A tenth had received from five to ten years of care. Four per cent had been under care for ten years or more. Nine persons had received care for between fifteen and twenty years, and four persons, twenty years or longer.

Ten per cent of the patients cared for by family agencies had been known to the agencies prior to the onset of chronic illness. Of those for whom both the length of time since the onset of the disease and the length of time since the agency's first contact with the client were reported, 22 per cent had been known to the agencies for the duration of the illness and 78 per cent

TABLE 63

ADMISSIONS OF CHRONICALLY ILL CLIENTS OF FAMILY SERVICE AGENCIES
TO INSTITUTIONS ON ACCOUNT OF CHRONIC ILLNESS

Admissions	Number	Per cent
Total	1,338[1]	100.0
One admission	482	36.0
Two admissions	259	19.4
Three admissions	110	8.2
Four admissions	49	3.7
Five admissions	27	2.0
Six admissions	17	1.3
Seven admissions	7	0.5
Eight admissions	2	0.1
More than 9 admissions	1	0.1
No admissions	384	28.7

[1] Number of admissions not reported for 714 persons.

had been known for a shorter period. Of those who had been known to the agency ten years or more, all had been ill for at least ten years. Of those ill ten years or more, 15 per cent had been known to the agency as long as ten years; and 35 per cent had been known less than a year. Of those ill between five and ten years, 21 per cent had been under the care of the agency for an equal period, and 28 per cent for less than a year. (See Appendix Table 9.)

That most of the chronically ill clients of the family agencies had at some time received institutional care for their illness is shown by Table 63 above.

Less than a third of those for whom the information was obtained had never been in an institution on account of chronic illness. A third had been admitted more than once to an institution for this reason. Over a third had received institutional care only once. Ten persons had been seven or more times in an institution. As many as 16 per cent had been admitted to an institution more than twice.

Home Conditions

Of all the adult patients reported by family service agencies, over two thirds were married. A much larger percentage of men than women in each age group were married. There were comparatively few unattached chronically ill men. The problems of chronic illness, therefore, with which the family service agencies deal are found chiefly in normal families or in families of single or widowed women.

A small percentage (3.9 per cent) of the chronically ill clients had no permanent home at the time of the census. They were either in an institution temporarily or in a temporary lodging. The home conditions of those who had homes were rated as satisfactory or unsatisfactory, in the opinion of the social worker responsible for the client's care, in respect to physical condition, the make-up of the family, and the family attitudes. The evaluation

TABLE 64

CHRONICALLY ILL CLIENTS OF FAMILY SERVICE AGENCIES WITH HOMES
CLASSIFIED BY HOME CONDITIONS

Situation reported	HOME CONDITIONS							
	All conditions		Physical condition		Family make-up		Family attitude	
	Number	Per cent	Number	Per cent	Number	Per cent	Number	Per cent
Total . .	1,973[1]	100.0[1]	1,973	100.0	1,973	100.0	1,973	100.0
Suitable . .	1,185	60.1	1,401	71.0	1,373	69.6	1,399	70.9
Unsuitable .	131	6.6	327	16.6	282	14.3	253	12.8
Unknown . .	211	10.7	245	12.4	318	16.1	321	16.3
[1]	446	22.6	. . . .	. . . .	. . . .	. . . .	. . . .	. . . .

[1] These are made up of homes in which there were various combinations of suitable, unsuitable, and unknown factors.

of the physical conditions of the home was based upon a judgment as to whether the surroundings were suitable for the patient's care in regard to sanitation, heat, light, fresh air, and space. The make-up of the family was judged from the standpoint of the ability of members of the family to provide for the needs of the sick person. A home in which the adult members were obliged to go out to work leaving a bedridden patient or a crippled child alone was considered unsatisfactory in this respect. In regard to family attitudes, both the attitude of other members of the household toward the patient and his attitude toward them were taken into consideration.

The home conditions of 60 per cent of those with homes were reported to be satisfactory in all these respects. All conditions were reported to be unsatisfactory in the homes of 7 per cent, or 131 persons. The information about home conditions was incomplete for 22 per cent. Some unsatisfactory condition was reported in the majority of these homes. No information about home conditions was reported for 11 per cent. In each age group, approximately the same proportion of unsuitable homes were reported.

The percentage of homes in which different conditions were found to be suitable or unsuitable for the patient's care is shown in Table 64. Approximately the same proportion of homes were reported unsuitable from the standpoint of each of the three conditions noted.

The judgment of the social worker responsible for the client in regard to the possibility of adjusting unsatisfactory home conditions was recorded whenever possible, but the information obtained on this subject is too slight to have much significance. The possibility of adjusting unsuitable conditions was judged to be favorable in the instances in which the information was reported as follows: in 58 of 68 homes in regard to physical condition; in 14 of 35 homes, in regard to family make-up; and in 17 of 40 homes in regard to family attitude. In 79 of the 90 homes in which the unsatisfactory conditions were not specified, the situation was not considered capable of being adjusted.

An analysis of the records of the 131 clients whose homes were reported to be unsuitable for their care in all respects showed that among them the average size of the family was nearly eight persons. A seventh of all the families with nine members or more reported by family service agencies were in this group. Nearly two thirds of these clients were foreign-born. Thirty-seven per cent of them showed some mental abnormality in contrast to 24 per cent of all patients reported by family service agencies. There was a larger proportion of persons between forty and sixty years of age in this group and a smaller proportion of adults under forty years of age than in the whole group of patients reported by family service agencies. The proportion of persons needing only attendant care was also larger. A fifth of the group were in institutions at the time of the census. A fourth of those at home lived alone or with relatives. Thirteen persons sixty years of age or over were living alone under unsuitable conditions. Thirty-seven persons, forty years of age or over, with a variety of diseases, were living under unsuitable conditions in homes where there were growing children, on an average four children between three months and fifteen years in each home.

The agencies having these 131 patients under care reported a possibility of adjusting the unsatisfactory home conditions in only ten families. In the family of a child who was the patient, it would be necessary to find the father employment and teach the mother how to keep house. For a woman of fifty-three years of age, the attitude of her children toward her care and support needed to be changed. Other adjustments indicated were moving to better living quarters, reëstablishing a broken home, and removing another member of the family suffering from a mental disease.

Financial Status

Income. The sources from which the chronically ill clients of family agencies derived their income are shown in Table 65 for persons of different ages. Nine per cent of the adults had no income at the time. Three children were working and had a personal income. Of the adults reported to have a personal income, 69 per cent were being subsidized by a social agency, 46 per cent were sharing the family income, 25 per cent were earning, and nearly 10 per cent were receiving income from compensation, insurance, pensions, savings, and other sources.

In the whole census, information in regard to income was reported for all but 7 per cent of the adults outside of homes for the aged. Only 40 per cent of them had some personal income derived from family income (57.9 per cent), subsidy from a social agency (38.3 per cent), earnings (25.2 per cent), or from all such sources as savings, pension, insurance, and workmen's compensation (9 per cent).

Of all the adult chronically ill clients of the family agencies, over a third were being assisted financially; less than a third had resources of their own;

TABLE 65

CHRONICALLY ILL ADULT CLIENTS OF FAMILY SERVICE AGENCIES WITH INCOMES CLASSIFIED BY SOURCES OF INCOME, EACH AGE GROUP

Source of income	Total	AGE GROUP			
		16–39	40–69	70 and over	Not reported
Total reporting sources[1] . . .	1,648	497	938	207	6
Subsidy, ...	69.2[2]	59.6	70.8	83.6	0
Family income	45.7	46.9	50.1	24.2	0
Earnings	24.7[3]	27.4	24.8	18.4	0
Savings	2.1	.8	1.6	7.2	0
Pensions	1.9	3.6	1.1	1.9	0
Compensation	1.8	2.2	2.0	0.0	0
Insurance	1.5	2.4	1.1	1.4	0
Other	2.2	2.0	1.9	4.3	0

[1] The percentages below are based on the number of persons reporting sources of income, and not on the total number of sources.

[2] Represents 55.6 per cent of total number of chronically ill persons under care of the agencies.

[3] Represents 20.0 per cent of total number of chronically ill persons under care of the agencies.

and a little over one half were receiving support from their families. Frequently, the patient's income was derived from several sources.

As would be expected, the proportion of persons receiving a subsidy from an agency was largest among the aged; and a smaller proportion of the aged were depending upon a family income. The proportion of persons who depended upon a family income was somewhat higher among persons forty to sixty-nine years of age than among the younger adults. The income of the 1,648 adults whose sources of income were reported came from 2,458 different sources, an average of 1.5 sources per person. The relative frequency of the various sources is shown in the following table.

The amount of the weekly family income is given in Appendix Table 10 for families of different sizes. A patient living alone was classified as a family of one. Information on the size of the family was obtained in all but twenty-one families; and the amount of the income was obtained for 65 per cent of the families with incomes. Small families of from one to three persons were 43 per cent of the whole number. Of the remaining families, approximately half were large families of over five members and the other half, families of four or five persons.

Of the families whose weekly income was reported at the time of the study, in the spring of 1928, nearly nine tenths had less than $35 a week; nearly two thirds, less than $25 a week; and nearly one fourth, less than $15 a week. There were 13 families in which 5 or more persons were dependent upon a family income of less than $15 a week. In 81 per cent of the families with $35 or more, there were at least 5 persons in the family. All of the 25 families with incomes of $50 or more had 4 or more members, and 12 of them had over 7 members.

The average size of the family among these chronically ill clients was a

TABLE 66

NUMBER AND PERCENTAGE DISTRIBUTION OF SOURCES OF INCOME
FOR 1,648 ADULT CLIENTS OF FAMILY SERVICE AGENCIES

Source of income	Number	Per cent
Total	2,458	100.0
Subsidy	1,140	46.4
Family	753	30.7
Earnings	407	16.5
Other	37	1.5
Savings	34	1.4
Pension	32	1.3
Compensation	30	1.2
Insurance	25	1.0

little more than 4 persons. The size of family found most frequently (18 per cent) was that of 2 persons. Of the families of one or 2 persons, 61 per cent had an income of less than $15, and 96 per cent had less than $25. Of families from 3 to 5 persons, 11 per cent had incomes below $15; 65 per cent had less than $25; 9 per cent had $35 or more. Of families of more than 5 persons, 27 per cent had incomes of less than $25; 70 per cent had less than $35; and 4 per cent had $50 or more.

Not more than 6 per cent of these families, whose income was known, had an income amounting if regular to $2,150 a year, which was estimated by the Labor Bureau Incorporated to be the amount necessary in 1928 to maintain a family of five at a level of health and decency in New York City. All but 1 per cent had incomes below $3,350, estimated by the same authority to be the standard budget for a skilled workman's family of 5 members.[12] The annual income of 87 per cent would amount to less than $2,000; of 63 per cent to less than $1,300; and of 23 per cent to less than $800. The median weekly family income was $21.20. The modal weekly family income falls within the $15–$19 group. The average weekly income was $23.30.

The families of the chronically ill children reported by family agencies had larger incomes than the families that reported older members as patients. For example, incomes of less than $15 were found in 6 per cent of the

[12] The Living Wage—June, 1928. *Facts for Workers:* A Monthly Review published by The Labor Bureau, Inc., vol. 6, No. 12, September, 1928, p. 1.

families in which the patient was a child; in 12 per cent of the families of those sixteen to thirty-nine years of age; in 23 per cent of the families of those forty to sixty-nine years of age; and in 66 per cent of the families of those seventy years of age or over. Incomes of $35 or more were found in 21 per cent of the families of children; in 15 per cent of those sixteen to thirty-nine years of age; 13 per cent of those forty to sixty-nine years of age; and only 1 per cent of those seventy years of age or over. Four per cent

TABLE 67

CHRONICALLY ILL CLIENTS OF FAMILY SERVICE AGENCIES CLASSIFIED BY
AMOUNT OF WEEKLY EARNINGS AND SEX

Weekly earnings	Total	Male	Female
Total	1,897[1]	1,094	803
No earnings	1,439	807	632
Total with earnings reported	419	260	159
Under $5	52	18	34
$5–$9	83	40	43
$10–$14	39	22	17
$15–$19	58	47	11
$20–$24	24	22	2
$25–$29	18	18	0
$30–$34	12	12	0
$35–$39	6	5	1
$40 and over	8	6	2
Amount not specified	119	70	49
Not reported	39	27	12

[1] Children under working age numbered 155.

of the families of children had incomes of $50 or more; 3 per cent of those sixteen to thirty-nine years of age; 2 per cent of those forty to sixty-nine years of age; and none of the families of the aged, seventy years of age or over.

Earnings and Employment

Although the census included only persons incapacitated for carrying on their usual occupations, over a fifth of the chronically ill adults, or 22 per cent, reported by family service agencies had some employment for which they were paid. Three children under sixteen years of age were also working. Eighteen per cent of the adults had never been employed. Housewives were regarded as being not employed, although their occupation was tabulated. Of those who had employment, a little over half were casually and not regularly employed. Among the aged, of seventy years of age or over, who were working, less than 4 per cent were regularly employed.

The earnings of 26 per cent of the men and 22 per cent of the women who had employment are shown in Table 67. The amounts earned were for the most part small. However, 4 per cent of all the men were earning $25 a week or over. Only 3 women earned as much as $25 a week.

The proportion of persons able to earn something was about the same among the younger and the older adults, approximately a fourth, as shown in Table 68. About a fifth of the aged, seventy years of age or over, were earning something.

TABLE 68

CHRONICALLY ILL CLIENTS OF FAMILY SERVICE AGENCIES CLASSIFIED BY
AMOUNT OF WEEKLY EARNINGS, EACH AGE GROUP

Weekly earnings	Total	AGE GROUP				
		Under 16	16–39	40–59	70 and over	Not reported
Total	1,897[1]	38	586	1,046	218	9
No earnings	1,439	35	431	787	178	8
Total with earnings reported . .	419	3	141	237	38	0
Under $5	52	2	8	28	14	0
$5–$9	83	1	21	50	11	0
$10–$14	39	0	14	23	2	0
$15–$19	58	0	23	35	0	0
$20–$24	24	0	12	11	1	0
$25–$29	18	0	5	13	0	0
$30–$34	12	0	5	7	0	0
$35–$39	6	0	4	1	1	0
$40 and over	8	0	4	4	0	0
Amount not specified	119	0	45	65	9	0
Not reported	39	0	14	22	2	1

[1] Children under working age numbered 155.

The period since the last employment was reported for about 900 of the 1,100 persons previously employed who were out of employment and is shown in Table 69 for different age groups:

TABLE 69

CHRONICALLY ILL CLIENTS OF FAMILY SERVICE AGENCIES NOT EMPLOYED
CLASSIFIED BY LENGTH OF TIME UNEMPLOYED, EACH AGE GROUP

Age group	Total	LENGTH OF TIME UNEMPLOYED						
		Less than 3 months	3 months and less than 1 year	1 year and less than 2 years	2 years and less than 3 years	3 years and less than 5 years	5 years and less than 10 years	10 years and over
Total	905[1]	5.1	27.3	20.9	14.1	16.7	10.9	5.0
16–39 years	236	8.5	34.3	24.1	10.2	13.1	8.9	.9
40–69 years	551	4.5	27.2	20.0	16.1	17.1	11.1	4.0
70 years and over . .	113	0.9	10.6	19.5	12.4	23.0	15.0	18.6
Not reported	5	0	4	0	1	0	0	0

[1] Length of time unemployed not reported for 206 persons.

Sixteen per cent had been unemployed five years or more. Of those 70 or over, 34 per cent had been out of employment for at least five years, and 18.6 per cent for at least ten years.

The customary occupation before the illness was recorded is shown in Table 70 below, and classified as "light" or "heavy" work of different types.

Nearly three fourths of the women, including the housewives, and more than a tenth of the men had done domestic work. A nearly equal propor-

TABLE 70

CHRONICALLY ILL CLIENTS OF FAMILY SERVICE AGENCIES
CLASSIFIED BY OCCUPATION AND SEX

Occupation	Male		Female	
	Number	Per cent	Number	Per cent
Total	1,013	100.0	685	100.0
Heavy work	417	41.2	513	74.9
Outdoor	196	19.4	5	0.8
Mechanical	86	8.5	1	0.1
Domestic	135	13.3	507	74.0
Light work	596	58.8	172	25.1
Outdoor	163	16.1	17	2.5
Non-sedentary mechanical . .	289	28.5	57	8.3
Sedentary mechanical	144	14.2	98	14.3

tion of men and women had done light mechanical work of a sedentary character. A small proportion of the women had done other light mechanical work. A larger percentage of the men (28.5 per cent) had done light mechanical work than any other type. The next largest percentage of the men (19.3 per cent) had done heavy outdoor work. Another 8.5 per cent had done heavy mechanical work. Therefore, 41 per cent of the men had done heavy work including domestic work, and nearly 59 per cent had done light work.

Dependency. All persons in the census were considered dependent, since they were receiving some form of care or assistance from a welfare agency. One fourth of the whole number of chronically ill clients of the family service agencies were wholly dependent—4 per cent on public agencies, 18 per cent on private agencies, and 3 per cent on the combined assistance of both. Besides the 18 per cent wholly dependent on aid from private agencies, 48 per cent were depending in part on private aid without other assistance from family or friends. Thirteen per cent in all were receiving some assistance from public sources, either through temporary care in hospitals or through mothers' pensions or other outdoor relief.

Of the 1,781 chronically ill adult clients for whom the information was reported, 36 per cent were wholly dependent and 64 per cent partly dependent for care and maintenance upon resources other than their own. Of the adults who were wholly dependent, more than a fourth and of those partly dependent, 8.4 per cent were receiving some assistance from relatives or friends. The number of persons of different ages dependent upon assistance from public and private sources appears in Table 71.

TABLE 71

CHRONICALLY ILL CLIENTS OF FAMILY SERVICE AGENCIES
CLASSIFIED BY TYPES OF DEPENDENCY, EACH AGE GROUP

Type of dependency	Total	AGE GROUP					
		Under 16	16–39	40–59	60–69	70 and over	Not reported
Total reporting	1,974	193	568	771	227	207	8
Patient wholly dependent	829	190	209	217	101	106	6
Public aid only	76	6	25	30	10	5	0
Private aid only	355	13	100	120	60	59	3
Private aid and family or friends .	291	148	41	37	25	37	3
Public and private aid	59	4	25	25	3	2	0
Public and private aid, family . .	48[1]	19[1]	18	5	3	3	0
Patient partly dependent	1,145	3	359	554	126	101	2
Public aid only	5	0	3	1	0	1	0
Private aid only	953	2	301	466	100	82	2
Private aid and family or friends .	87	1	24	36	14	12	0
Public and private aid	90	0	28	46	12	4	0
Public and private aid, family . .	10	0	3	5	0	2	0
Not reported	78	0	18	38	10	10	2

[1] Includes one person who was receiving public aid and aid from family or friends.

Of the 193 children reported by family agencies, 23 were entirely dependent upon welfare agencies, 3 were working, and the remainder were mainly dependent upon their families or friends. The smallest percentage of persons wholly dependent, except children, is found in the age group, forty to fifty-nine years of age (28 per cent) and the largest percentage among persons sixty years of age or over (47 per cent).

The amount granted by the family agency as a regular allowance in a family in which there is a chronic invalid is given on the census schedule. This information was tabulated in two representative agencies in order to indicate the cost of chronic illness through amounts granted in relief alone. The amount spent by the agency for workers' services and overhead expenses in assisting those families would be difficult to estimate. (See also pp. 276–277.)

An analysis of the allowances of 212 families assisted by these two agencies, which reported 33 per cent of all the chronically ill clients of family service agencies, is shown in Table 72 below. In each family, there was at least one chronic patient; and in one family there were four. Eight hundred and eighty-eight persons were members of these 212 families. They received a total of $2,371 in weekly allowances. This represents an average allowance of $11.18 per family per week.

In more than half of these families, the weekly allowance amounted to nearly half of the total weekly income. The amounts allowed ranged from under $5.00 in 21 per cent of the families to between $30 and $35 for 1 per cent. The largest number, 27.8 per cent, received between $10 and $15. Nearly one third of all the persons in the 212 families were in the families receiving allowances of between $10 and $15.

TABLE 72

FAMILIES UNDER CARE, PERSONS IN FAMILIES, AND WEEKLY ALLOWANCES
REPORTED BY TWO FAMILY SERVICE AGENCIES

Agencies	Number of families	Number of persons in families	Weekly allowances
Total	212	888	$2,370.89
First agency	54[1]	263	507.90
Second agency . . .	158[2]	625	1,862.99

[1] One family, number of persons not reported; one family had 2 chronic sick patients reported.

[2] Eleven families had 2 chronic sick patients; one family had 3 chronic sick patients; one family had 4 chronic sick patients.

INADEQUACIES IN PRESENT CARE

Types of Care Needed

For 82 per cent of the chronically ill clients of the family agencies active medical treatment, or "A," care was required. Nursing, or "B," care was required for 1 per cent. Attendant, or "C," care was required for 17 per cent. Nearly a third of those needing "C" care were aged infirm persons without a specific chronic disease who required only the simplest form of attendant care.

A comparison of the type of care needed with the type of care the client was receiving is presented in Chart 17. Of those needing "A" care, 88.5 per cent were receiving it; over half of those needing "B" care were receiving it; and 37.5 per cent of those needing "C" care were receiving it. Of those who required "B" or "C" care, 34.6 per cent were receiving "A" care and 18.3 per cent no care at all for the chronic illness. Of those who needed "A" care, 0.5 per cent received "B" care, 4.4 per cent "C" care, and 6.6 per cent no care.

There were 178 persons, or 9.2 per cent of the whole number, whose illness was not receiving any special attention, of whom 171 were adults and 7 children. Of this number, 97 adults and 7 children were in need of medical treatment and 64 adults needed nursing or attendant care. The care needed for the remainder was not indicated.

Nearly two thirds of the clients were getting clinic care, and another 8 per cent care from a private physician. Of the whole number, 73.6 per cent

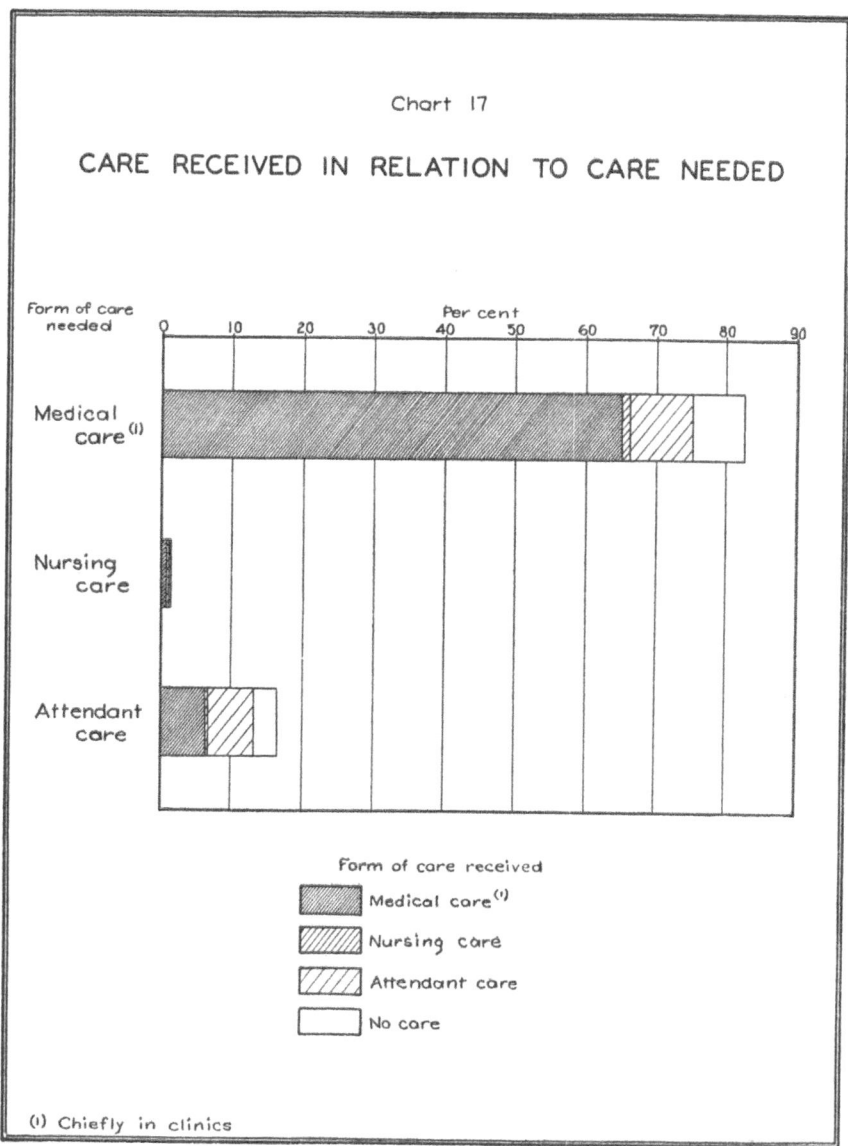

Chart 17

CARE RECEIVED IN RELATION TO CARE NEEDED

(1) Chiefly in clinics

were receiving either clinic or private medical care and 5.6 per cent were in hospitals. It was found, however, that 11.9 per cent of the whole number were in need of hospital care and 69.9 per cent in need of private or clinic care.

TABLE 73

CHRONICALLY ILL CLIENTS OF FAMILY SERVICE AGENCIES CLASSIFIED BY
CARE NEEDED, EACH AGE GROUP

Age group	Total	Medical			Nursing	Attendant
		Total	Hospital	Clinic		
Total	2,023[1]	81.8	11.9	69.9	1.0	17.2
Under 16 years	193	93.8	14.0	79.8	1.0	5.2
16–39 years	583	88.0	11.0	77.0	0.5	11.5
40–69 years	1,020	86.6	14.1	72.5	1.5	11.9
70 years and over	218	31.2	2.8	28.4	0.4	68.4
Not reported	9	7	1	6	0	2

[1] Care needed not reported for 29 persons.

A small number of those needing clinic care were in hospitals, perhaps temporarily or possibly they were sent to hospitals because clinics were not accessible. One tenth were receiving other forms of care or no care. Of those needing hospital care, one fifth were not receiving any medical treatment, and one half of those who were receiving it were having it from clinics or private physicians.

TABLE 74

CHRONICALLY ILL CLIENTS OF FAMILY SERVICE AGENCIES CLASSIFIED BY
CARE RECEIVED, EACH AGE GROUP

Age group	Total	Medical			Nursing	Attendant	No care
		Total	Hospital	Clinic			
Total	1,937[1]	79.2	5.6	73.6	1.3	10.3	9.2
Under 16 years	187	87.1	9.1	78.0	2.1	7.0	3.8
16–39 years	556	84.3	6.5	77.8	1.1	6.5	8.1
40–69 years	987	79.4	5.2	74.2	1.3	9.7	9.6
70 years and over . . .	199	56.3	1.5	54.8	1.0	27.1	15.6
Not reported	8	6	0	6	0	2	0

[1] Care received not reported for 115 persons.

The proportion of the clients of family service agencies who needed and received each form of care is shown in Tables 73 and 74.

The largest proportion of persons needing medical, or "A" care, was found among the children and a decreasing proportion in each age group.

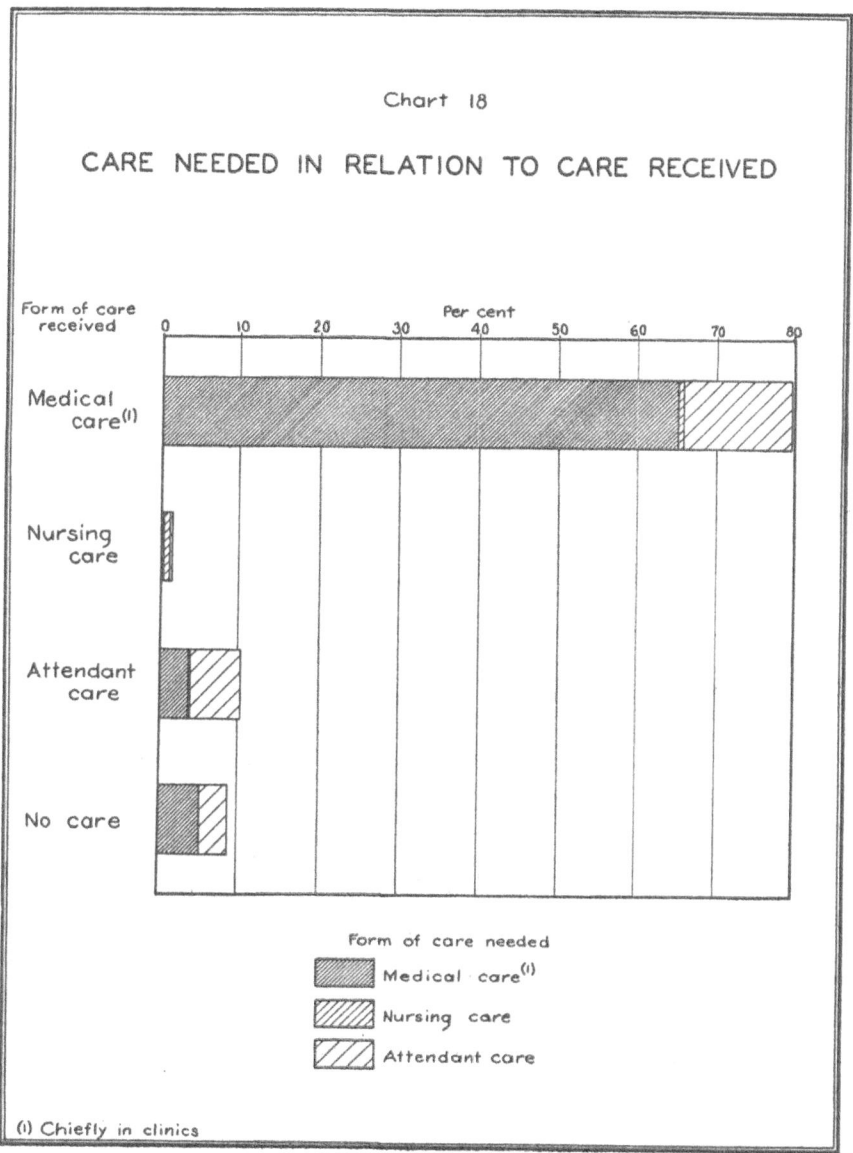

Chart 18

CARE NEEDED IN RELATION TO CARE RECEIVED

The number receiving "A" care was larger than the number who needed it among the aged seventy years and over, and smaller among all other age groups. The proportion of all persons needing the form of care they were receiving is represented in Chart 18.

Attendant, or "C" care, was required for a small percentage of the children and over a tenth of the adults under seventy years of age. Over two thirds of the aged required only attendant care, of whom nearly three fourths were infirm aged persons without a particular chronic disease needing the simplest form of care.

Among 36 younger adults in need of medical or nursing care, 14 were receiving only "C" care. Forty-two among 95 older adults, up to seventy years of age, needing "A" or "B" care, were receiving "C" care. Ten children receiving "B" or "C" care needed "A" care.

Persons Receiving Unsuitable Care

Of the 1,568 patients for whom the family service agencies had a responsibility not shared with another service, over a third (37.4 per cent) were not getting suitable care for one reason or another. Some patients were getting no care for their illness, others were receiving a different form of care from the type they required, and some were receiving care that was inadequate although of the type required. In some instances, as explained above, a more skilled form of care was being given than was necessary. A small number of patients getting unsuitable care were in institutions at the time of the census.

There was no report on the home conditions of 15.4 per cent of the whole group of patients but since two thirds of them were reported to be receiving satisfactory care from a medical standpoint, presumably the majority were getting satisfactory care. It seems improbable that the family agencies did not actually know the home conditions of so many clients, and the lack of this information is probably due to the agency's visitors' failure to record it and the recorders' failure to obtain the information by other means.

The highest percentage (54.0 per cent) of unsuitable care at home appeared in the group of 113 persons seventy years of age and over. Among persons between sixty and seventy years of age, the percentage of unsuitable care was lower (44 per cent). The lowest percentage (36 per cent) appeared among the 122 children at home. The proportion of clients, however, whose home conditions were not reported although their medical care was said to be satisfactory was smaller among the children and aged than among the other groups. Therefore, if it should be assumed that most of these homes were satisfactory, the percentage of unsuitable care among children still remains lower than among older persons.

Among the 105 adults in institutions at the time of the census, 10 were reported to be receiving unsuitable care, in that they were getting more skilled care than they required. All of the 13 children in institutions were receiving suitable care.

In Chart 19 is shown the proportion of persons in each age group whose

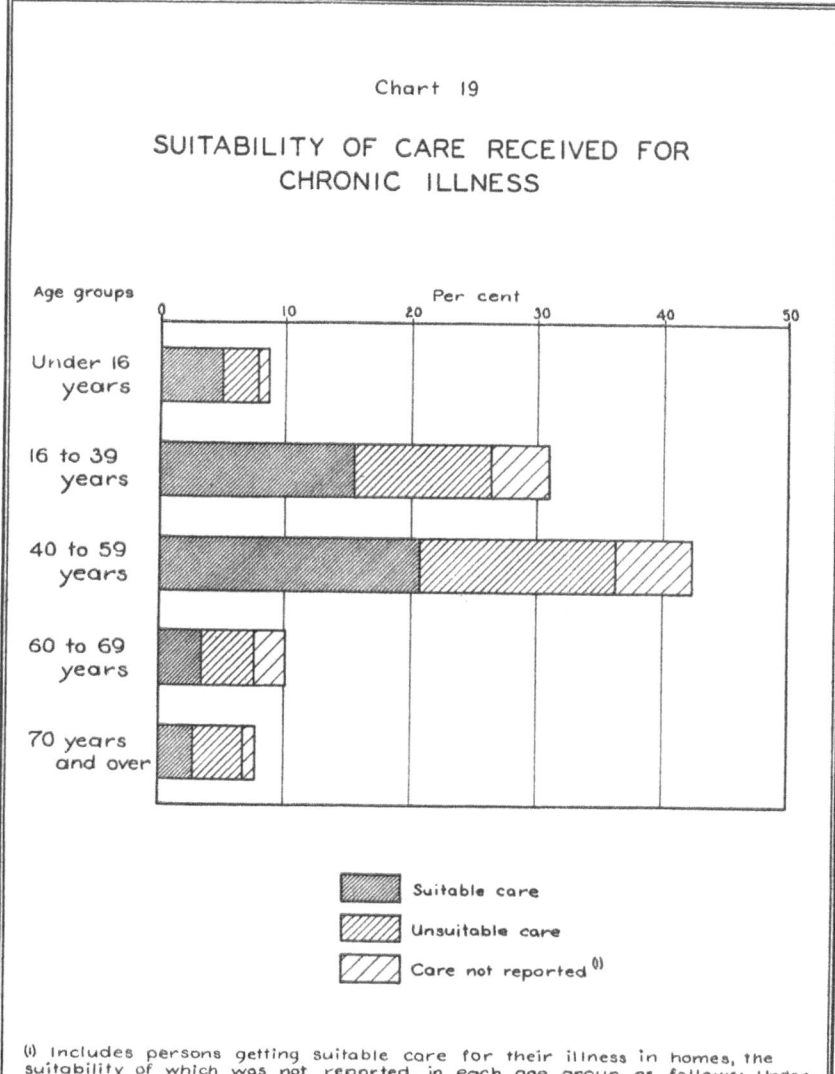

Chart 19

SUITABILITY OF CARE RECEIVED FOR
CHRONIC ILLNESS

Age groups — Per cent

(i) Includes persons getting suitable care for their illness in homes, the suitability of which was not reported, in each age group as follows: Under 16 yrs., 8; 16 to 39 yrs, 80; 40 to 59 yrs., 68; 60 to 69 yrs., 16; 70 yrs. and over, 9.

care was not satisfactory. The proportion of unsuitable care reported among the clients of family service agencies (39.3 per cent) is higher than among the total number of persons in the census (33.4 per cent). For the children, it is considerably higher, 34.6 per cent against 21.2 per cent in the total census. For the younger adults the proportion of unsuitable care reported is very little higher, 36.6 per cent against 34.0 per cent of the total census. For the older adults up to sixty years of age, it is approximately the same, 38.0 per cent as against 39.5 per cent in the total census. For those between sixty and seventy years of age, it is the same, 46.7 per cent as against 46.8 per cent in the total census. For those seventy years of age or over, it is decidedly higher, 52.6 per cent as against 37.8 per cent in the total census.

Lack of Institutional Beds

The patients who needed institutional care but were not receiving it numbered 227 or 15.3 per cent of all patients reported by family agencies as primarily their responsibility. The highest percentage of the chronically ill clients of any one family agency needing admission to an institution was 25 per cent; the next highest was 18 per cent. The family agencies had the largest proportion of patients at home needing institutional care; but among the patients of nursing agencies, the proportion was only slightly lower, 12.6 per cent.

The reason that patients were not in a suitable institution was given for 165 patients, of whom one was in an unsuitable type of institution and the remainder at home. Opposition to institutional care by the patient or his family was given as the reason more frequently than the lack of facilities. It was not recorded whether this was opposition to a particular institution or resistance to institutional care of any kind. The number of persons for whom this information was recorded, however, is too small to be significant.

Of the total of 227 persons in need of institutional care and not receiving it, 116 needed hospital care. Of the remainder, 100 required the custodial type of care, 7 only because of the infirmities of old age. Two persons needing " B " care and 9 needing clinic care should have been in institutions because of unsatisfactory home conditions. There were only 2 clients of family agencies in institutions who could have received proper care at home. A need for 225 additional institutional beds, therefore, is indicated for suitable care for chronically ill clients of family service agencies—approximately half hospital beds and the other half custodial beds.

In the total census a need was indicated for nearly 1,000 additional beds for patients requiring institutional care but not receiving it, of which 76 per cent were hospital beds; nearly 14 per cent, custodial beds; and 9 per cent, beds in institutions able to arrange clinic care for the patient. The demand for nearly a fourth of the additional beds needed comes from the family service agencies; and the remainder are needed for patients under the care of nursing services.

In considering the institutional facilities needed for the care of the chronic sick, not only the number of patients in need of institutional care must be taken into account but also the number of those in institutions not equipped to give them the form of care needed and of those improperly placed in general hospitals. (See pp. 2; 32–36.)

SUMMARY

Number and Proportion of Chronically Ill Clients

Eleven family service agencies, that is, all of the larger voluntary agencies of this type in the city, reported 2,052 persons with chronic illness causing disability for at least three months, who represent a tenth of all the chronically ill persons in the care of medical and social agencies.

Over three fourths of these 2,052 patients were reported by agencies serving Manhattan and the Bronx, which had 46 per cent of the population. Nearly one fourth were reported by agencies in Brooklyn which had 37 per cent of the population and a small percentage were reported by agencies in Queens, which had 15 per cent of the population.

In six family service agencies, reporting all but 8 per cent of the chronic patients in the census there was a person incapacitated by chronic illness in 15 per cent of the families served, varying from 11 per cent to 23 per cent in different agencies.

It is estimated on the basis of available figures that at least half of the families served by family welfare agencies present a problem of chronic illness of the type, though not of the degree of severity, with which this study deals, in one or more members of the family. If the actual figures were available, they would probably show an even larger proportion of families with members suffering from chronic illness of greater or less severity.

Age, Sex, and Marital Status

Over a fourth of the chronically ill clients of family service agencies were in the earlier productive period of life, between sixteen and forty years. Nearly a tenth were children. A tenth were in the period of old age. Two fifths were in the middle years between forty and sixty, of whom more than a third (15 per cent of the whole number) were between forty and forty-five years. Over a tenth were in the period between sixty and seventy years.

Males predominated to an even greater degree than in the total census, particularly in the period between forty and sixty years. There were more women than men among the aged. Married men were nearly three times as numerous as married women. Over two thirds of the whole number were married and nearly one third were single, widowed, or divorced.

Medical Condition

The chief causes of illness were heart diseases and diseases of the nervous system. Rheumatism and respiratory diseases came next. The chronic diseases usually thought of in connection with older persons were found also in younger adults.

The highest percentage of mentally abnormal persons in any group of agencies included in the census was reported by the family agencies. This is probably due to more frequent recognition of mental abnormality by the family service agencies, as they are obliged to evaluate the personality and mental capacity of the client in order to plan for his rehabilitation.

Duration of the Care Required

Persons of all ages had been under the care of the family service agencies for chronic illness for long periods. Nearly two fifths had been under care two years or more; nearly one third, three years or more. Periods of care from five to twenty years or over were reported for more than one tenth.

Over three fourths had been ill for two years or more; nearly half, for five years or more; a fifth, for ten years or more; a tenth, for fifteen years or more; and 72 persons, for twenty years or more.

The prognosis for recovery from the chronic illness was favorable for a third of the children, nearly a sixth of the younger adults, a twelfth of the older adults, and 1 per cent of the aged.

Social and Economic Conditions

The homes of three fifths of the patients were satisfactory from the standpoint of their care. There were about 4 per cent who had no permanent home. Unsuitable homes were found with about the same frequency in each age group. The three factors noted, physical condition, family make-up, and family attitudes were found to be unsatisfactory with about the same frequency. The figures obtained bearing on the possibility of adjusting unsatisfactory home conditions were not large enough to be significant.

Over half of all the chronically ill clients were being subsidized by a social agency. Nearly half of those with an income, omitting children and a few who had no regular income, received all or part of their income from their families; and about a fourth, from earnings. A somewhat larger percentage of these clients than of the total number in the census were receiving income from pensions, compensation, insurance, and savings.

The weekly family income of three fifths of the families of these patients, in the spring of 1928 was less than $25 a week, less than $15 for nearly a fourth. Larger incomes were found in families where the patient was a child than in the families of adult patients. For a large majority of the families, the income was not over $35, even in families of five or more persons. The average size of the family was over four persons. The average weekly income was $23.30.

Nearly a fourth of the adult patients, although incapacitated for their ordinary occupations, were employed, more than half of them irregularly. The amounts earned were naturally small; however, a small percentage of all earned as much as $25 a week. A fourth of the adult patients with the exception of the aged and a fifth of the aged had earnings. Persons of all ages beyond childhood were among those employed.

Over one sixth of the persons of working age had never been employed.

Sixteen per cent of those who had worked had been unemployed five years or more; over half, between one and five years; over a fourth, between three months and a year; and 5 per cent, less than three months.

The occupation of the majority of the women had been domestic work. The majority of the men had been employed in the lighter forms of outdoor or mechanical work.

Forms of Care Needed and Received

Over a third of these chronically ill clients were not having suitable care for their illness, which is a larger proportion than the proportion found among all persons in the census having unsuitable care. Nearly a tenth were not receiving any care with reference to their illness. In the total census, those receiving no care for their illness were less than 2 per cent.

Over four fifths of the chronically ill clients needed active medical treatment; but more than a tenth of those who needed it were not receiving it. On the other hand, the number receiving medical care was larger than the number needing it. Some needing only nursing or attendant care were receiving medical care from clinics or private physicians. Some whose condition called for medical study and treatment were receiving only attendant care or were getting no care at all for their illness.

Clinic care was being given to over a fourth of those who needed only custodial care.

Two fifths of those needing hospital care were receiving clinic care.

The use of 225 additional institutional beds would be required for these patients—half of the "A," or hospital, type and the other half of the "C," or custodial, type.

THE FACILITIES OF FAMILY SERVICE AGENCIES IN
RELATION TO THE CARE OF THE CHRONIC SICK

AGENCIES INCLUDED IN THE STUDY

In the census of the chronic sick the 2,052 records were secured from
eleven family service agencies, the Charity Organization Society, the Jewish Social Service Association, the Association for Improving the Condition
of the Poor, the Catholic Charities, the New York Chapter and the Brooklyn Chapter of the American Red Cross, the Brooklyn Bureau of Charities,
the United Jewish Aid Societies of Brooklyn, the Brooklyn Association for
Improving the Condition of the Poor, the Family Welfare Society of
Queens, the Associated Charities of Flushing. These are all the family welfare agencies working in the five boroughs represented in the Family Service Section of the Welfare Council with the exception of the Staten Island
Social Service Association and four chapters of the American Red Cross,
three of which are located in Queens and one in Richmond. From these
agencies, all of which have a small case load, it was not possible to secure a
record of chronically ill clients.

All of the larger organizations for family service under private auspices
are, therefore, included. Two family service agencies under public auspices, not at that time represented in the Family Section of the Welfare
Council, were not studied—the Board of Child Welfare of the City of New
York and the After-Care Service of the State Department of Labor's Bureau of Workmen's Compensation.

Relief societies and free loan associations were not included among
the agencies in which the census was taken because accurate data were
not available in regard to chronic illness among their clientele. Relief societies usually give aid in money or in material goods but do not provide
other forms of organized service. Their case work and follow-up work
are not as a rule systematic and their records are apt to be incomplete and
unstandardized.

In regard to Jewish relief societies the Jewish Communal Survey says,
"In Brooklyn and New York are hundreds of relief societies, of which
approximately 300 were listed by the Survey. The combined expenditures
of these unaffiliated agencies exceed the relief budgets of the large family
welfare societies."[13] It is impossible to tell how much of this expenditure is
in behalf of persons with chronic illness. An effort has been made by the
Jewish Social Service Association to bring these relief societies into the field
of professional social service. It has taken the leadership in organizing the
Cooperative Council in Manhattan and the Bronx, which is an organization
of many of these relief societies working in close coöperation, with the Jewish Social Service Association in their relief giving.

[13] The Jewish Communal Survey, Family Welfare Section, summary statement. The Bureau of
Jewish Social Research, 1929, pp. 5–6, mimeographed copy.

SPECIAL FACILITIES FOR THE CHRONIC SICK

Some of the family service agencies provide special facilities for their chronically ill clients.

The Association for Improving the Condition of the Poor provides sheltered employment in the Crawford Shops for a limited number of persons with disabilities connected with old age. Institutional care is provided for old persons in Ward Manor, a home for the aged, with a capacity of 100 beds. A unique apartment house for aged persons is conducted by this association. The building and management of the house are specially adapted to the needs of the aged, many of whom are suffering from chronic illnesses; and a nurse in charge has general oversight of the health of the residents. The house, overlooking one of the city parks, "provides a comfortable home in a modern fire-proof apartment for about sixty aged men and women, single or married. Those who wish prepare their own meals in kitchens provided for the purpose; those who prefer may get simple, inexpensive but nourishing meals in the cafeteria provided to meet this need. All pay their own rent and cost of living either from their own earnings or from allowances if need be from the Relief Bureau. They lead their own independent lives—or if not completely independent, they live normal self-controlled lives which is what they wish more than anything else."[14] The Association has a staff of graduate nurses who provide educational nursing service for clients who need such care; and it maintains a number of health clinics for its clients. One of its health examination clinics is for business women, and moderate fees are charged. In its medical clinics, nearly 5,000 persons were examined in the year 1927–1928. In addition the Association maintains dental clinics which, in the same year, treated 6,500 patients. Its mental hygiene clinic gave service in that year to nearly 150 families.[15]

The Brooklyn Association for Improving the Condition of the Poor, by appropriating substantial sums to the Orthopedic Department of the Long Island College Hospital, takes care indirectly of many crippled children.[16]

The Brooklyn Bureau of Charities has a Committee for the Crippled whose special concern is the care and training of crippled children and adults. This Committee conducts sheltered workshops with provision for the sale of the articles made. In addition it provides vocational instruction and work for homebound cripples.

The Jewish Social Service Association has conducted for several years a Visiting Housekeepers' Service to provide assistance to families in which the mother is ill in bed or in a hospital.[17] Usually the visiting housekeeper spends a full day in the family but she may give more or less time if the

[14] The New York Association for Improving the Condition of the Poor, Eighty-eighth Annual Report, 1930–1931, p. 32.
[15] The New York Association for Improving the Condition of the Poor, Eighty-fifth Annual Report, 1927–1928, pp. 6, 23.
[16] The Brooklyn Association for Improving the Condition of the Poor, Eighty-fifth Annual Report: Eighty-five Years of Community Service, 1843–1928, p. 5.
[17] Visiting Housekeepers' Service of the Jewish Social Service Association, New York, Annual Report, January 1, 1931, to December 31, 1931.

situation requires it. From half to a third of the clients who receive this service are suffering from chronic conditions.

The American Red Cross, through its Home Service Department, gave service, in 1928, to 2,862 disabled ex-service men and their families.[18] Working through the Veterans' Bureau of the Government it secures hospital care in the United States Veterans' Hospital for disabled veterans.

Mental diseases were excluded in this study since the extent of illness from this cause has been the subject of other investigations and the problem of care for such conditions is fairly well understood. However, the mental hygiene clinic may have a relation to the prevention of chronic illness in helping to distinguish between physiological and psychological causes of ill health and in promoting the proper functioning of the body. Many case-working agencies now maintain a mental hygiene service for their clients. "There has not been enough mental hygiene service in the community to provide the type of examination and treatment that the agencies need in their casework."[19] The Association for Improving the Condition of the Poor, the Brooklyn Bureau of Charities, and the State Charities Aid Association maintain jointly a mental hygiene clinic under the direction of a psychiatrist assisted by a psychologist and by a psychiatric social worker on the staff of each agency. The Jewish Social Service Association has had for some years a mental hygiene department with a psychiatrist and a psychiatric social worker. The United Jewish Aid Societies of Brooklyn has added a mental hygiene department to its services.

USE OF COMMUNITY RESOURCES FOR THE CHRONIC SICK

The family service agencies draw upon all the facilities of the city for the benefit of their clients. They coöperate with all the agencies that provide any form of care or service for the chronically ill in the interests of different clients. Among the agencies upon which they must rely particularly for coöperation in caring for the chronic sick are clinics, hospitals, medical social service departments, convalescent homes, employment services for the handicapped, sheltered workshops, and nursing services. For nearly one fourth of their patients the family service agencies shared with nursing services the responsibility for the care of the chronic illness. The law for old age assistance[20] brought the family agencies into a close relation with the municipal Department of Public Welfare in behalf of their aged clients.

Through the Board of Child Welfare, families in which the father is permanently incapacitated by chronic disease and in an institution, may receive a pension.[21]

[18] The New York County Chapter of the American National Red Cross, Annual Report, 1928, p. 9.
[19] Davis, Michael M., and Jarrett, Mary C., A Health Inventory of New York City: A Study of the Volume and Distribution of Health Service in the Five Boroughs. The Welfare Council of New York City, 1929, p. 217.
[20] Article XIV-A of the Public Welfare Law entitled Security Against Old Age Want. Chapter 387, Laws of 1930.
[21] State of New York Department of Social Welfare, Law Governing Boards of Child Welfare, 1929, Section 153.

Clinics, which do not come into the present study, are the main resource of family agencies in dealing with the health problems of their clients. A discussion of the interrelations of these two groups of agencies, referred to above (p. 244), points out that in chronic conditions it is particularly difficult to obtain adequate medical attention.[22]

A discussion of the lack of institutional facilities of different types for the care of chronic patients appears above (pp. 268–269).

The relationship between family service agencies and the medical social service departments of hospitals is under consideration by a Joint Committee of the Medical Social Service Section and the Family Service Section of the Welfare Council. Both sections are concerned in defining better methods of coöperation in order to give better medical service to the client or patients.

No study has been made of the relation of the family service agencies to other services upon which they must rely for coöperation in the care of clients with chronic illness, such as, visiting housekeeper service, visiting doctor service, and sheltered workshops. Further study should be given to the extent to which various resources are needed and are available.

PERSONNEL

In 1928, the eleven agencies studied had 274 case workers and 25 executives and supervisors directing the case work, in addition a clerical staff and volunteers. The agencies varied in the number of case workers employed from two persons in one agency to 73 case workers and 136 volunteers in another agency. The Charity Organization Society has developed a consultant personnel for its case workers, in addition to the supervisory staff, consisting of consultants in mental hygiene, home economics, and industrial problems. The case work staff of the Association for Improving the Condition of the Poor includes nurses who do all the case work in tuberculosis families.

The larger family service agencies carry on a variety of activities, which require an administrative staff in addition to their case workers. The varied activities of the Association for Improving the Condition of the Poor include a home for the aged, an apartment house for aged persons, a mental hygiene clinic, an educational nursing service, a tuberculosis prevention service, convalescent homes, fresh air camps, day nurseries, health centers, a nutrition bureau, and sheltered workshops. It conducts jointly with the Charity Organization Society, a Joint Application Bureau for homeless men. Its Bureau of Educational Nursing had 56 nurses who gave general nursing service, prenatal care, maternity instruction, and did preschool work and preventive and educational nursing for tuberculous clients. The section of this study dealing with nursing services contains a more detailed account

[22] Bryant, Louise Stevens, Better Doctoring—Less Dependency: A Study of the Relations Between Medical and Non-Medical Agencies, with Special Reference to Clinic and Family Services. Committee on Dispensary Development of the United Hospital Fund of New York, 1927, p. 11.

of these activities. (See p. 218.) The activities of the Charity Organization Society include a Bureau of Advice and Information, a Tenement House Committee, a Committee on Home Economics, and a Criminal Courts Committee. The Society conducts a wood yard and laundry and has always emphasized the training aspects of its work and is a center for training of social workers. One of its departments is the New York School of Social Work. The Jewish Social Service Association is a training center for the School of Jewish Social Work. It conducts mental hygiene and nutrition clinics, a Visiting Housekeepers' Service, and a Homeless Men's Department. One of its activities is the coördination of the smaller Jewish

TABLE 75

FAMILIES RECEIVING AN ALLOWANCE AND AMOUNTS OF THE ALLOWANCES
RECEIVED CLASSIFIED BY CHIEF CAUSE OF NEED[1]

Chief cause of need	FAMILIES		ALLOWANCES	
	Number	Per cent	Amount	Per cent
Total	458	100.0	$195,254	100.0
Illness of chief wage earner	161	35.2	87,118	44.6
Widows with dependent children . .	61	13.3	21,510	11.0
Desertion, non-support	111	24.2	43,606	22.3
Mental illness of wage earner	39	8.5	18,841	9.7
Old age	69	15.1	18,911	9.7
Others	17	3.7	5,269	2.7

[1] The Charity Organization Society of the City of New York, Annual Report, Forty-seventh Year, October 1, 1928, to September 30, 1929, p. 21.

relief organizations, referred to above. The Brooklyn Bureau of Charities conducts sheltered workshops for both the crippled and the blind; maintains the Brooklyn Tuberculosis and Health Association which carries on health education, health examination and mental hygiene clinics, and fresh air work; conducts a day nursery; and has a Housing Committee. It also receives workers for training in affiliation with the New York School of Social Work.

COSTS

From the financial statements of the agencies, it is not possible to gain any indication of the amounts spent for chronically ill clients. The entire expenditure for relief and the cost of administration and service by the family service agencies over a period of years ending with the year 1929 is given in the Study of Financial Trends of Organized Social Work in New York City, made in the Research Bureau of the Welfare Council.[23] In 1929, fourteen family service agencies, that is, all the family service agencies represented in the Family Service Section of the Welfare Council

[23] Huntley, Kate E., Financial Trends of Agencies Engaged in Giving Outdoor Relief in New York City. The Welfare Council of New York City, November, 1931.

spent directly for relief $1,825,000. The cost of administration and service of the departments of these agencies that administered the relief was $1,394,000.

The Charity Organization Society was the only one of these agencies that had published statistics showing the chief causes of need in families receiving allowances. This agency follows the usual practice of family agencies of giving interim financial relief for two months until a plan is made for the family. If the situation requires relief for a long period, a regular allowance, based on an estimated budget, is granted the family. Table 75 above shows the number of allowance families, together with the amounts of allowances granted, in the year 1928–1929, classified under the main causes of the need.

The families in which the principal cause of need was the illness of the chief wage earner were over a third of all the families receiving allowances. The percentage of money expended for such families was even higher, 45 per cent. Because, in the practice of the agency, families are not classed as allowance families unless there is a long-time problem, these cases of illness of the chief wage earner are probably cases of chronic illness as defined in this study.

CHAPTER 9

Agencies for Sheltered Work in Relation to the Care of the Chronic Sick

DEVELOPMENT OF SHELTERED WORK AGENCIES

SHELTERED work for persons unable by reason of a permanent or temporary handicap to secure employment in regular industry may be provided either in a workshop or, in the case of persons whose handicaps prohibit regular attendance at a shop, in their homes. In the latter type of sheltered work, occupation at home, mental therapy is usually a more important objective than self-support, although the attempt is usually made to have the work contribute something to the patient's support.

A sheltered workshop furnishes an opportunity for work to those who cannot compete with others in regular employment either temporarily or permanently. It employs either large or small groups for wages paid on a per diem, hourly, or piece basis. The product may be sold to a manufacturer, retailed at market prices, or sold directly to the consumer; but such a shop is not a profit-making enterprise. It is understood that in an agency bearing this name, the work shall be directed by a paid person and that the workers shall be under competent supervision and required to work for definite periods, which may vary if necessary from day to day. It is expected that the shop shall observe all the minimum requirements of the factory law. Most of the shops in New York have facilities for medical care, recreation, and financial aid, if necessary, through the organizations by which they are maintained.

Sheltered workshops serve various purposes: (1) The workshop may be a laboratory in which the work tolerance of a person is tested preparatory to his return to his usual occupation in industry; (2) it may furnish protection from competitive industry and a means of livelihood during a period of readjustment when he is unable to do full-time work; (3) it may give training in an occupation in which the handicap will not be a bar to successful competition; or, if this is impossible, (4) it may provide occupation that will protect him permanently from the strain of competition; (5) it may afford an opportunity for "industrial convalescence," that is, for recovery through work graduated as to time spent and tasks undertaken until a person is able to do full-time work or the maximum amount that he is capable of doing. This is a primary object of sheltered workshops for tuberculous and cardiac patients in danger of suffering a relapse by returning to full-time work too soon. This type of sheltered work has been stimulated by the development of occupational therapy.

It is essential that a sheltered workshop shall have good medical service. "Most shops require a medical diagnosis before registering a patient. The physician determines the working capacity of the individual and prescribes the number of hours he can work. Subsequent increases of working hours are made only after examination by the physician. Periodic medical examinations are insisted on by many of the sheltered shops, and these serve not only as a measurement of the progress the patient is making, but also act as a guide in the formulation of vocational plans. Finally the physician determines the length of the curative period and makes the recommendation for discharge."[1]

The conception of sheltered work as a public welfare measure has been influenced by the efforts at industrial rehabilitation that have accompanied the administration of workmen's compensation laws, the widespread interest in the care and training of young cripples, and finally the need for vocational reëducation of handicapped war veterans and the provision made by the federal government for their vocational rehabilitation. Workmen's compensation laws, inaugurated in Germany in 1884, were first put in operation in the United States in 1911; and many states in quick succession adopted such legislation. The necessity for expert medical care and vocational guidance was recognized; and physical and vocational rehabilitation became an inseparable part of the operation of the compensation laws. In 1917, Congress established the Federal Board for Vocational Education, which, the following year, was charged with the administration of the act for vocational rehabilitation of those handicapped in the war. The federal law was amended in 1920 to enable the states to establish bureaus for the rehabilitation of those disabled in industry and in other ways. Official vocational rehabilitation agencies by 1930 were in operation in forty-four states.

The movement for sheltered workshops in New York City gained impetus from the post-war efforts to rehabilitate the disabled soldier. Several workshops for special groups had been opened earlier. The Crippled Children's East Side Free School had started a workroom for hand sewing for girls in 1903. For several years, from 1913 to 1916, the Trade School for Cardiac Convalescents was conducted as a workshop for men who had been patients in a cardiac convalescent home at Sharon, New York. The Altro Work Shops for the tuberculous were opened in 1915. The Association for Improving the Condition of the Poor, in 1916, as a part of its program for the care of aged persons, opened the Crawford Shops, where toy making and other work is given to aged persons no longer employable in industry. The first sheltered workshop in the city for adults suffering from various forms of physical handicap was the Red Cross Institute for Crippled and Disabled Men. This was started soon after the United States entered the war by personal contributions from Mr. Jeremiah Milbank with the definite object of serving as an experimental laboratory for the rehabilitation of civilian handicapped, in order that there might be a body of experience ready later on for the planning of a program for disabled soldiers. The American Red Cross was asked to assume charge of the Institute and did so until 1919, when it was turned over to the private

[1] Leavitt, Moses A., Handicapped Wage Earners—As Studied by a Family Welfare Agency. Jewish Social Service Association, New York, 1928, p. 59.

board that has since directed it. In 1928, its name was changed to the Institute for the Crippled and Disabled and its activities were extended to handicapped women. It opened a sheltered workroom, in 1927, for employment of handicapped persons who could not be expected to return to industry.

An outstanding example of an agency for sheltered work, the Altro Work Shops, conducted by the Committee for the Care of Jewish Tuberculous, was opened in 1915 to provide employment for persons handicapped with tuberculosis; but its activities are not discussed below, as tuberculosis is not included in the study. The Vab Workshops conducted by the Vocational Adjustment Bureau for the rehabilitation of nervous women and girls, opened in 1922, also serve a group not included in the study.

The Curative Workshop, designed particularly to test the employability of the handicapped under actual working conditions, was started in 1924. The New York City Visiting Committee, in 1925, opened a convalescent workshop to give employment and work therapy to convalescents. In 1927, the Committee for the Crippled of the Brooklyn Bureau of Charities opened its sheltered workshop. This committee had previously experimented, in the winter of 1926, with a curative workshop to bridge the gap between a new job and the old job made impossible by the physical handicap, which was given up as it was found to be too expensive in proportion to its benefits; and its work for homebound cripples had been going on for a number of years. The committee was organized in 1913 and in the beginning worked largely with children. A sheltered workshop for cardiac girls, known as the New York Cardiac Shop, was opened in 1928 by a committee of Irvington House.

As a part of the program to meet the unemployment emergency, about twenty-five workrooms for women were established by the Emergency Work Bureau, during the winter of 1929-1930, to provide sewing and wages for unemployed women. These workrooms are still continued in the winter of 1932-1933. They are conducted in churches, settlements, and other neighborhood agencies; and some agencies of these types have established and supported their own workrooms.

An experiment in providing work for aged persons resident in homes for the aged, conducted jointly by the sections of the Welfare Council concerned with the care of the aged and with sheltered workshops, has been described above. (See p. 110.) The products made by residents in a number of homes for the aged have been sold through a central office, under the trade-mark "Dega" (aged reversed). The experiment is believed by those who sponsored it to have demonstrated the value of employment in bringing satisfaction and renewed interest in life, together with the benefits of a small amount of money to spend, to the aged men and women in institutions. It is thought that for economical administration, a service for this purpose should be conducted as a coöperative enterprise along with other sheltered work services.

Agencies providing sheltered work organized in June, 1928, as the Sub-section on Sheltered Workshops of the Section on Employment and Vocational Guidance of the Welfare Council, with the purpose of coördinating their activities and having a meeting ground for discussion of their common problems. They remained as an organized sub-section for three years, until in May, 1931, they decided to discontinue their separate organization and to become a part of the Employment and Vocational Guidance Section along with other agencies interested in vocational guidance and employment. Among the projects of this section has been the development in the Research Bureau of the Welfare Council of a system of central reporting by sheltered workshops of the city. Since December, 1928, twelve sheltered workshops have reported their monthly statistics to the Research Bureau which has analyzed them and prepared monthly summaries of the work of the reporting agencies. The figures reported care for enrollment, admissions, withdrawals, vacancies, total hours worked, and total wages paid.

The sheltered work agencies organized in the Welfare Council requested the Research Bureau, in 1930, to undertake a study of these agencies in New York City that should cover the functions and classification of present sheltered work facilities, the management of existing shops, the number and types of handicap needing sheltered work, and the ways in which these needs should be supplied. This study has not been undertaken; but early in 1932, the Research Bureau undertook a more limited study of the possibilities of central purchasing and central marketing by sheltered workshops. A sheltered workshop as a rule is not self-supporting but on the contrary is usually an expensive service. It is possible to support such a service by the sale of its products only in rare instances under special conditions. With a view to possible reduction of the expense, the sheltered work agencies initiated the study to determine whether the buying of materials and marketing of products might be improved through some coöperative action.[2]

The cost of the service depends upon its objectives, which may be therapeutic, vocational, or productive. The problems of organization and personnel are very different if the primary object of the workshop is to maintain morale, to teach a trade, or to afford opportunity for earnings.

The provision of sheltered work for the aged is another separate problem, for the cost of maintaining a service for persons of sixty years of age and over, such as the toy shop conducted by the Crawford Shops, is at least twice as great as its returns. Occupational work for the residents of homes for the aged is much less expensive. A workshop for the aged conducted upon the premises of a home for the aged, possibly with some assistance from the regular staff of the home, would cost considerably less than a shop paying overhead charges.

The possibilities of municipal coöperation in furnishing sheltered work services to the various groups who need them have not yet received sufficient attention. It has been suggested that the city might coöperate by using the products of the existing shops and by providing buildings and

[2] Rosenthal, Clarice A., A Limited Study of the Sheltered Workshops of New York City with Special Reference to Marketing of Their Products. The Welfare Council of New York City, October, 1932, MS.

equipment for other shops. In this connection, consideration should also be given to the need for opportunities to work among the thousands of chronically disabled persons whom the city maintains in its hospitals and homes.

The study of purchasing and marketing, just referred to, found that "the general trend of the present workshops is strongly away from the informal shop making a sentimental appeal, toward commercial type of production. This is modified to meet the clients' needs, but the products made are those for which there is a genuine commercial demand. The finding of such products is a marked problem for some of the workshops."[3]

One of the values of the sheltered workshop, which should be mentioned, is that it demonstrates what it is possible for industry to do in retaining employees suffering from physical handicaps. It may even suggest that an industry similarly organized might advantageously employ handicapped persons. It is desirable that greater publicity should be given to the ways in which sheltered work services have dealt with different types of handicap, so that industry may become acquainted with these experiences. Certain industrial and business firms do have plans for employing the handicapped in jobs for which they are qualified. The American Telephone and Telegraph Company tries to arrange a program of work for convalescent employees in accordance with their condition; and those who are handicapped either after they become employees or before seeking employment are engaged wherever it is possible to adjust them to the available jobs in the organization. The Western Electric Company reëmploys tuberculous employees who have received sanitarium care and attempts to readjust them either to their own jobs or to other jobs, often starting them on part time when they return to work. The Metropolitan Life Insurance Company reëmploys physically handicapped employees and gives them medical supervision.

There is still much confusion as to the objectives of different shops, which is recognized by those responsible for the development of this service. It is primarily important to have a definite policy as to whether the object of a particular shop is to give permanent or temporary care. In the shop that is intended for temporary care, the tendency to keep good workers longer than necessary in order to increase the production of the shop is almost inevitable unless checked by a firm policy, particularly as every shop requires a nucleus of dependable, experienced workers. The consensus of opinion among those offering this service is that every shop at intervals should evaluate its activities in order to see to what extent they accomplish the objects for which the service exists and to determine what changes need to be made.

There is also a recognized need for ascertaining the cost of services for different purposes and for determining in the light of costs and values of different types of service to what extent they should be extended or reduced. The question whether there may be ways of accomplishing the same results more effectively and economically by coöperation or combination of a

[3] *Ibid.*, p. 34.

number of workshops or of workshops and certain institutions is also being considered by those engaged in providing this service.

The recent study of the marketing of products points out the need for evaluation of the cost of sheltered work service in relation to its results: "because of the recent rapid growth of sheltered workshops and because of the large expenditures of effort and money being put into them, workshops would also probably find it advantageous to make an evaluation of their own work; an evaluation showing (1) the extent to which a satisfactory adjustment has been made for the individual clients and (2) the cost to the community as compared to the cost of other methods of care."[4]

THE CHRONIC SICK REPORTED BY SHELTERED WORK AGENCIES

Facilities of all types providing sheltered work for the chronically ill as defined in this study, were as follows:

a) Six workshops for the physically handicapped: the Curative Workshop, equipped primarily to test work tolerance; the Institute for the Crippled and Disabled and the Brooklyn Bureau of Charities' Committee for the Crippled, both training the handicapped for industry and giving permanent employment to those unable to reënter industry; the Workroom of the Crippled Children's East Side Free School, giving permanent employment to a group of handicapped women; the Convalescent Shop, for a temporary period of convalescence during readjustment to work habits; and the Crawford Shops for permanent employment of the aged. These six agencies had altogether shop facilities for about 250 persons.

b) Three agencies that, although they may have the physically handicapped under care, are serving primarily the socially handicapped who for any reason are unable to find employment: the Goodwill Industries of Brooklyn and of the New York Protestant Episcopal City Mission Society of Manhattan, employing both men and women in shops for the repair of clothing and furniture; the Salvation Army, with one branch in Brooklyn and one in Manhattan, which gives work to anyone who wants food and lodging and will work at whatever there is to do in the institution. These agencies were able to give work to about 400 persons at a time.

c) Four agencies furnishing work and training in their own homes to those who are too handicapped to travel to a workroom: the Committee for the Crippled of the Brooklyn Bureau of Charities, the Institute for the Crippled and Disabled, the Fraternity for Friendly Service, and the Shut-In Society. The last two are organized to furnish various kinds of friendly service to the homebound crippled, such as, visiting, reading aloud, letter writing, and providing reading matter. Among other services, they furnish handwork of various kinds to the homebound and find a market for the products.

In addition to these agencies, there are also the Altro Work Shops for the tuberculous, several workshops for the blind, and the Vocational Ad-

---

[4] *Ibid.*, p. 36.

justment Bureau's shops for mentally maladjusted women and girls, which were not within the scope of the study.

The nine sheltered work agencies that reported chronic patients in the census had over 500 chronically ill persons under care, of whom about a fourth were also under the care of other agencies. Less than a fourth were

TABLE 76

CHRONIC PATIENTS UNDER THE CARE OF EACH SHELTERED WORK AGENCY

Agency	Number
Total	537
Committee for the Crippled, Brooklyn Bureau of Charities	61
Convalescent Workshop, New York City Visiting Committee	7
Crawford Shops, Association for Improving the Condition of the Poor	25
Crippled Children's East Side Free School, Workroom	34
Curative Workshop	21
Fraternity for Friendly Service	144
Goodwill Industries of Brooklyn	5
Salvation Army, Manhattan	5
Shut-In Society	235

in shops and the rest were receiving service in their own homes or in institutions. The number reported by each agency is given in Table 76. Seventy per cent were reported by the two agencies for home service, the Fraternity for Friendly Service and the Shut-In Society. The Institute for the Crippled and Disabled was not able at the time to supply its records for the census; and the Goodwill Industries of the New York Protestant Episcopal City Mission Society reported no chronically ill persons under care at that time.

TABLE 77

PATIENTS UNDER THE CARE OF SHELTERED WORK AGENCIES CLASSIFIED BY AGE

Age	Number	Per cent
Total	537	100.0
Under 16 years	33	6.5
16–39 years	182	35.7
40–59 years	151	29.7
60–69 years	81	15.9
70 years and over	62	12.2
Not reported	28	. . . . .

There were about 2,500 ambulant adults under seventy years of age in the census under the care of nursing and family agencies. Probably among them were at least as many as the number already receiving sheltered work who would have been benefited by this service if facilities had been available.

A large proportion, 68 per cent, of the patients under the care of sheltered work agencies were women. Even among those working in shops, women were nearly two thirds of the whole number. This is partly explained by the fact that the shop conducted by the Institute for the Crippled and Disabled which serves largely men was not included in the census.

The age distribution of the patients of sheltered work agencies is shown in Table 77. Adults under sixty years of age were nearly two thirds of the whole number. Sheltered work is apparently in demand for young and middle-aged adults even more than for older persons.

The chief diagnoses of the patients of sheltered work agencies were orthopedic and neurological diseases, which together accounted for more than half of the patients. Over half of the orthopedic disorders were caused by poliomyelitis. Table 78 shows the chief diagnoses reported.

TABLE 78

PATIENTS UNDER THE CARE OF SHELTERED WORK AGENCIES
CLASSIFIED BY DIAGNOSES, EACH AGE GROUP

Diagnosis	Total		AGE GROUP					
	Number	Per cent	Under 16	16–39	40–59	60–69	70 and over	Not reported
Total	537	100.0	33	182	151	81	62	28
Orthopedic disorders . .	139	25.9	16	92	23	5	1	2
Neurological diseases . .	132	24.6	9	39	47	17	11	9
Rheumatism	95	17.7	0	14	38	26	9	8
Circulatory diseases . .	46	8.6	7	12	13	8	5	1
Diseases due to external causes	29	5.4	0	6	12	3	6	2
Old age	22	4.1	0	0	0	0	21	1
Ill-defined diseases . . .	22	4.1	0	7	4	6	2	3
Other diseases	52	9.7	1	12	14	16	7	2

The agencies that provide work for the homebound also give this service to patients in institutions; and 125 persons reported by the sheltered work agencies were in institutions—over half in hospitals, nearly half in homes for incurables, and a few in homes for the aged.

Of the 412 patients living at home reported by sheltered work agencies, about a fourth were not receiving suitable care, that is, they were not getting proper medical care or their home conditions were not satisfactory. The remainder were almost evenly divided between those who received suitable care in all respects and those whose medical care was suitable but whose home conditions were not reported. The presumption is that a large proportion of the latter group were suitably cared for in all respects.

What proportion of all the chronic sick needing sheltered work, the 500 persons under the care of sheltered work agencies in the census may represent cannot be inferred. Sheltered work, as described above, serves a number of different purposes in the care and treatment of chronic patients. The needs of each type of patient requiring such facilities calls for special study. Some are patients needing medical, or "A," care in clinics; others need attendant, or "C," care in their homes or in institutions supplemented by occupation. The organization of shop and home services for providing sheltered work obviously present very different problems.

While no conclusion in regard to the need for this type of care for the chronic sick can be drawn from the fact that the number of chronic patients in the census receiving sheltered work service was comparatively small, general evidence of the need for increased facilities for the care of the chronically ill is not lacking. The Sub-section on Sheltered Workshops of the Welfare Council organized an Employment Case Committee, in 1928, to discuss types of patients presenting special problems and the extent to which they are employable. After several months of study and discussion, the Committee, in June, 1928, recommended that sheltered work should be provided for many more types of disability and for a much larger number of persons than could then be accommodated.[5] The benefits of such an extension of this service the committee outlined as: (a) improving the economic standing of the patient, so that less charitable relief would be necessary; (b) relieving the employment bureaus of persons found to be unemployable; (c) improving the mental health and morale of the patient, which profoundly affects his physical health and his family and social relationships.

Among the disease conditions discussed by this Employment Case Committee as those in which a need for sheltered work is likely to occur were heart disease, thromboangiitis obliterans, epilepsy, encephalitis, and amputations. Many persons in each of these groups otherwise unemployable are capable of doing some work, provided it is properly supervised. In the course of these discussions, the Employment Center for the Handicapped reported its experience with persons suffering from such disabilities who cannot be placed in regular industry but could be placed at sheltered work if there were suitable facilities. The director of the Center stated, at the time of the census of the chronic sick, that her organization could place 200 persons in sheltered work immediately if facilities were available. Among nearly 9,400 applicants registered in three years, there were 350 persons in need of sheltered employment.[6] There are also undoubtedly many ambulant patients in hospitals, many of whom have been there for years, able to do some work but not enough to get regular employment.

SUMMARY

1. Sheltered work agencies included in the study are of two kinds, those that provide work for invalids at home, in which mental therapy is usually the principle objective, and those that provide work, in special workshops, for persons who cannot compete with other workers in regular industry either temporarily or permanently.

[5] The Section on Employment and Vocational Guidance of The Welfare Council of New York City, First Annual Report, June, 1928. Mimeographed copy.
[6] Information received by letter from Miss Louise C. Odencrantz, Director of the Employment Center for the Handicapped.

2. Various purposes may be served by sheltered workshops—testing work tolerance, protection during a period of readjustment, training for a new occupation, permanent employment without the strain of competition, or "industrial convalescence" through graded work.

3. The movement has received impetus from a number of sources—rehabilitation work connected with workmen's compensation, training of young cripples, vocational reëducation of war veterans, and occupational therapy.

4. The agencies furnishing sheltered work service in New York City have been organized since 1928 in the Welfare Council, and have joined in a central reporting system for recording monthly statistics in the Research Bureau of the Council.

5. Recognition of the functions of sheltered work agencies, the number of those needing sheltered work, and the ways in which these needs should be met led to a proposal for a complete study of the situation, which has not yet been possible; but a limited study of the possibilities of central purchasing and marketing has been made by the Welfare Council.

6. Special study of the cost of sheltered work service in relation to the results is needed.

7. Particularly the economy and effectiveness of coöperation or combination by certain shops or by certain institutions and shops should be studied.

8. The possibilities of municipal coöperation in the use of products and provision of buildings and equipment should be investigated.

9. The objectives of the workshops should be more clearly defined; and from time to time each shop should evaluate its activities in relation to its objectives.

10. The influence of sheltered workshops on industry, in showing the way for the employment of physically handicapped persons, should be given more weight through greater publicity for the experience of the shops.

11. The census in agencies providing sheltered work for persons with the types of chronic illness included in the study reported about 500 patients, of whom three fourths were at home or in institutions and one fourth in workshops.

12. There are general indications that in addition to the persons employed in sheltered workshops in 1928, a time of favorable economic conditions, there were at least as many again, and probably many more, in need of this service.

TABLE I. CAPACITY, NUMBER OF CHRONIC PATIENTS, AND DAILY COST PER PATIENT
IN PRIVATE INSTITUTIONS FOR THE SICK IN WHICH A CENSUS OF THE
CHRONIC SICK WAS MADE, 1928

Hospital	Capacity		Number of chronic patients	Daily cost per patient	
	Total beds	Ward beds		Total	Ward
Total	11,037	7,584	2,707	. . . .	. . . .
CHRONIC[1]	1,946	1,679	1,244	. . . .	. . . .
Beth Abraham Home for Incurables . .	224	224	160	3.75	3.75
Home for Incurables '	307	170	184	2.47	2.47
House of Calvary	100	100	74	. . . .	. . . .
House of the Holy Comforter	100	100	65	2.57	2.57
Memorial Hospital	104	52	40	8.26	7.48
Montefiore Hospital	614	569	393	3.68	3.67
New York Skin and Cancer Hospital[2] .	98	65	18	9.29	8.93
St. Francis Home	250	250	193	. . . .	. . . .
St. Joseph's Hospital (chronic wards) .	60	60	54	. . . .	. . . .
St. Rose's Free Home	89	89	63	. . . .	. . . .
ORTHOPEDIC	1,019	835	462	. . . .	. . . .
Hospital for Joint Diseases	277	180	75	6.36	5.33
Hospital for Ruptured and Crippled . .	273	230	65	5.94	5.16
House of St. Giles the Cripple	45	45	31	2.85	2.92
New York Orthopedic Hospital	132	90	60	4.92	4.48
St. Charles Hospital	42	40	18	. . . .	. . . .
St. Charles Hospital and Home[3] . . .	250	250	213	. . . .	. . . .
GENERAL AND OTHER SPECIAL	8,072	5,070	1,001	. . . .	. . . .
Babies Hospital	80	69	5	5.02	4.69
Beth Israel Hospital	137	121	40	6.94	6.39
Bethany Deaconess Hospital	90	8	2	. . . .	. . . .
Booth Memorial Hospital	52	33	0	. . . .	. . . .
Bronx Hospital	86	47	7	6.01	6.01
Brooklyn Hospital	260	164	25	5.87	5.66
Caledonian Hospital	110	21	1	. . . .	. . . .
Flushing Hospital	135	88	11	. . . .	. . . .
Holy Family Hospital	110	56	10	. . . .	. . . .
Jewish Hospital	288	210	55	6.65	6.35
Knickerbocker Hospital	155	97	18	6.25	6.25
Lenox Hill Hospital	318	194	35	6.86	6.09
Long Island College Hospital	440	333	91	4.51	4.38
Lutheran Hospital Association	110	16	4	. . . .	. . . .

[1] The census was not taken in Faith Home for Incurables.
[2] Now the Stuyvesant Square Hospital.
[3] Known also as Brooklyn Home for Blind, Crippled, and Defective Children.

TABLE I—(*Continued*)

Hospital	Capacity		Number of chronic patients	Daily cost per patient	
	Total beds	Ward beds		Total	Ward
Mary Immaculate Hospital	90	61	7	. . . .	. . . .
Midtown Hospital	41	24	0	. . . .	. . . .
Mt. Sinai Hospital	669	517	177	7.65	6.65
Neurological Institute	86	43	24	8.13	5.99
New York Hospital	320	187	40	6.72	5.65
New York Infirmary for Women and Children	103	67	7	5.26	4.58
New York Nursery and Child's Hospital	170	96	6	5.19	5.42
New York Post-Graduate Hospital . .	420	238	45	7.81	6.64
Norwegian Lutheran Deaconess Hospital	171	78	16	3.67	3.25
Reconstruction Hospital	63	40	5	7.38	6.96
Rockefeller Institute	50	50	17	. . . .	. . . .
Roosevelt Hospital	377	292	21	6.32	5.45
St. Catherine's Hospital	296	170	16	. . . .	. . . .
St. John's Hospital, Brooklyn	86	60	10	5.77	5.74
St. John's Hospital, Long Island City .	235	71	21	. . . .	. . . .
St. Joseph's Hospital	101	57	3	. . . .	. . . .
St. Luke's Hospital	474	340	111	7.35	5.42
St. Mary's Free Hospital for Children .	134	134	0	2.99	2.99
St. Mary's Hospital, Brooklyn	278	156	34	. . . .	. . . .
St. Peter's Hospital, Brooklyn	225	180	24	. . . .	. . . .
St. Vincent's Hospital, Manhattan . .	355	234	67	. . . .	. . . .
St. Vincent's Hospital, Richmond . . .	100	59	7	. . . .	. . . .
Samaritan Hospital	60	45	0	. . . .	. . . .
Staten Island Hospital	225	122	15	. . . .	. . . .
Sloane Hospital	163	114	12	. . . .	. . . .
Unity Hospital	200	58	8	. . . .	. . . .
Woman's Hospital	209	120	4	6.69	6.12

TABLE 2

NUMBER AND PERCENTAGE DISTRIBUTION OF TOTAL BEDS AND WARD BEDS IN ALL GENERAL HOSPITALS AND IN THOSE STUDIED, EACH BOROUGH, 1928

Borough	ALL HOSPITALS						HOSPITALS STUDIED					
	Hospitals		Beds		Ward beds		Hospitals		Beds		Ward beds	
	Number	Per cent	Number	Per cent	Number	Per cent	Number	Per cent	Number	Per cent	Number	Per cent
Total	77	100.0	13,539	100.0	7,971	100.0	41	100.0	8,072	100.0	5,070	100.0
Manhattan	40	51.9	7,465	55.1	4,522	56.7	20	48.8	4,376	54.2	3,010	59.4
Bronx	4	5.2	753	5.6	581	7.3	1	2.4	86	1.1	47	0.9
Brooklyn	24	31.2	4,181	30.9	2,261	28.4	14	34.1	2,724	33.7	1,555	30.7
Queens	7	9.1	815	6.0	421	5.3	4	9.8	561	6.9	277	5.4
Richmond	2	2.6	325	2.4	186	2.3	2	4.9	325	4.0	181	3.6

TABLE 3

CAPACITY,[1] NUMBER OF CHRONIC PATIENTS, AND DAILY COST[2] PER PATIENT
IN PUBLIC HOSPITALS, 1928

Hospital	Beds	Number of chronic patients	Daily cost per patient
Total	12,063	2,849	. . . .
General hospitals	4,729	747	. . . .
Bellevue	2,106	401	3.58
Coney Island	358	41	5.21
Cumberland Street Hospital[3]	400	99	3.96
Fordham	264	8	3.53
Gouverneur	210	17	5.64
Greenpoint	264	1	4.41
Harlem	346	71	4.32
Lincoln	331	109	4.84
Morrisania (Opened in July, 1929) . . .	450	. . . . .	4.23
General hospitals with chronic services . . .	4,053	1,258	. . . .
City	1,060	401[4]	2.31
Kings County	1,660	639	3.16
Metropolitan	1,333[5]	218[4]	2.83
Special hospitals	2,806	356	. . . .
Brooklyn Cancer Institute[3]	100	53	3.96
Kingston Avenue	400	22	5.87
Neponsit Beach	120	112	2.61
New York City Cancer Institute	192	139	1.39[6]
Queensboro	74	0	9.71
Riverside	540[7]	5	5.40
Sea View	1,000	25	3.28
Willard Parker	380	0	9.71
Chronic hospitals	475	488	. . . .
Neurological	475	488	1.39[6]

[1] Figures are those submitted by the institutions to the State Department of Social Welfare for the year 1928.

[2] The published figures of the Department of Hospitals for the year 1929 are given; they represent total operating and maintenance costs.

[3] Cumberland Street Hospital and Brooklyn Cancer Institute were an administrative unit and their cost figures were not separated.

[4] This institution reported only chronic sick who had been in the hospital three months.

[5] The official bed capacity as reported to the State Department of Social Welfare was 1,665. In this instance the actual bed capacity was used, as it appears in the 1926 report of the Department of Public Welfare and in the 1928 inspection reports of the New York City Visiting Committee.

[6] In the report of the Department of Hospitals the daily cost per patient for Neurological Hospital and Cancer Institute is given as a unit.

[7] Although this was the official reported bed capacity, only 336 beds were in use during 1928, because some of the buildings were unfit for use.

TABLE 4

CHRONICALLY ILL GUESTS OF PRIVATE HOMES FOR THE AGED
CLASSIFIED BY DIAGNOSIS, EACH AGE GROUP

Diagnosis	Total	AGE GROUP			
		40–59	60–69	70 and over	Not reported
Total	2,822	65[1]	642	2,090	25
Epidemic diseases	25	4	9	12	0
General diseases	363	15	108	233	7
Cancer and other malignant tumors	48	1	6	40	1
Arthritis and rheumatism	230	11	73	141	5
Diabetes	61	2	21	38	0
Other	24	1	8	14	1
Diseases of nervous system and of organs of special sense	360	24	108	224	4
Diseases of spinal cord	24	4	10	10	0
Cerebral hemorrhage and shock	44	2	7	34	1
Other paralysis	244	8	87	147	2
Other diseases of the nervous system	43	9	4	29	1
Diseases of eye and ear	5	1	0	4	0
Diseases of circulatory system	600	14	199	378	9
Diseases of the heart	403	6	113	279	5
Arteriosclerosis	136	3	60	69	4
Other	61	5	26	30	0
Diseases of respiratory system, non-tuberculous . .	160	7	42	110	1
Diseases of the digestive system	114	2	36	75	1
Hernia, intestinal obstruction	54	1	14	38	1
Cirrhosis and other diseases of liver	12	0	6	6	0
Other	48	1	16	31	0
Non-venereal diseases of genitourinary system . .	131	1	17	112	1
Chronic nephritis	70	1	11	58	0
Diseases of prostate	23	0	4	18	1
Other	38	0	2	36	0
Diseases of skin and cellular tissue	39	1	9	29	0
Diseases of bones and organs of locomotion. . . .	43	15	12	26	0
Malformations	5	0	3	2	0
Old age	821	0	7	813	1
Old age	763	0	0	763	0
Senile dementia	58	0	7	50	1
External causes	89	2	18	68	1
Ill-defined diseases	72	0	64	8	0

[1] Includes one person 34 years of age.

TABLE 5

CHRONICALLY ILL GUESTS OF PRIVATE HOMES FOR THE AGED CLASSIFIED BY
MENTAL ABNORMALITY, EACH AGE GROUP

Age group	Persons	MENTAL ABNORMALITY			Per cent reporting
		None	Diagnosed	Suspected	
Total	2,673[1]	84.8	8.6	6.6	94.7
40–59 years	64	59[2]	3	2	98.5
60–69 years	616	90.4	3.9	5.7	96.0
70 years and over . . .	974	82.9	10.1	7.0	94.4
Not reported	19	16	2	1	76.0

[1] Mental abnormality not reported for 149 persons.
[2] This includes one patient thirty-four years of age.

TABLE 6

CHRONICALLY ILL GUESTS OF PRIVATE HOMES FOR THE AGED CLASSIFIED BY
DURATION OF THE ILLNESS AND TIME SINCE THE FIRST INSTITUTIONAL CARE

Duration of illness	Total	TIME SINCE THE FIRST INSTITUTIONAL CARE						
		Less than 1 year	1 year under 2 years	2 years under 3 years	3 years under 4 years	4 years under 5 years	5 years under 10 years	10 years and over
Total	428[1]	77	64	56	67	42	88	34
Under 3 months	12	12	..	..	..	..	..	..
3 months under 1 year . . .	36	36	..	..	..	..	..	..
1 year and under 2 years . .	52	12	40	..	..	..	..	..
2 years and under 3 years . .	58	6	6	46	..	..	..	..
3 years and under 4 years . .	64	5	6	4	49	..	..	..
4 years and under 5 years . .	32	..	2	2	3	25	..	..
5 years and under 10 years .	105	4	6	3	8	13	71	..
10 years and over	69	2	4	1	7	4	17	34

[1] Neither the duration of illness nor the time since the earliest institutional care were reported for 1,561 persons; one of these items was not reported for 833 persons.

TABLE 7

CHRONIC PATIENTS OF NURSING SERVICES CLASSIFIED BY DIAGNOSIS, EACH AGE GROUP

Diagnosis	Total	AGE GROUP					
		Under 16	16–39	40–59	60–69	70 and over	Not reported
Total	6,401	4,318	945	544	284	264	46
Epidemic diseases	2,740	2,200	483	48	4	0	5
Poliomyelitis	2,223	1,881	337	1	0	0	4
Tuberculosis, spine	173	103	55	14	0	0	1
Tuberculosis, bones and joints . .	238	175	54	8	1	0	0
Other forms of tuberculosis . . .	22	15	6	1	0	0	0
Syphilis	73	20	28	22	3	0	0
Other	11	6	3	2	0	0	0
General diseases	948	392	109	246	107	75	19
Cancer and other malignant tumors	274	2	32	118	62	47	13
Benign tumors, cysts, etc.	30	9	13	4	1	3	0
Arthritis and rheumatism	256	68	52	84	32	16	4
Rickets	307	307	0	0	0	0	0
Diabetes . . '	51	0	5	24	12	8	2
Other	30	6	7	16	0	1	0
Diseases of nervous system and of or- gans of special sense	657	458	65	49	47	29	9
Diseases of spinal cord	392	367	22	3	0	0	0
Cerebral hemorrhage and shock .	26	3	1	4	11	5	2
Other paralysis	145	57	10	27	26	21	4
Other diseases, nervous system . .	70	15	26	14	10	2	2
Diseases of eye and ear	14	6	6	1	0	0	1
Diseases of circulatory system	239	50	46	61	49	30	3
Diseases of the heart	193	49	37	46	37	22	2
Other	46	1	9	15	12	8	1
Diseases of respiratory system, non- tuberculous	74	14	15	21	11	11	2
Diseases of the digestive system . .	48	5	5	23	10	3	2
Diseases of genitourinary system . .	71	2	12	29	17	8	3
Chronic nephritis	33	1	6	15	7	3	1
Other	38	1	6	14	10	5	2
Diseases of skin, cellular tissue . . .	47	11	4	10	13	9	0
Diseases of bones and organs of loco- motion	801	633	135	29	1	2	1
Malformations	416	392	24	0	0	0	0
Old age	83	0	0	0	0	83	0
External causes	238	150	38	25	11	12	2
Fractures	205	132	30	20	10	11	2
Other	33	18	8	5	1	1	0
Ill-defined diseases	25	5	4	3	13	0	0
Undiagnosed or diagnosis not reported	14	6	5	0	1	2	0

TABLE 8

CHRONICALLY ILL CLIENTS OF FAMILY SERVICE AGENCIES CLASSIFIED BY
DIAGNOSIS, EACH AGE GROUP

Diagnosis	Total	AGE GROUP					
		Under 16	16–39	40–59	60–69	70 and over	Not reported
Total	2,052	193	586	809	237	218	9
Epidemic diseases	212	47	80	71	11	2	1
Poliomyelitis	26	13	11	1	1	0	0
Tuberculosis, spine	12	3	3	6	0	0	0
Tuberculosis, bones and joints	14	8	4	1	1	0	0
Other forms of tuberculosis	11	3	6	2	0	0	0
Syphilis	127	20	42	55	8	2	0
Other	22	0	14	6	1	0	0
General diseases	473	33	120	225	63	30	2
Cancer and other malignant tumors	63	0	8	36	14	5	0
Benign tumors, cysts, etc.	13	0	4	7	2	0	0
Arthritis and rheumatism	172	4	49	75	27	16	1
Rickets	14	13	1	0	0	0	0
Diabetes	89	3	17	49	14	6	0
Anemia, pernicious, secondary	10	1	2	6	1	0	0
Chronic alcoholism	50	0	17	30	2	0	1
Chronic drug poisoning	8	0	3	3	0	2	0
Other	54	12	19	19	3	1	0
Diseases of nervous system and of organs of special sense	282	23	98	110	33	15	3
Encephalitis	34	1	18	15	0	0	0
Tabes dorsalis	17	0	4	11	2	0	0
Other diseases of spinal cord	17	4	7	6	0	0	0
Cerebral hemorrhage and shock	12	0	0	4	4	3	1
Other paralysis	95	6	19	40	20	9	1
Epilepsy	37	2	22	11	1	1	0
Chorea	5	4	1	0	0	0	0
Other diseases, nervous system	47	2	20	18	5	2	0
Diseases of eye and ear	18	4	7	5	1	0	1
Diseases of circulatory system	406	47	108	179	49	22	1
Diseases of the heart	298	47	82	118	34	16	1
Arteriosclerosis	51	0	11	33	5	2	0
Other	57	0	15	28	10	4	0
Diseases of respiratory system, non-tuberculous	150	14	45	67	15	8	1
Diseases of the digestive system	125	6	43	62	9	5	0
Ulcers of stomach	40	0	18	21	0	1	0
Hernia, intestinal obstruction	27	1	6	15	4	1	0
Cirrhosis and other diseases of liver	20	0	4	12	2	2	0
Other	38	5	15	14	3	1	0

TABLE 8—*(Continued)*

Diagnosis		AGE GROUP					
	Total	Under 16	16–39	40–59	60–69	70 and over	Not reported
Non-venereal diseases of genitourinary system	73	4	22	28	12	7	0
Chronic nephritis	24	3	7	9	4	1	0
Diseases of prostate	6	1	1	2	2	0	0
Other	43	0	14	17	6	6	0
Diseases of skin and cellular tissue	35	2	6	16	7	4	0
Leg ulcers	20	0	3	10	3	4	0
Other	15	2	3	6	4	0	0
Diseases of bones and organs of locomotion	60	11	25	20	2	2	0
Malformations	10	4	4	2	0	0	0
Old age	114	0	0	0	2	112	0
Old age	110	0	0	0	0	110	0
Senile dementia	4	0	0	0	2	2	0
External causes	52	1	22	14	5	10	0
Fractures	32	1	12	8	4	7	0
Other	20	0	10	6	1	3	0
Ill-defined diseases	43	0	4	10	28	0	1
Undiagnosed	7	0	3	3	0	1	0
Diagnosis not reported	10	1	6	2	1	0	0

TABLE 9

CHRONICALLY ILL CLIENTS OF FAMILY SERVICE AGENCIES CLASSIFIED BY DURATION OF ILLNESS AND PERIODS OF CARE RECEIVED

Duration of illness	Persons	PERIOD OF CARE RECEIVED									
		Under 3 months	3 months under 1 year	1 year under 2 years	2 years under 3 years	3 years under 4 years	4 years under 5 years	5 years under 10 years	10 years under 15 years	15 years under 20 years	20 years and over
Total	1,351	12.5	28.5	19.7	11.0	9.5	5.3	9.9	2.7	0.6	0.3
Less than 3 months	13	100.0	...	...	...	...	...	...	...	...	...
Three months under 1 year .	111	22.5	77.5	...	...	...	...	...	...	...	...
1 year under 2 years . . .	177	11.3	39.5	49.2	...	...	...	...	...	...	...
2 years under 3 years . . .	154	18.9	29.2	25.3	26.6	...	...	...	...	...	...
3 years under 4 years . . .	149	12.8	22.8	16.1	17.4	30.9	...	...	...	...	...
4 years under 5 years . . .	120	8.4	19.2	15.8	10.8	23.3	22.5	...	...	...	...
5 years under 10 years . . .	349	7.2	17.5	16.6	11.7	9.2	8.9	28.9	...	...	...
10 years under 15 years . .	154	11.0	23.4	13.0	9.7	6.5	5.2	15.6	15.6	...	...
15 years under 20 years . .	59	8.5	27.1	10.2	11.9	10.2	5.1	8.5	15.3	3.4	...
20 years and over	65	9.2	21.5	20.0	9.2	9.2	3.1	7.7	4.7	9.2	6.2

TABLE 10

CHRONICALLY ILL CLIENTS OF FAMILY SERVICE AGENCIES CLASSIFIED BY WEEKLY FAMILY INCOME AND NUMBER OF PERSONS DEPENDENT

Weekly family income	Persons	PERSONS DEPENDENT									
		1	2	3	4	5	6	7	8	9	More than 9
Total, family income reported	1,999	12.4	18.0	12.8	14.6	13.9	9.6	7.2	5.8	2.9	2.8
Amount reported	1,306	11.7	18.1	12.5	15.3	12.2	9.4	8.0	6.3	3.2	3.3
Amount.											
Under $5	4	3	1	....	....	....	....	....	....	....	....
$5-$9	90	71	18	1	....	....	....	....	....	....	....
$10-$14	205	28.3	42.4	12.7	10.2	4.9	0.5	0.5	0.5	....	0.8
$15-$19	266	3.8	30.5	21.8	19.9	13.5	5.6	3.0	1.1	1.6	....
$20-$24	258	2.7	15.1	15.5	23.2	14.3	12.8	7.4	7.4	5.7	3.1
$25-$29	192	0.5	3.2	8.3	15.6	21.5	15.1	16.1	10.9	4.8	9.7
$30-$34	124	0.8	3.2	11.3	12.1	14.5	16.2	14.5	12.9	13.0	14.2
$35-$39	77	2.6	....	3.9	10.4	9.2	14.2	15.6	16.9	4	5
$40-$44	43	....	....	5	2	7	9	7	4	2	2
$45-$49	22	....	1	....	4	1	2	7	3	5	5
$50 and over	25	....	....	....	7	2	3	1	2	....	5
Amount not specified	693	13.8	17.6	13.3	13.3	17.2	10.1	5.8	4.7	2.3	1.9

APPENDIX II

"The course as planned by this Committee offers two academic years. Approximately half of this time is given to practice, approximately one-quarter to classroom work, and approximately one-quarter to reading and other preparation.

"In general, the plan advocated by the Committee for the curriculum is as follows:

"A. Primary: to establish technique of work
   Social case work
   Problems of medical social work
   Psychiatric and psychological principles of human behavior
   Statistics

"B. Secondary: to establish background
   Medical
      Physiology and hygiene
      Certain physical diseases
      History and organization of medical practice
      Public health
   Social
      Government
      Community organization
      Industrial organization

"The subjects listed under 'B' are necessary to give the student medical and sociological background and an orientation in his field.

"An understanding of the normal functioning of the body, the chief causes of its disturbance, and the means of maintaining health is a necessary part of the equipment of any social worker. A course in physiology and hygiene should be taught as much as possible by means of practical demonstration. It should cover the principles of growth, development, nutrition, and infection.

"The hospital social worker needs to know the social significance of the common diseases, especially the chronic infections and those diseases which cause permanent or long-continued social disability. She needs to know their social causes and results, the conditions necessary to recovery, and the means of protecting others from infection and undue burden of care. Courses in disease should, like courses in hygiene, be taught by clinical demonstration and by classroom discussions, as well as by lecture.

"A course in the history and organization of medicine and nursing and of medical institutions is advised for the purpose of giving the hospital social worker an intelligent understanding of the habits, ethics, and instruments of the professions with which he must be associated in his work. The hospital social worker has to interpret physicians to members of the community, and has, moreover, often to guide individuals in the securing of proper medical care. He should, therefore, have some basis for judging the reliability of medical practice, as well as for intelligent cooperation in a medical plan."

[1] Report of the Committee on Training for Hospital Social Work. The American Hospital Association, *Bulletin No. 55*, 1923, pp. 20–22.

APPENDIX III

LIST OF FIFTY-FIVE HOSPITALS IN WHICH A SURVEY OF THE SOCIAL SERVICE
WAS MADE, CLASSIFIED BY TYPE OF HOSPITAL, 1928

Total 55

Public 16

  General 11
    Bellevue Hospital
    City Hospital
    Coney Island Hospital
    Cumberland Street Hospital
    Fordham Hospital
    Gouverneur Hospital
    Greenpoint Hospital
    Harlem Hospital
    Kings County Hospital
    Lincoln Hospital
    Metropolitan Hospital

  Special 5
    Kingston Avenue Hospital
    New York City Cancer Institute
    Riverside Hospital
    Sea View Hospital
    Willard Parker Hospital

Private 39

  Chronic 2
    Montefiore Hospital
    New York Skin and Cancer Hospital

  Orthopedic 3
    Hospital for Joint Diseases
    Hospital for Ruptured and Crippled
    House of St. Giles the Cripple

  General and other special 34
    Babies Hospital
    Beth David Hospital
    Beth Israel Hospital
    Beth Moses Hospital
    Bronx Hospital
    Brooklyn Hospital
    Fifth Avenue Hospital
    Jewish Hospital of Brooklyn
    Knickerbocker Hospital
    Lebanon Hospital
    Lenox Hill Hospital
    Long Island College Hospital
    Lutheran Hospital
    Methodist Episcopal Hospital
    Mt. Sinai Hospital
    Neurological Institute
    New York Hospital
    New York Infirmary for Women and Children

APPENDIX III—(*Continued*)

New York Nursery and Child's Hospital
New York Polyclinic Hospital
New York Post Graduate Hospital
Presbyterian Hospital
Reconstruction Hospital
Rockefeller Institute
Roosevelt Hospital
St. John's Hospital of Brooklyn
St. John's Long Island City Hospital
St. Luke's Hospital
St. Mark's Hospital
St. Mary's Hospital
St. Vincent's Hospital
Staten Island Hospital
United Israel-Zion Hospital
Woman's Hospital

APPENDIX IV

OFFICIAL LIST OF PRIVATE HOMES FOR THE AGED OF THE CENTRAL INFORMATION BUREAU FOR
THE CARE OF THE AGED, NOVEMBER 1, 1929

Manhattan

A. Clayton Powell Home for the Aged
Association for Relief of Respectable, Aged, Indigent Females
Baptist Home for the Aged
French Home for the Aged[1]
Grace Home for Aged Protestants[1]
Hebrew Home for Aged of Harlem[2]
Home for Aged and Infirm Hebrews of New York
Home for Old Men and Aged Couples
Home of Old Israel
Home of the Daughters of Israel
Home of the Sons and Daughters of Israel
Isabella Home
Little Sisters of the Poor, 213 E. 70
Little Sisters of the Poor, 135 W. 106
Methodist Episcopal Church Home
Presbyterian Home for Aged Women
St. Joseph's Home for the Aged
St. Luke's Home for Aged Women
St. Philip's Parish Home
Samaritan Home for the Aged

Bronx

Andrew Freedman Home
Braker Memorial Home[2]
Home of the Daughters of Jacob
Little Sisters of the Poor, 660 E. 183
New York Baptist Home[2]
Old People's Home of Eastern Missionary Association
Peabody Home for Aged and Indigent Women
Trinity Chapel for Aged Church Women
United Odd Fellow's Home and Orphanage Association[1]
Waiting Home, Protestant Unity League[2]
Webb Institute of Naval Architecture[2]

Brooklyn

Baptist Home of Brooklyn
Bethany Home for the Aged
Brooklyn Hebrew Home and Hospital for the Aged
Brooklyn Home for Aged Colored People
Brooklyn Home for Aged Men and Couples
Brooklyn Methodist Episcopal Church Home for the Aged
Church Charity Foundation of Long Island
Danish Home for the Aged
German Evangelical Home for the Aged
Graham Home for Old Ladies
Greenpoint Home for the Aged
Little Sisters of the Poor, Bushwick and DeKalb[2]
Little Sisters of the Poor, 8th Ave. and 16th St.
Marien-Heim of Brooklyn
Menorah Home for Aged and Infirm

[1] Not included in the census of the chronic sick.
[2] Not included in either the study of facilities or the census of the chronic sick.

New York Congregational Home for the Aged[1]
Norwegian Christian Home for the Aged
Swedish Augustana Home for the Aged
Wartburg Home for Aged and Infirm[1]

Queens

Chapin Home for Aged and Infirm
Far Rockaway Home for the Aged[2]
Long Island I. O. O. F. Association

Richmond

Carl Michel Eger Norwegian Lutheran Home for Aged
Home of Divine Providence
Mariner's Family Asylum
Sailor's Snug Harbor
Swedish Home for Aged People Association

Outside of New York City

Actors' Fund Home, New Jersey
Actors' Fund, Percy Williams Home, Long Island
A. I. C. P., Ward Manor, Dutchess County
Bethel Swedish Methodist Episcopal Home for Aged People, Westchester
Eventide Home, Salvation Army, Rockland County
German Masonic Home, Rockland County
Independent Order B'nai B'rith Home for Aged, Westchester
Little House of Divine Providence, Westchester
Margaret A. Howard Home, Westchester[1]
Mary Louise Heins Memorial Home, Westchester
Miriam Osborne Home Association, Westchester
Plattdeutsches Altenheim, Long Island
St. Catherine's Infirmary for the Aged, Long Island[2]
Seabury Memorial Home, Westchester
Sinnott Memorial Home for the Aged, Westchester[2]
Society of St. Johnland, Long Island[1]
Sons and Daughters of Liberty Home, Long Island[2]
Swiss Home for Aged, Westchester
United Home for Aged Hebrews, Westchester
Victoria Home for Aged British Men and Women, Westchester[2]

[1] Not included in the census of the chronic sick.
[2] Not included in either the study of facilities or the census of the chronic sick.

APPENDIX V

General

Bikur Cholim Convalescent Home
Burke Foundation
Campbell Cottages
Children's Aid Society, Elizabeth Milbank Anderson Home for Convalescent Children
Children's Aid Society, Milbank Memorial Home for Convalescent Boys
Children's Aid Society, Martha Home for Convalescent Boys
Hebrew Convalescent Home
Isabella Home
Jewish Home for Convalescents
Reed Farm
St. Luke's Convalescent Hospital
Surprise Lake Camp

Orthopedic

Blythedale Home
Brooklyn Children's Aid Society, Wave Crest Convalescent Hospital Home
Convalescent Home for Hebrew Children
Evelyn Goldsmith Home for Crippled Children
Hospital for Joint Diseases, Natalie and Louis Heinsheimer Memorial Home
House of St. Giles the Cripple, Convalescent Home and School
New York Orthopedic Hospital, Country Branch
Robin's Nest

Cardiac

Irvington House
Martine Farm
Nichols Cottage
Pelham Home for Children

Name	CAPACITY		
	Total	Adults	Children
Total	1,591	735	627
Arthur Pitney Comfort Home	30	...	...
Association for Improving the Condition of the Poor, Caroline Rest	117	31	86
Association for Improving the Condition of the Poor, Nurses' Home	30	30	...
Bishop McDonnel Hall for Convalescent Women	16	16	...
Catholic Charities, Loretto Rest	16	16	...
Catholic Charities, St. John's Convalescent Home	25	25	...
Children's Aid Society, Goodhue Home	25	...	25
Children's Country Home Association	50	...	50
Daisy Fields Home and Hospital	18	...	18
Gould Farm	45	45	...
Holiday Farm	50	...	50
Incarnation Convalescent Home	60	35	25
Josephine Home	50	...	50
Little Mothers' Aid Association, Ernst Bliss Memorial	50	...	...
Margaret and Sarah Switzer Foundation, Sunnyside Farm	52	52	...
Mary Zinn Home for Convalescent Children	41	...	41
Montclair Fresh Air and Convalescent Home	32	...	32
Neustadter Foundation	58	40	18
New York Protestant Episcopal City Mission Society, Edgewater Creche	44	...	44
New York Protestant Episcopal City Mission Society, Sarah Schermerhorn	75	...	...
New York Urban League, Nepperhan Heights	12	12	...
Posner Brooklyn Jewish Home	60	60	...
Rest for Convalescents	72	72	...
St. Andrew's Convalescent Hospital	30	...	...
St. Eleanora's Home for Convalescents	50	28	22
St. Elizabeth's Convalescent Home	45	45	...
St. James' Convalescent and Rest Home	22	...	...
St. Mary's Free Hospital for Children, Noyes Memorial	30	...	30
St. Phebe's Mission and Convalescent Home	22	...	...
Solomon and Betty Loeb Memorial Home	108	74	34
Speedwell Society	102	...	102
Union Settlement, House-by-the-Sea	20	20	...
Valeria Home	125	125	...
Working Girls' Vacation Society	9	9	...

APPENDIX VI

LIST OF NURSING AGENCIES CLASSIFIED BY TYPE OF SERVICE AND BOROUGH IN WHICH SERVICE IS RENDERED, 1928

Agencies	Nursing personnel	Educational nursing	Specialized nursing	Community nursing and bedside care	Manhattan	Bronx	Brooklyn	Queens	Richmond
Association for the Aid of Crippled Children	18		X		X	X			
Association for Improving the Condition of the Poor	39	X			X	X			
Columbus Hill Center	5	X			X				
Mulberry Health Center[1]	12	X			X				
Bowling Green Neighborhood Association[1]	6	X			X				
Christodora House	1				X				
Dominican Sisters of the Sick Poor	22			X	X	X			
East Harlem Nursing and Health Service	24			X	X				
Henry Street Visiting Nurse Service[2]	236			X	X	X			X[2]
Jamaica District Nursing and Social Service Committee[3]	1			X				X	
John Hancock Life Insurance Company[4]	3			X				X	
Judson Health Center	13	X			X				
Little Sisters of the Assumption	24	X			X				
Maternity Center Association[5]	22		X		X				
Maternity Center Association of Brooklyn[5]	3		X				X		
Memorial Hospital	6		X		X		X		
Metropolitan Life Insurance Company[4]	30			X	X	X	X	X	X
Missionary Cononesses of St. Augustine	9			X	X	X	X	X	
New York City Mission Society, Woman's Branch	12			X	X				
New York Orthopedic Dispensary and Hospital	18		X		X	X	X	X	
North Shore Public Health Nursing Association	1			X				X	
Norwegian Lutheran Deaconess Hospital	3			X			X		
Nursing Sisters of the Sick Poor, Brooklyn	30			X			X		
Nursing Sisters of the Sick Poor, Queens	8			X				X	
Recreation Rooms and Settlement	2	X			X				
Sisters of Bon Secours	11			X	X	X			
Visiting Nurse Association of Brooklyn	133			X			X	X	

[1] Discontinued in June, 1932.

[2] The Richmond center of the Henry Street Visiting Nurse Service, on January 1, 1929, became the Visiting Nurse Association of Staten Island, an independent organization; and the Henry Street Visiting Nurse Service has now extended its service into Queens.

[3] In 1929, this organization gave up its nursing service.

[4] The life insurance companies actually include all the boroughs in their service, but in the boroughs other than Queens, they gave the service entirely through the community visiting nurse services; and the John Hancock Life Insurance Company since 1930 has done so in all boroughs.

[5] Not included in the survey of facilities for the care of the chronic sick.

APPENDIX VII

a) *Schedule used in Chronic Hospitals*

Name of hospital..........................Bed capacity.....................
Address...................................Occupancy.......................
Superintendent............................Average duration of stay.........
Services...

ADMISSION

Types of patient accepted...
Source of reference of patients...
Number of refusals, 1927, and reasons.....................................
Who accepts patients for admission?.......................................
Is there medical investigation?...................Social investigation?....
Are patients accepted merely on recommendation?...Whose?..................
Is a waiting list kept?........Number on waiting list $\begin{cases} \text{Free}............\\ \text{Part-pay}..........\\ \text{Pay}............. \end{cases}$
Average time from the date of application to date of admission.............
If city charges are taken, how long do these wait for admission?...........

CHARGES AND COSTS

Full pay: number of beds........Amount charged.....................
Part pay: number of beds........Amount charged.....................
Free: number of beds........May be used by whom?.................
Daily cost per patient...

DISCHARGE

Are patients discharged to public institutions?......Specify which?.........
Number of patients so discharged, 1927....................................
Does the hospital seek to make available to the patient before discharge facilities for further treatment?...............................
Does the hospital investigate the conditions of the patient's home before discharge?...
Who makes the decisions in regard to discharges?..........................

TRANSFER

Is the hospital equipped to give patients complete medical treatment?.......
If not, has it specific arrangements for transfer?.........................
Specify types of patient transferred......................................
Does it agree to take them back on discharge from other institutions?.....

MEDICAL STAFF	NURSING STAFF
Number on visiting staff.........	Number of:
Specialties represented..........	Graduates......................
	Pupil nurses...................
	Attendants....................
	Ward maids...................
Frequency of visits.............	Orderlies.....................
Number of internes.............	Hospital helpers.................
Number of residents............	Is there a training school for nurses?....

[1] It seems unnecessary to print the very simple form of schedule used in the survey of certain other types of agency.

PHYSICAL PLAN

    Are patients for hospital care and attendant care separated?...............

    Does the building plan permit all patients to get out-of-doors?..............

    Are the buildings adapted to use of wheelchairs?........................

    Number of elevators..............Do they accommodate wheelchairs?....

    Are recreation rooms provided?.......................................

SPECIAL SERVICES

    Is there provision for special dietetic care?..........................

    Is there an occupational therapy unit?........Number of workers..........

      Average daily attendance, 1927.......................................

    Is there a social service department?..........Number of workers..........

    Is recreation provided?..

      Through the social service or otherwise?...........................

      Specify...

    Are religious services provided?.....................................

    Is there an out-patient department?..................................

    Does the hospital send out an electrotherapy unit?...A physiotherapy unit?..

    Are any changes in purpose or organization contemplated?.....Specify......

    Arrangements for the census of the chronic sick......................

    Name of interviewer......................Date.....................

b) *Schedule used in General Hospitals*

Name of hospital.........................Capacity.....................

Address............................. Total......................

                                           Ward beds.................

Ward rates............................Occupancy.....................

                                       Average duration of stay........

ADMISSION

    Types of patient accepted..

    Types of patient excluded..

    Number of refusals, 1927, and reasons................................

    Estimated number of weekly requests for admission of chronic patients who

      cannot be received..

    Is any responsibility assumed for the medical guidance of those refused?....

      Specify..

    Are they referred elsewhere?...

    Is a waiting list kept?........................Remarks...............

DISCHARGE

    Are patients discharged to public institutions?.......................

    Number of patients so discharged, 1927............Reasons..............

    Does the hospital make arrangements for further care of patients who need it?.

      Refer to out-patient department?................................

      Refer to other institutions?.................Specify...............

      Refer to other agencies?....................Specify...............

SPECIAL SERVICES

    Has the hospital:

      Visiting doctor service?...

      Traveling electrotherapy unit?....................................

      Traveling physiotherapy unit?.....................................

    Are any changes contemplated that would affect the hospital's provision for

    the chronic sick?...

CENSUS OF THE CHRONIC SICK:

How was information secured for schedules of chronic patients?............

How many schedules were filled out?................................

Total number of patients on the wards on date of census?................

Name of interviewer.......................Date......................

c) *Schedule used in Private Homes for the Aged*

Name of home...

GUESTS TRANSFERRED FOR MEDICAL CARE

Number and description...

Where transferred...

Advantages and disadvantages of transferral............................

GUESTS GIVEN MEDICAL CARE IN THE HOME

Infirmary or hospital

Number of beds...................Number in use...................

Equipment of infirmary...

Cost per patient per day..

Person in charge..

Number of nurses...

Number of attendants..

Physicians:

Resident........................Number......................

On call.........................Number......................

General........................Number......................

Special........................Number......................

Special diets..

Average length of stay...

Discharge from infirmary...

Volume of chronic illness in Home...................................

No infirmary or hospital

Number of nurses.....................Resident........On call........

Number of attendants..

Physicians:

On call.........................Number......................

General........................Number......................

Special........................Number......................

Special diets..

Volume of chronic illness in Home...................................

MEDICAL SERVICE

On what basis are physicians chosen?..................................

How long do physicians stay with the institution?.......................

What is the procedure in case of sickness of any guest?...................

What examinations are regularly given?...............................

Routine physical...................Dental.............X-ray......

Laboratory tests...................Mental......................

Is the physician affiliated with a scientific institution?......................

Are patients used for teaching purposes?..............................

ADMISSION REQUIREMENTS

Charter and endowment limitations....................................

Other limitations on admissions and by what authority modifiable..........

With whose consent can census records be released?.........................

Method of procedure...

REMARKS

d) *Schedule used in Nursing Services*

Name... .

Address... .

Director.. .

Number of supervisors... .

Number of registered nurses.........Number of practical nurses......... .

Nursing centers and territory covered by each. (List on reverse side of this
    sheet).. .

Types of patients accepted for care of:

    Registered nurse... .

    Practical nurse.. .

Types of patients refused... .

    Are such patients referred elsewhere?.............................. .

    Number of refusals, 1927... .

Is any responsibility taken for the care of the household?.................. .

    Specify... .

Patients and visits, 1927.. .

MONTH	PATIENTS		VISITS	
	Total	*Chronic*	*Total*	*Chronic*
January				
February				
March				
April				
May				
June				
July				
August				
September				
October				
November				
December				

COLUMBIA UNIVERSITY PRESS
COLUMBIA UNIVERSITY
NEW YORK

———

FOREIGN AGENT
OXFORD UNIVERSITY PRESS
HUMPHREY MILFORD
AMEN HOUSE, LONDON, E.C.